# DENTAL ANATOMY

## Its Relevance to Dentistry

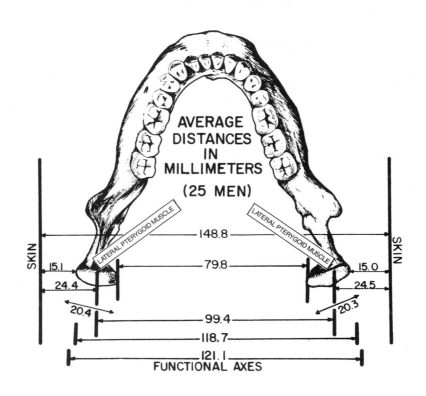

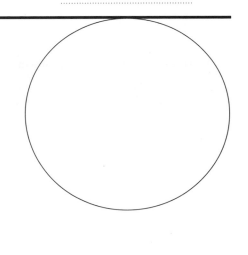

# DENTAL ANATOMY

## Its Relevance to Dentistry

### fifth edition

**JULIAN B. WOELFEL, D.D.S.**

Professor Emeritus, Divisions of Prosthodontics,
Dental Materials, and Dental Hygiene
The Ohio State University College of Dentistry
Columbus, Ohio

**RICKNE C. SCHEID, D.D.S., M.A.**

Associate Professor
Department of Primary Care,
Division of Dental Hygiene and
Department of Restorative Dentistry,
Prosthodontics and Endodontics
The Ohio State University College of Dentistry
Columbus, Ohio

## Williams & Wilkins

### A WAVERLY COMPANY

BALTIMORE • PHILADELPHIA • LONDON • PARIS • BANGKOK
BUENOS AIRES • HONG KONG • MUNICH • SYDNEY • TOKYO • WROCLAW

*Editor:* Sharon R. Zinner
*Managing Editor:* Tanya Lazar
*Production Coordinator:* Cindy Park
*Book Project Editor:* Robert D. Magee
*Designer:* Ellen B. Zanolle
*Illustration Planner:* Cindy Park
*Cover Designer:* Tom Sheuerman
*Typesetter:* Peirce Graphic Services, Inc.
*Printer:* RR Donnelley & Sons Company
*Digitized Illustrations:* Peirce Graphic Services, Inc.
*Binder:* RR Donnelley & Sons Company

The front cover concept was designed and contributed for the fifth edition by Dr. Ralph Rosenblum, Professor Emeritus, The Ohio State University College of Dentistry.

351 West Camden Street
Baltimore, Maryland 21201-2436 USA

Rose Tree Corporate Center
1400 North Providence Road
Building II, Suite 5025
Media, Pennsylvania 19063-2043 USA

*Printed in the United States of America*

**Library of Congress Cataloging-in-Publication Data**

Woelfel, Julian B.
    Dental anatomy : its relevance to dentistry. — 5th ed. / Julian B. Woelfel, Rickne C. Scheid.
      p.    cm.
    Includes bibliographical references and index.
    ISBN 0-683-30044-X
    1. Teeth—Anatomy.  2. Mouth—Anatomy.  I. Scheid, Rickne C.  II. Title
    [DNLM: 1. Tooth—anatomy & histology—outlines.  2. Mouth—anatomy & histology—outlines.
  3. Jaw—anatomy & histology—outlines.  WU 18.2 W842d 1997]
    QM311.W64  1997
    611'.314—dc20
    DNLM/DLC
    for Library of Congress                         96-41063
                                                    CIP

*The publishers have made every effort to trace the copyright holders for borrowed material. If they have inadvertently overlooked any, they will be pleased to make the necessary arrangements at the first opportunity.*

To purchase additional copies of this book, call our customer service department at **(800) 638-0672** or fax orders to **(800) 447-8438.** For other book services, including chapter reprints and large quantity sales, ask for the Special Sales department.

Canadian customers should call **(800) 268-4178,** or fax **(905) 470-6780.** For all other calls originating outside of the United States, please call **(410) 528-4223** or fax us at **(410) 528-8550.**

**Visit Williams & Wilkins on the Internet: http://www.wwilkins.com** or contact our customer service department at **custserv@wwilkins.com.** Williams & Wilkins customer service representatives are available from 8:30 am to 6:00 pm, EST. Monday through Friday, for telephone access.

98 99
3 4 5 6 7 8 9 10

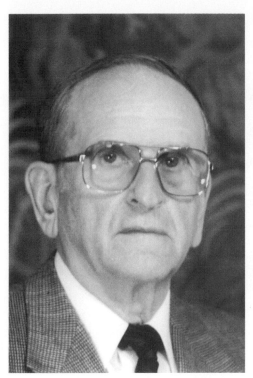

## JULIAN B. WOELFEL, D.D.S

Professor Woelfel, known primarily for his expertise on complete dentures, research and occlusion, taught clinical dentistry for 40 years in the College of Dentistry, The Ohio State University, Columbus, Ohio. He served as an Army prosthodontist for 2 years and a visiting professor in Japan, Taiwan, England and Brazil. He has published over 70 scientific articles, four editions of Dental Anatomy and chapters in five books.

In 1967, he was the first recipient of the International Association of Dental Research Award for Research in Prosthodontics. In 1972, the New York Prosthodontic Society selected him for the Jerome and Dorothy Schweitzer Award for Outstanding and Continuing Research in Prosthodontics. In 1992, the Ohio Dental Association chose Dr. Woelfel for the prestigious Callahan Award.

He has lectured in fifteen foreign countries. Dr. Woelfel holds patents on his two inventions widely used in Europe for accurately recording jaw relations. In addition to his love for students and teaching, he conducted a part-time private practice limited to partial and complete dentures for 33 years. One of his proudest accomplishments is this textbook.

## RICKNE C. SCHEID, D.D.S., M.ED.

Dr. Rickne Scheid received his D.D.S. in 1972 at The Ohio State University, and was inducted into the dental honorary, Omicron Kappa Upsilon. After serving in the U.S. Navy Dental Corps, he went into part-time practice and has taught at his alma mater since 1974. His appointments at the College of Dentistry have been in the Department of Operative Dentistry, The Division of Dental Hygiene, and, most recently, the Section of Restorative Dentistry, Prosthodontics and Endodontics, and the Section of Primary Care. While teaching, he received his Masters in Education in 1980. He has been responsible for revising and directing twelve different courses throughout his teaching career, and has been the recipient of student teaching awards on three different occasions. His responsibilities now include course director of the dental anatomy course in which he teaches both dental and dental hygiene students.

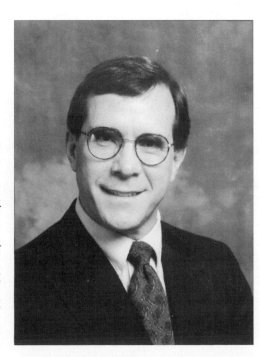

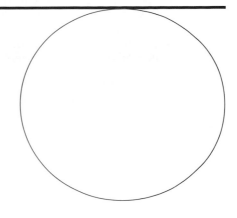

# Preface to the 5th Edition

My natural curiosity and dislike for ambiguous terms stimulated my original research based on personal observations of thousands of teeth, diagnostic casts, and mouths. I have included the results of my research, in brackets, throughout this and previous editions. You will find such information as the average mandibular hinge opening, the average gingival sulci depths, the frequency of Carabelli cusp formation, the frequency of two- and three-cusp mandibular second premolars, the frequency of marginal ridge grooves, comparative size of deciduous and permanent teeth, which muscles move the jaw (determined by electrography), and more.

I retired from the Ohio State University in 1988 after 40 years of teaching. While completing the changes for the 4th edition, I decided it would be wise to select a coauthor for the 5th edition. I chose Associate Professor Rickne Scheid because of my great respect for his integrity, intellect, and abilities. I have known him as an outstanding dental student and later as a faculty member who had codirected many dental courses with me. Dr.

Scheid has a Master's Degree in Education in addition to his dental degree, and since 1974 has taught in the Departments of Restorative and Prosthetic Dentistry and Dental Hygiene Expanded Functions. This background contributes to his excellent teaching capabilities and he has a wonderful rapport with students. Both of us have used this textbook for a total of 22 years. We have gained considerable insight as to where additional information was needed, and where study guides would improve clarity and understanding.

Both of us have worked diligently for many hours on the revisions for this edition. These revisions include a reorganization of existing material to make it easier to learn, the incorporation of more learning exercises that stimulate active learning, and an appendix that includes over 90 new computer-generated illustrations with learning guides that are referenced throughout the text. Where appropriate, chapters have been combined to help the learner better correlate related material. The reorganization and changes for this edition were done so as to keep the text science-based, while making it as student-friendly as possible. The reorganization is described fully in the Introduction.

A very special thanks goes to the many dental hygiene students in the years 1971 to 1987 who brought in unique tooth specimens and suggested where changes would improve this text. Further, for their help on this 5th edition, much thanks goes to Cherie Golowin and Jan Smith from the Department of Primary Care, and Connie Mason and Terri Pheister from the Department of Restorative and Prosthetic Dentistry and Endodontics for their many hours of transcribing this edition onto the computer discs, and to Ron McLean from University Technology Services for his help in developing new computer-generated graphics for this edition. Finally, special thanks to my wife, Marcile, for much love and care and editorial assistance.

Julian B. Woelfel

# Contents

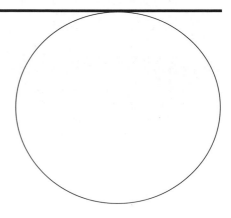

# Introduction to Fifth Edition

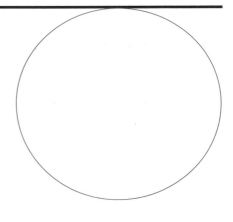

*Dental Anatomy: Its Relevance to Dentistry* is primarily intended as a guide for dental students, dental hygiene students, dental assistants, and dental laboratory technicians in the study of tooth morphology and related structures. It is designed to help them understand the relationship of teeth to one another, and to the bones, muscles, and nerves closely associated with the teeth. It is intended to be used by instructors of dental anatomy courses as a teaching manual for use during lectures, discussion periods, laboratory sessions, and early clinical experiences. *Dental Anatomy: Its Relevance to Dentistry* can also serve as a ready reference for many other dental courses and in a dental office.

This book is for those who may not have had a formal course in head anatomy. Therefore, descriptions of the skull, craniomandibular articulation, muscles of mastication, and nerves and blood vessels associated with the teeth are included, along with a contemporary overview of occlusion, restorative dentistry, endodontics, and periodontics. The intent is to help the student study in a way that will make learning a use-ful, interesting, and hopefully memorable experience.

Dental anatomy in the broadest sense includes the surface form of the oral cavity, the external and internal morphology of the individual teeth, and the relationship of the teeth to each other (within an arch and between arches). It also includes the relationship of the skull bones in which the teeth are set, the complex joints that enable and control movement of the lower jaw relative to the cranium, the muscles that bring about this movement, and the nerves and blood vessels that supply these structures.

This book provides an organized way to learn and study oral anatomy. Throughout the text are numerous *learning exercises,* which suggest ways to think about and apply the topics in each chapter. These exercises suggest using extracted teeth or tooth models, skulls (or skull models), and self and partner examinations. More advanced exercises (in Chapter 13) provide methods for drawing and carving teeth from wax, allowing the student to become intimately familiar with tooth shape and terminology. As each topic is presented in words, examine the study aids in order to identify and relate each structure to the surrounding head and neck. It is well to keep in mind that some human skulls have had missing or damaged teeth replaced by teeth from other sources. This substitution will not affect the study of skull structures, but beware, since this substitution could affect your study of occlusion.

Also, with every new topic, reference is made to drawings, tables, and photographs within the text. Since a picture is worth a thousand words, it is critical that you take advantage of the various figures to assure your understanding of each concept or structure. Many figures are designed so you can cover up the names of structures with a card and test yourself.

As you begin learning the characteristics differentiating each type of tooth as described in Chapters 4 through 7, you need to be aware of the considerable variation in tooth morphology that can occur from one patient to the next. Relative tooth sizes and characteristics cited within the text do *not* apply to *all* patients' teeth, but are based on average dimensions, or morphology that occurs with the greatest frequency. This text is unique in providing you with both original and reviewed research findings based on the study of thousands of teeth, casts, and mouths. The original research data are presented throughout the text in *brackets* [like this] and provides a scientific basis for understanding the frequency and extent to which differences from the norm occur. For example, the text states that "a mesial marginal groove is a distinguishing characteristic of the maxillary first premolar [but this occurred in only 97% of the 600 premolars checked, which means that, on the average, 3% may not have this groove], whereas the maxillary second premolar is not nearly as likely to have this groove [but 37% do have it]."

Relative to tooth morphology, this text is designed to prepare you to be able to:

1. Identify and differentiate each type of tooth.

2. Communicate with instructors, peers, and patients using understandable terminology and sketches when appropriate.

3. Describe existing restoration contours.

4. Describe and draw root and crown contours in order to properly adapt instruments required to clean these surfaces.

5. Describe the relationship of vital nerves and blood supply of the pulp to tooth morphology and function.

6. Reproduce acceptable tooth contours as required when eventually finishing and polishing, or placing, restorations.

For learning the form of individual teeth, the best learning resource is a collection of as many intact extracted teeth as you are able to acquire. A dentist, if presented with a quart jar of formalin, will remember his or her own student days and will probably be glad to put extracted teeth in the jar. Do not expect these teeth to be clean or sorted out; sorting is your job. While handling these teeth, it is critical that the guidelines for infection control be followed:

Using protective gloves, tooth specimens should be scraped clean with a knife. Soaking for several hours in hydrogen peroxide before scraping is helpful. After scraping to remove hard deposits and soft tissue, tooth specimens should be further cleansed by soaking for 20 minutes in 4 ounces of household bleach containing 2 tablespoons of Calgon (a water softener). Once cleaned, they should be stored in fresh 10% neutral formalin for days or weeks. If formalin has not been buffered, formic acid will form and dissolve tooth enamel. If teeth dry out, they will become fragile and easily break.

Buffered neutral formalin (pH 7) is made up of formalin, full strength (100 ml of 40% formaldehyde), distilled water (900 ml), sodium phosphate dibasic (anhydrous) (6.5 g), and sodium phosphate monobasic (4.0 g). An easier *alternative* is to buffer a mixture of 9 parts water and 1 part full strength formalin by adding a few marble chips to prevent accumulation of formic acid.

As you read the description of tooth morphology, identify each structure not only visually, but also using a dental explorer to feel the contours being described, since you will eventually be required to evaluate and reproduce these same contours with other dental instruments. As you become interested in the many simi-larities and differences of tooth morphology, you can later apply this information expeditiously during patient treatment or evaluation.

New in this edition is an appendix with many tearout study pages, designed to be taken out and kept available in a separate loose-leaf notebook. It is hoped that the drawings in the appendix will provide you with an easier mechanism for relating the narrative in the text to the actual shapes of structures seen on each tooth. These pages will be referred to throughout the chapters on tooth morphology, and will minimize the time required to search out figures often placed on other pages. The appendix pages can also be used as separate study guides since all concepts or structures are referenced on the back of each page. Reference will be made to the appendix pages and specific items on each page as follows: "Appendix" followed by the page number and letter to denote items being discussed (for example, "Appendix 1a" denotes page 1, item "a" in the appendix). Many new illustrations were added, and some 40 old ones were revised, making a total of close to 400 illustrations.

Your study within this text begins in Chapter 1 with a very brief overview of tooth types and location to prepare you to understand their relationship with the skull. A short glossary is provided to help relate new terms to those you already know. Next, an overview of key landmarks on the skull, including the jaw joints, muscle connections, and passageways of nerves and blood vessels, are described. This is followed in Chapter 2 by a guided clinical examination on a partner, which involves identifying all soft tissue landmarks which cover the bones and surround the teeth. After this overview of surrounding structures, Chapter 3 provides you with the terminology that must be mastered to understand tooth morphology and ideal occlusion relationships. This is

followed by Chapters 4–7 with an in-depth description of each type of tooth emphasizing and comparing the similarities and differences of one tooth to another so you do not have to memorize 32 different sets of facts for each of the 32 permanent teeth.

In subsequent chapters, we present the clinical implications of internal and external root anatomy, an overview of deciduous tooth morphology, and the more advanced aspects of jaw movement and malocclusion. The final chapters are designed to provide an overview of tooth anomalies (again reinforcing the variety in tooth morphology), an overview of restorative dentistry and how it relates to tooth morphology, a step-by-step method for drawing and carving teeth, and, finally, an interesting discussion of the importance of tooth morphology in forensic dentistry.

Hopefully, you will spend some time thinking about the concepts as you are learning. After all, you are learning the "foreign" language of dental anatomy that you will be using for the rest of your professional lives. Have fun looking at teeth as though you were a tooth detective. Take notes, sketch different views of each tooth, take advantage of all learning exercises and references to figures and the appendix, and ask questions until your curiosity is satisfied. Most importantly, we hope this book will stimulate your interest and involvement in the wonderful and fascinating field of dentistry, and that you will consider it to be worthwhile addition to your library even after your formal education is complete.

Julian B. Woelfel
Rick C. Scheid

# Structures That Form the Foundation for Tooth Function

This chapter discusses structures that form the foundation for tooth function with an emphasis on gross anatomy of the bones, muscles, nerves, and blood supply, which are also important to the functioning of the jaws and teeth.

## SECTION I. TEETH: A BRIEF OVERVIEW

Prior to a discussion of the structures that support the teeth, it is necessary to familiarize yourself with a *brief* description of the classes of teeth and their location in the jaws. This overview is necessary to appreciate and understand the full description of the bones, nerves, and blood vessels described in this chapter, as well as the description of oral landmarks described in Chapter 2. A more in-depth description of all teeth begins in Chapter 3.

The word *dentition* refers to all of the teeth in the upper jaw bones (called the maxillae) and the lower jaw bone (called the mandible). Due to their location, the upper teeth are called *maxillary* teeth, and together form an arch shape known as the *maxillary arch* of teeth. In contrast, the lower teeth are called *mandibular* teeth, collectively forming the *mandibular arch* of teeth. Humans have two dentitions throughout life: one during childhood, called the primary dentition, and one for most or all of adulthood, called the permanent teeth.

**DECIDUOUS TEETH**

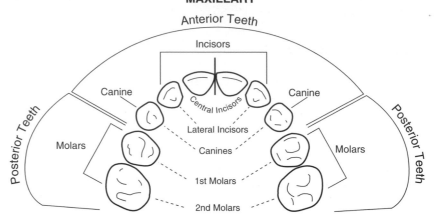

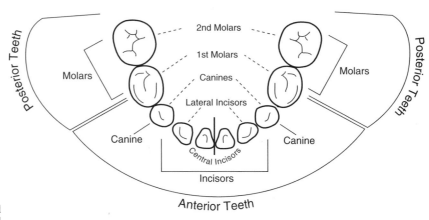

**Figure 1.1.** Maxillary and mandibular primary dental arches.

## A. Primary Dentition

There are only 20 teeth in the primary dentition (Fig. 1.1): 10 in the maxillary arch and 10 in the mandibular arch. This dentition is also called the *deciduous dentition,* referring to the fact that these teeth are eventually shed or exfoliated by age 12 or 13, being replaced by the permanent dentition. The complete primary dentition has five teeth in each quadrant (half of each arch). The two front teeth in each quadrant are the central and lateral incisor (I), followed posteriorly by one canine (C), then a first and second primary molar (M).

A dental formula can be used to briefly indicate this information for the maxillary and mandibular teeth on one side of the mouth:

$$I \frac{2}{2} C \frac{1}{1} M \frac{2}{2} = 10 \text{ teeth on either side; 20 teeth in all.}$$

Each tooth in a category can be differentiated from others in that category by the location in a specific quadrant (e.g., the canine in the upper right quadrant vs. the canine in the lower right quadrant). Further, the two deciduous incisors and two deciduous molars in each quadrant can be differentiated as follows: incisors closest to the midline between the right and left quadrants are called central incisors, whereas incisors next to (or lateral to) central incisors in that quadrant are called lateral incisors. Deciduous molars that are closest to the midline in each quadrant are called *first* deciduous molars, whereas last molars in each quadrant are called second deciduous molars.

### LEARNING EXERCISE

*Using models of the primary dentition and referring to Figure 1.1, identify each tooth by name and quadrant.*

## B. Permanent Dentition

Permanent dentition (Fig. 1.2) is also called the *secondary* dentition or that which follows the primary dentition. It is composed of 32 teeth: 16 maxillary and 16 mandibular. The complete permanent dentition has eight teeth in each quadrant. The two front teeth

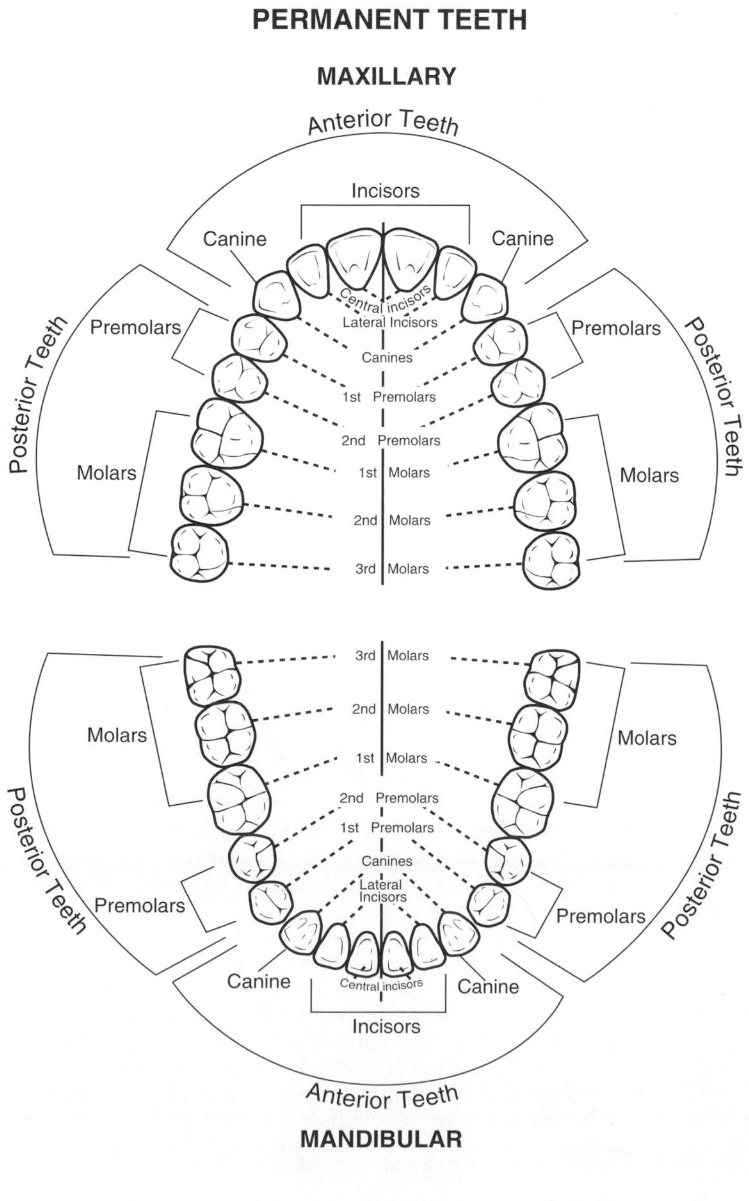

**Figure 1.2.** Maxillary and mandibular permanent dentition.

in a quadrant are the central and lateral incisors (I), followed by one canine (C), a first and second premolar (PM), then the first, second, and third molars (M). The dental formula is:

$$I\ \frac{2}{2}\ C\ \frac{1}{1}\ PM\ \frac{2}{2}\ M\ \frac{3}{3} = 16 \text{ teeth on either side; 32 teeth in all.}$$

As noted by comparing the formulas for deciduous and permanent teeth, differences exist. Although central and lateral incisors and canines are similarly positioned in both denti-

**Table 1.1.** Some Dental Formulae (Order of Teeth Per Quadrant) and Interesting Facts About Teeth in Animals[33-35]

| Animal | Formula | | | | Animal | Formula | | | |
|---|---|---|---|---|---|---|---|---|---|
| Humans, Old World monkeys, and apes | $I\ \frac{2}{2}$ | $C\ \frac{1}{1}$ | $P\ \frac{2}{2}$ | $M\ \frac{3}{3}$ | Porcupines and beavers | $I\ \frac{1}{1}$ | $C\ \frac{0}{0}$ | $P\ \frac{1}{1}$ | $M\ \frac{3}{3}$ |
| New World monkeys | $I\ \frac{2}{2}$ | $C\ \frac{1}{1}$ | $P\ \frac{3}{3}$ | $M\ \frac{3}{3}$ | Bears and pandas | $I\ \frac{3}{3}$ | $C\ \frac{1}{1}$ | $P\ \frac{4}{4}$ | $M\ \frac{2}{3}$ |
| Dogs, wolves, and foxes | $I\ \frac{3}{3}$ | $C\ \frac{1}{1}$ | $P\ \frac{4}{4}$ | $M\ \frac{2}{3}$ | Squirrels | $I\ \frac{1}{1}$ | $C\ \frac{0}{0}$ | $P\ \frac{2}{1}$ | $M\ \frac{3}{3}$ |
| Cats | $I\ \frac{3}{3}$ | $C\ \frac{1}{1}$ | $P\ \frac{3}{2}$ | $M\ \frac{1}{1}$ | Rabbit‡ | $I\ \frac{2}{1}$ | $C\ \frac{0}{0}$ | $P\ \frac{3}{2}$ | $M\ \frac{3}{3}$ |
| Cows | $I\ \frac{0}{3}$ | $C\ \frac{0}{1}$ | $P\ \frac{3}{3}$ | $M\ \frac{3}{3}$ | Mice and rats | $I\ \frac{1}{1}$ | $C\ \frac{0}{0}$ | $P\ \frac{0}{0}$ | $M\ \frac{3}{3}$ |
| Horses and zebra* | $I\ \frac{3}{3}$ | $C\ \frac{1}{1}$ | $P\ \frac{4}{4}$ | $M\ \frac{3}{3}$ | Moles | $I\ \frac{3}{3}$ | $C\ \frac{1}{1}$ | $P\ \frac{4}{4}$ | $M\ \frac{3}{3}$ |
| Walruses | $I\ \frac{1}{0}$ | $C\ \frac{1}{1}$ | $P\ \frac{3}{3}$ | $M\ \frac{0}{0}$ | Vampire bats | $I\ \frac{1}{2}$ | $C\ \frac{1}{1}$ | $P\ \frac{2}{3}$ | $M\ \frac{0}{0}$ |
| Elephants | $I\ \frac{1}{0}$ | $C\ \frac{0}{0}$ | $Dm†\ \frac{3}{3}$ | $M\ \frac{3}{3}$ | Shrews | $I\ \frac{3}{1}$ | $C\ \frac{1}{1}$ | $P\ \frac{3}{1}$ | $M\ \frac{3}{3}$ |

*Pigs and hippopotami have the same formula, except that they have two or three upper and two or three lower incisors.

†Elephants have deciduous molars but no premolars. An elephant's skull is larger than necessary to house his brain. The size is needed to provide mechanical support for the tusks (one-third of their length is embedded in the skull) and the enormous molars. Each molar weighs about 9 pounds and is nearly a foot long mesiodistally on the occlusal surface. Tusks (the central incisors) can be as long as 11½ feet and weigh 440 pounds (42).

‡Guinea pigs have the same formula, except that they have only one maxillary incisor.

The beaver has four strong curved incisors. They have very hard, bright orange enamel on their labial surface and much softer exposed dentin on the lingual surface. As the dentin wears off, this leaves very sharp cutting edges of enamel. The incisors continue to grow throughout life. The posterior teeth have flat, rough edges on the occlusal surface, and they stop growing at 2 years of age. There is a large diastema immediately posterior to the incisors, and flaps of skin fold inward and meet behind the incisors to seal off the back part of the mouth during gnawing. Therefore, splinters are kept out. The flaps of skin relax for eating and drinking. Most of the wood beavers gnaw as nonedible.

The shrew has two hooked cusps on the upper first incisor. Their deciduous dentition is shed in utero. Their 1–1½-year life span is limited by the wear on their molars. Death occurs by starvation once the molars wear out. Also their small body can store only enough food for 1 to 2 hours, so they must feed almost continually. Their diet consists of small invertebrates, woodlice, and fruit.

The vampire bat has large canines, but it is its highly specialized upper incisors, which are V-shaped and razor-edged, that remove a piece of the victim's skin. The bat's saliva contains an anticoagulant, and its tongue rolls up in a tube to suck or lap the exuding blood.

Some vertebrates do not have any teeth (complete anodontia) but have descended from ancestors that possessed teeth. Birds have beaks but depend on a gizzard to do the grinding that molars would usually perform. Turtles have heavy jaw coverings, which are thin-edged in the incisor region and wide posteriorly for crushing. The duck-billed platypus has its early-life teeth replaced by keratinous plates, which it uses to crush aquatic insects, crustaceans, and molluscs. The whalebone whale and anteaters also have no teeth, but their diets do not require mastication.

tions, permanent dentitions have a new category of teeth called premolars which are just behind the canines. Premolars are positioned in the spaces left where the molars had been in the deciduous dentition. Premolars closest to the midline are called *first* premolars, followed behind by *second* premolars. Behind the premolars, there are now three instead of two molars. As in the deciduous dentition, molars closest to the midline are *first* molars, followed next by *second* molars. The farthest back molars in each quadrant of the permanent dentition are called *third* molars.

(The animal dentition is represented by the same type of formula. Cows have no upper incisors or upper canines. They have three upper and three lower premolars on each side. Can you write the formula for a cow? If not, look at the formulas for several animals in Table 1.1. Did you know that dogs have twice as many premolars as humans? How many do you suppose this is? Do not forget to include uppers and lowers, as well as the right and left sides.)

## LEARNING EXERCISE

*Using models of the permanent dentition, identify each tooth by name.*

Note that permanent incisors and canines replace primary incisors and canines respectively, whereas permanent premolars replace primary molars. In the strict sense, succedaneous teeth would exclude the permanent molars, because they erupt posterior to the deciduous molars, having no predecessors or precursors in the primary dentition.

## C. Dentition: Anterior and Posterior Teeth

The anterior teeth are the incisors and the canines; the posterior teeth are the premolars and the molars. (Figs. 1.1 and 1.2.)

# SECTION II: THE HUMAN SKULL

## LEARNING EXERCISE

*To obtain a clear understanding of these bones and their relationship to one another and to the teeth, it is almost necessary to have a skull at hand to examine while reading the outline. If you touch or trace each bone with your fingers as you read, you are not apt to forget its characteristics.*

There are 208 bones in our skeleton, 22 of which are in the skull. If we count the malleus, stapes, and incus bones in each ear, there are 28 bones in the skull. The skull bones can be divided into two parts: the neurocranium and the facial or visceral apparatus.

## A. Neurocranium

The neurocranium is the portion which functions to support, house (surround and cover), and protect the brain (Fig. 1.3). It is made up of replacement bone (i.e., there is a cartilaginous precursor or model for these bones). Other names for this type of bone are cartilage bone and endochondral bone.

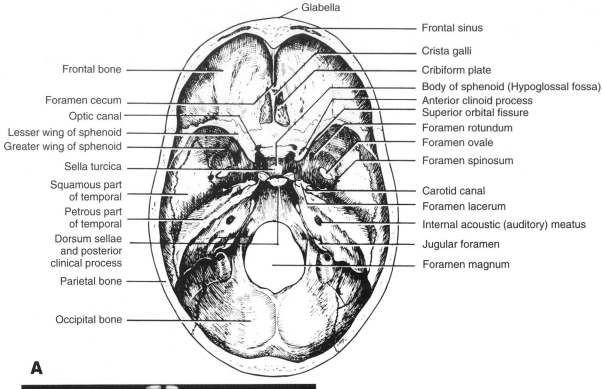

Glabella

Frontal sinus

Crista galli

Frontal bone — Cribiform plate

Body of sphenoid (Hypoglossal fossa)

Foramen cecum — Anterior clinoid process

Optic canal — Superior orbital fissure

Lesser wing of sphenoid — Foramen rotundum

Greater wing of sphenoid — Foramen ovale

Sella turcica — Foramen spinosum

Squamous part of temporal —

Petrous part of temporal — Carotid canal

Foramen lacerum

Dorsum sellae and posterior clinical process — Internal acoustic (auditory) meatus

Jugular foramen

Parietal bone — Foramen magnum

Occipital bone

**A**

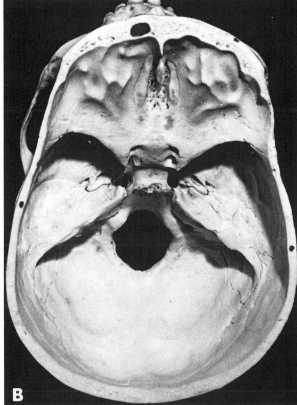

**B**

**Figure 1.3. A.** Base of the skull, the superior surface depicting many important structures. Those portions of the bones shown here comprise the neurocranium and develop from replacement type of bone (having a cartilaginous precursor). **B.** Photograph of the same structures shown in **A** with five anterior teeth and the left zygomatic arch projecting beyond the skull outline. Cover up **A** and try to identify many of the same structures in **B** (foramen rotundum is hidden in the shadow cast by the lesser wing of the sphenoid bone).

The eight bones of the neurocranium are:

| Single bones | Paired bones (one on each side) |
| --- | --- |
| Sphenoid<br>Occipital<br>Ethmoid<br>Frontal | Temporal<br>Parietal |

Muscles that attach from the neurocranium to the mandible have their *origin* or immovable attachment on the neurocranium bones, and their *insertion* on the movable lower jaw. The sphenoid and temporal bones are most significant when discussing jaw movement since they serve as the origin for three of the four major pairs of muscles of mastication (chewing). These bones also serve as part of the attachment for ligaments, bands of tough tissue (fascia) that limit the movement of the lower jaw.

## 1. BONES OF THE NEUROCRANIUM

### a. Sphenoid Bone

This midline bone is an irregular shaped bone that cradles the base of the brain and pituitary gland (see body and greater and lesser wings of the sphenoid bone in Fig. 1.3), and forms the posterior part of the orbit. There are two wing-shaped *pterygoid processes* that project downward from the base of skull, posterior to the palatine bones of the hard palate (see the pterygoid process [lateral pterygoid lamina or plate can be seen] in Fig. 1.5). (Since this pterygoid process is somewhat shaped like a wing with a scalloped border, to remember pterygoid, cf. *ptero*dactyl = winged dinosaur.) The space between the pterygoid plate and palatine bones is the *pterygopalatine space or canal* (see probe in Fig. 1.5). This fossa is the passage way for the major nerves and blood vessels of the jaws and muscles of mastication.

Each pterygoid process is the origin of two muscles of mastication that extend from the base of the skull to the lower jaw:

The *lateral pterygoid plate or lamina* is the origin for the lateral pterygoid muscle (Fig. 1.5).

The *pterygoid fossa* is the origin for the medial pterygoid muscle; you can place your little finger in this depression (Fig. 1.6**A**).

The *greater wing* (external surface) is part of the origin of the temporalis muscle (Fig. 1.4).

The *foramen ovale* is the skull opening for the mandibular division of the fifth cranial nerve (CN V), a major nerve for the teeth and jaws (Fig. 1.3).

The *foramen rotundum* is the opening for the maxillary division of fifth cranial nerve (Fig. 1.3).

The *angular spine* (sharp small process on the sphenoid bone just posterior to foramina ovale and spinosum) serves as the attachment for the sphenomandibular ligament which extends to the medial surface of lower jaw or mandible (Fig. 1.6).

### b. Temporal Bones (Paired)

The temporal bones (Fig. 1.4) are a pair of complex bones which form part of the sides and base of the skull. The temporal fossa is a large shallow depression in the temple region made up primarily of the temporal bone, along with a portion of the sphenoid (greater wing), parietal, and frontal bones (mentioned below). The temporalis muscle has its origin in this temporal fossa.

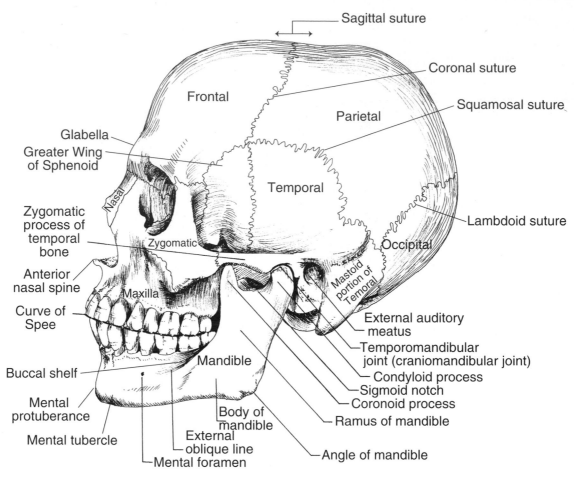

**Figure 1.4.** Left side of a human skull. Try to find these structures and suture lines on a skull. The temporal fossa is the shallow depression on the right or left side of the cranium that includes the temporal bone and greater wing of the sphenoid, as well as the adjacent portions of the frontal and parietal bones.

The temporal bones are important to dental professionals since they contain the fossae where the lower jaw (or mandible) articulates (joins) with the base of the neurocranium. *An articular (mandibular) fossa* and *articular eminence* located bilaterally on the inferior aspect of the temporal bone provide this articulating area for the lower jaw (Fig. 1.6). (Since the lower jaw is also known as the mandible, this joint is known as the craniomandibular joint [CMJ], or, in some current literature, the temporomandibular joint [TMJ].)

The *mastoid process,* inferiorly and posteriorly, serves as the attachment of a major neck muscle, the sternocleidomastoid muscle (Fig. 1.6).

The *styloid process,* shaped like a small skinny pencil (or stylus), is one attachment of the stylomandibular ligament which extends to the angle of the lower jaw (Fig. 1.6).

c. **Frontal Bone**

This singular midline bone forms the "forehead" and eyebrow region (Fig. 1.7). A small portion of this bone in the temporal fossa region serves as part of the origin of the temporalis muscle (Fig. 1.4).

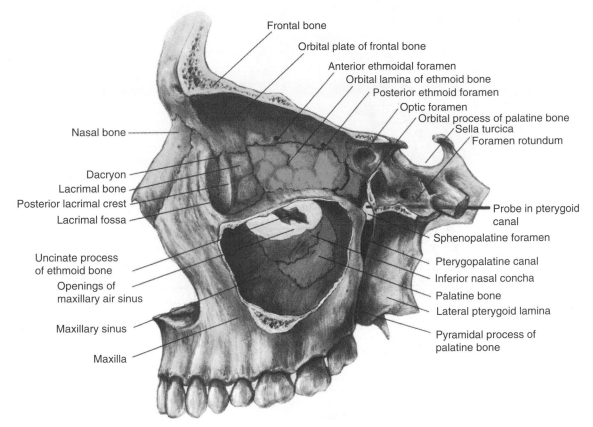

Frontal bone
Orbital plate of frontal bone
Anterior ethmoidal foramen
Orbital lamina of ethmoid bone
Posterior ethmoid foramen
Optic foramen
Orbital process of palatine bone
Sella turcica
Foramen rotundum
Nasal bone
Dacryon
Lacrimal bone
Posterior lacrimal crest
Lacrimal fossa
Probe in pterygoid canal
Sphenopalatine foramen
Uncinate process of ethmoid bone
Openings of maxillary air sinus
Maxillary sinus
Maxilla
Pterygopalatine canal
Inferior nasal concha
Palatine bone
Lateral pterygoid lamina
Pyramidal process of palatine bone

**Figure 1.5.** The external wall of the body of the left maxillary bone has been removed and the large maxillary sinus is exposed. The floor of the sinus is above the maxillary posterior teeth, but it does not extend as far forward as the maxillary anterior teeth. The floor of the nasal cavity, not the floor of the sinus, is above the anterior teeth. Notice the openings into the nasal chamber in the medial wall of the sinus. The part of the palatine bone indicated in the illustration is not the part that makes up the posterior fourth of the hard palate; it is the vertical part of the palatine bone. The posterior quarter of the hard palate is the horizontal part of the palatine bone. (Reproduced by permission from Clemente CD, ed. Gray's anatomy of the human body. 30th ed. Philadelphia: Lea & Febiger, 1985:166.)

### d. Parietal Bones

These paired bones protect the brain laterally and posteriorly (Fig. 1.4). Like the frontal bone, a small portion of this bone in the temporal fossa is a portion of the origin of the temporalis muscle.

### e. Occipital Bone

This bone provides the articulating surface between the skull and vertebral column at the occipital condyle (Fig. 1.6). The large *foramen magnum* serves as the passageway for the spinal cord.

### f. Ethmoid Bone

This midline bone is visible on the inside of the brain case above the nasal passageway as the *cribriform* (sieve-like) *plate* (Fig. 1.3). It also extends downward to form the superior part (*along with the vomer*) of the *nasal septum* which separates the right and left nasal cavities. This bone also forms part of the medial aspect of each orbit (Fig. 1.5).

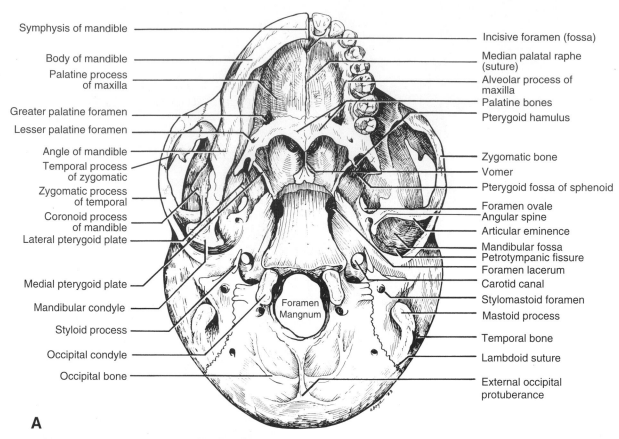

Symphysis of mandible

Body of mandible

Palatine process
of maxilla

Greater palatine foramen

Lesser palatine foramen

Angle of mandible

Temporal process
of zygomatic

Zygomatic process
of temporal

Coronoid process
of mandible

Lateral pterygoid plate

Medial pterygoid plate

Mandibular condyle

Styloid process

Occipital condyle

Occipital bone

Incisive foramen (fossa)

Median palatal raphe
(suture)

Alveolar process of
maxilla

Palatine bones

Pterygoid hamulus

Zygomatic bone

Vomer

Pterygoid fossa of sphenoid

Foramen ovale

Angular spine

Articular eminence

Mandibular fossa

Petrotympanic fissure

Foramen lacerum

Carotid canal

Stylomastoid foramen

Mastoid process

Temporal bone

Lambdoid suture

External occipital
protuberance

Foramen
Mangnum

**A**

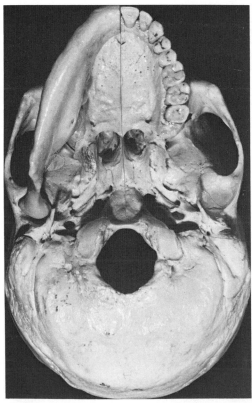

**B**

**Figure 1.6. A.** External surface of the skull with half of the mandible removed on one side. Cover up the structures on one side with a card and test yourself. **B.** Photograph of same structures shown in **A**. You should be able to find most of the structures labeled in **A** in the photograph (**B**).

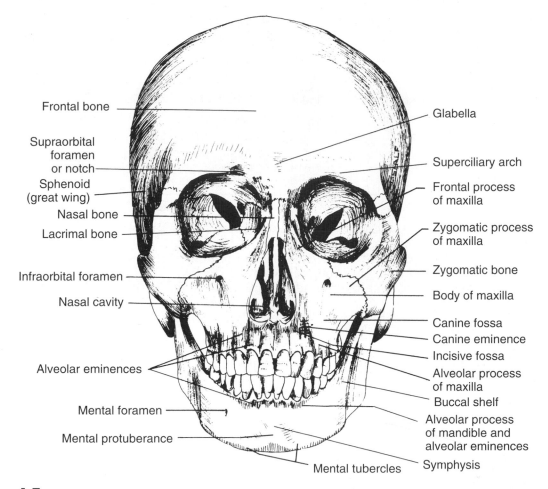

Frontal bone

Supraorbital foramen or notch

Sphenoid (great wing)

Nasal bone

Lacrimal bone

Infraorbital foramen

Nasal cavity

Alveolar eminences

Mental foramen

Mental protuberance

Glabella

Superciliary arch

Frontal process of maxilla

Zygomatic process of maxilla

Zygomatic bone

Body of maxilla

Canine fossa

Canine eminence

Incisive fossa

Alveolar process of maxilla

Buccal shelf

Alveolar process of mandible and alveolar eminences

Mental tubercles    Symphysis

**Figure 1.7.** Frontal aspect of a human skull. Try to find all of the labeled structures on a dry human skull.

## 2. SUTURES

Several major lengthy suture lines (Fig. 1.4) (i.e., lines where adjacent bones connect) are named as follows:

*coronal* between the frontal and two parietal bones;

*squamosal* between the temporal and parietal bones;

*sagittal* (best seen on the top of the skull) between the right and left parietal bones on the top midline of the skull;

*lambdoid* suture, joins the occipital bone with the parietal bones.

## B. Facial or Visceral Apparatus

These facial bones give us our appearance and function in both respiration and digestion. They are made up of dermal or intramembranous bone, the type which has no cartilaginous precursor. The facial apparatus is located anteriorly below the forehead and is a major part of the skull.

The mandible and maxillae are most important when discussing teeth and tooth movement. The mandible is the largest bone in the face. Each maxilla is the second largest bone in the face or facial apparatus.

These 14 bones make up the face or facial apparatus:

| Single bones | Paired bones (one on each side) |
|---|---|
| Mandible | Maxillae |
| Vomer (divides nose) | Palatine |
| | Zygomatic |
| | Nasal |
| | Lacrimal |
| | Inferior turbinates (concha) (The middle and superior turbinates are processes of the ethmoid bone, one of the bones of the neurocranium.) |

The *hyoid bone* is associated with the skull but is not connected to it except via soft tissue. It has a cartilaginous model precursor, so it is of replacement type bone (i.e., it forms as cartilage but it is eventually replaced with, and becomes, bone). The hyoid bone lies deep to and just above the laryngeal prominence of the thyroid cartilage. This laryngeal prominence has sometimes been called the Adam's apple (see Fig. 2.10).

All of the bones of the skull except the mandible and hyoid are firmly attached to one another via irregular sutures.

## 1. BONES OF THE VISCERAL APPARATUS (FACE)

### a. Maxillae (Right and Left Maxilla)

Each maxilla (right and left) consists of one large central mass, the *body*, and four smaller projecting *processes* (the frontal, zygomatic, alveolar, and palatine). (Study the drawings in Figure 1.7 for three of these processes, and Figure 1.8 for the palatine processes.)

#### (1) Body

The body of the maxilla is shaped like a four-sided hollow pyramid with the base oriented vertically next to the nasal cavity and the apex or peak extending laterally into the zygomatic process (part of the cheek bone).

It contains a large cavity—the *maxillary sinus* (Figs. 1.5 and 1.9).

The *infraorbital foramen* is on the anterior surface of the body just above the canine fossa (Fig. 1.7). It is an opening for the infraorbital nerve and vessels. The *alveolar canals*, where the superior alveolar nerves enter the maxilla, are located on the posterolateral or infratemporal surface behind the third molar, seen as a small opening (but not labelled) in Fig. 1.5.

Alveolar eminences are raised areas of bone overlying tooth root convexities. One of the alveolar eminences over the canine tooth on each side is called the *canine eminence* (Fig. 1.7). Anterior to the canine eminence is a fossa over the root of the maxillary lateral incisor called the *incisive fossa*. Posterior to the canine eminence is a fossa over the roots of maxillary premolars named the *canine fossa* (Fig. 1.7).

#### (2) Processes on Each Maxilla

##### (a) Frontal (or Nasofrontal) Process

Its anterior or medial edge articulates with the nasal bone, extending superiorly to articulate with the frontal bone (Fig. 1.7). The

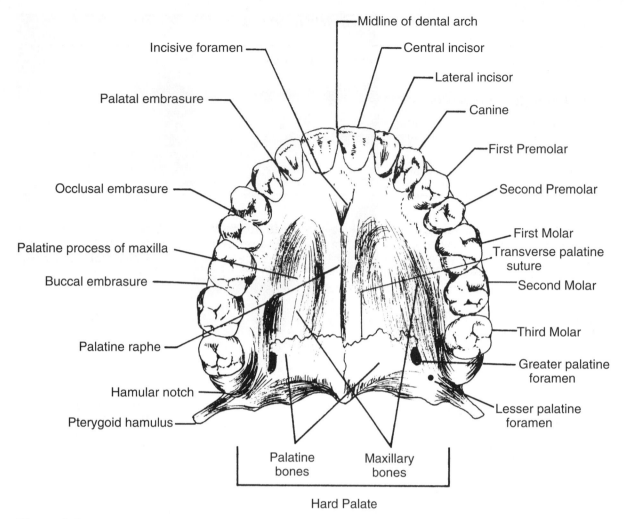

**Figure 1.8.** Maxillary dental arch and the bones of the hard palate. Compare this illustration with Figure 2.9. The transverse palatine suture is between the palatine and the maxillary bones.

nasal or medial surface is toward the nasal cavity and forms the lateral wall of the nasal cavity and half of the opening of the nasal cavity (piriform aperture).

*(b) Zygomatic Process (Elongated and Rough)*

This process (Fig. 1.7) extends laterally to articulate with the zygomatic bone. This process, along with the zygomatic bone and the zygomatic process of the temporal bone (Fig. 1.4), form the zygomatic arch. This arch serves as the origin of the masseter muscle.

In front, the zygomatic process forms part of the anterior or facial surface of the maxilla.

*(c) Alveolar Process*

It extends inferiorly, forming half of the maxillary dental arch, with eight sockets (alveoli), one for each tooth (Fig. 1.7). The *dental arches* of bone which surround and support the teeth are the alveolar processes of the upper and lower jaws. The roots of the teeth are embedded in *alveoli* (pits or sockets) in the maxillary and

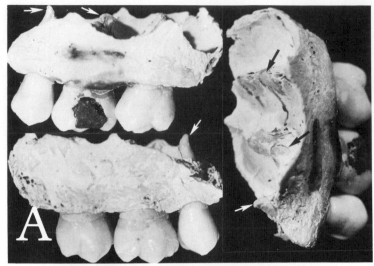

**Figure 1.9. A**. Three views of a left maxillary alveolar process and three teeth showing the close relationship between the root apices (*arrows*) to the maxillary sinus. *Top left:* Buccal view with two of the pneumatized portions of the sinus well below the roots tips (there is a poorly shaped large amalgam restoration in the first molar). *Lower left:* Lingual view with the second premolar root well above the floor of the sinus; right, superior view showing three concavities in the floor of the sinus that project as low as the middle portions of the molar roots, and no bony covering to the root apices (*arrows*).

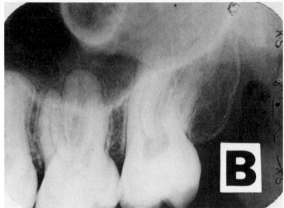

**B.** Radiograph of the maxillary molar region showing all three roots of the first molar several millimeters deep into the maxillary sinus (*dark area*). Part of the roots of the second molar are also within the sinus cavity. The apex of the second premolar root is in the sinus as well. This is a common relationship.

mandibular bones and are attached to the bone by the fibers of the periodontal ligament (see Figs. 1.10 and 1.11).

The alveolar process consists of bony layers which surround each tooth (Fig. 1.11). In the mouth, the alveolar process is covered by mucous membrane with the various regions named as shown in Figure 2.3.

**The Alveolar process is made up of the following bony layers (Fig. 1.11):**

(1) Lamina dura

Synonyms for lamina dura include: alveolar bony socket, alveolar bone, true alveolar bone, alveolar bone proper, cribriform plate of the alveolar process. The lamina dura is the thin, compact bone that forms the wall of each tooth socket or the alveolus where the periodontal ligament is attached. The shape of each alveolus or thin bony socket naturally corresponds exactly with the shape of the roots of the tooth it surrounds. The only space between the outer layer of tooth root (cementum) and this alveolar bone is that occupied by the periodontal ligament, which suspends and attaches each tooth to the bone. The periodontal ligament is between 0.12 and

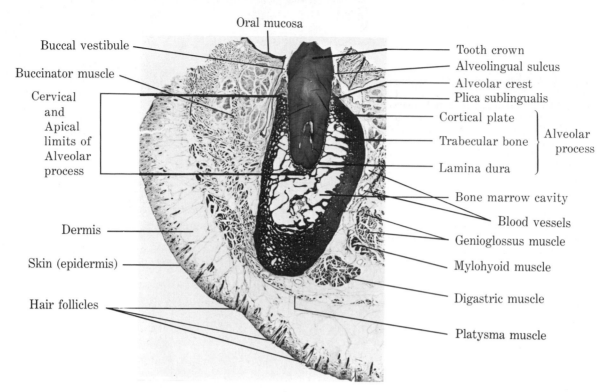

**Figure 1.10.** A buccolingual section, about 30 μm thick, of a human mandible and a posterior tooth. The tooth enamel was destroyed by the decalcification of the specimen with nitric acid preparatory to embedding and sectioning. Only a small part of the pulp cavity is in this section. The cortical plate is thick and the trabecular bone is less dense than in some specimens. The periodontal ligament is seen as the very thin, white line between the tooth root and the lamina dura. Its average thickness is only 0.2 mm (twice as thick as this page). The alveolar process comprises all of the bone surrounding the tooth from the alveolar crest to the root apex. To the left of the mandibular bone is the soft tissue of the cheek. For further information on the histology of these structures, refer to references 11, 23, 37–41.

0.33 mm thick and is composed of cells and fibrous intercellular substance. The periodontal ligament also contains *proprioceptive (sense of position) nerve endings,* which continually send messages to the brain as to the location at the mandible in space. This has a tremendous influence on jaw position, movement, and occlusion (the fitting together) of the teeth. Canines are reported to have the richest supply of proprioceptive nerve endings.

(2) Supporting Bone

Supporting bone is made up of an inner and outer cortical plate with trabecular bone sandwiched in between (Fig. 1.11). The *cortical plate* is made up of the thickened outer facial and inner lingual surfaces of the alveolar process. Bulges of cortical plate bone overlying the roots of teeth on the facial side are called alveolar eminences.

*Trabecular bone* (synonyms: cancellous bone, spongy bone) is composed of many platelike bone partitions that separate the irregularly shaped bone marrow spaces located within this trabecular or spongy bone (Figs. 1.10 and 1.11).

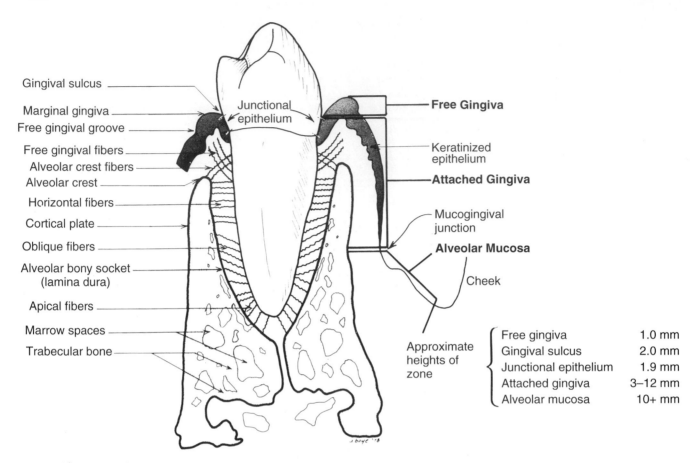

Gingival sulcus

Marginal gingiva

Free gingival groove

Free gingival fibers

Alveolar crest fibers

Alveolar crest

Horizontal fibers

Cortical plate

Oblique fibers

Alveolar bony socket
(lamina dura)

Apical fibers

Marrow spaces

Trabecular bone

Junctional
epithelium

**Free Gingiva**

Keratinized
epithelium

**Attached Gingiva**

Mucogingival
junction

**Alveolar Mucosa**

Cheek

Approximate
heights of
zone

| | |
|---|---|
| Free gingiva | 1.0 mm |
| Gingival sulcus | 2.0 mm |
| Junctional epithelium | 1.9 mm |
| Attached gingiva | 3–12 mm |
| Alveolar mucosa | 10+ mm |

**Figure 1.11.** Mesial side of a mandibular left first premolar suspended in its alveolus by the five groups of fibers of the periodontal ligament. (Periodontal ligament fibers include the apical, oblique, horizontal, alveolar crest, and free gingival fibers.) A sixth group, called transseptal fibers, runs directly from the cementum of one tooth to the cementum of the adjacent tooth at a level between the free gingival and alveolar crest fibers. The fibers of the periodontal ligament are much shorter than depicted here, averaging only 0.2 mm long (see actual size in Figure 1.10). (Compare the various zones of gingiva (*right side*) with those in Figure 2.3.) All of these structures supporting the teeth (including cementum) comprise the periodontium. Cover the names and see how many of the structures you are able to identify.

### (d) Palatine Process of the Maxilla

This process (Fig. 1.8) projects horizontally and medially from the inner surface of each maxilla as a thin, bony plate that meets the palatine process of the opposite maxilla at the median or *midpalatine suture line* of the hard palate.

### (3) Hard Palate

The inferior surfaces of the right and left palatine processes form the anterior three-fourths of the hard palate (Fig. 1.8). The superior surfaces form the floor of the nasal cavity. Part or all of the palatine processes are absent in a person who was born with a cleft palate.

The palatine process of each maxilla articulates posteriorly with the horizontal plate of each *palatine bone*, which forms the posterior one-fourth of the hard palate. This junction or suture line is called the *transverse palatine suture* (Fig. 1.8).

The shape of the palate and the shape of the maxillary arch vary in length, breadth, and height. The hard palate blends smoothly with the palatal portion of the maxillary alveolar process. The *incisive foramen* (Fig. 1.8) is on the midline just posterior to the central incisors. It transmits the anterior branches of the descending palatine artery and nasopalatine nerve.

The anteroposterior line of fusion (*median palatine suture*) between the right and left palatine processes of the maxillae and the horizontal plates of the palatine bones, runs at the midline posterior from the incisive foramen. In the mouth, this is the *palatine raphe* (pronounced rā'fē), which is frequently an obvious ridge when you look into the mouth (Fig. 2.2).

The *greater palatine foramina* (Fig. 1.8) are located posteriorly at the angle where the palatine bones and alveolar process of the hard palate meet. They transmit the descending palatine vessels and greater (anterior) palatine nerve.

The embryonic premaxilla cannot be distinguished in the adult. It is the anterior part of the maxillary bone, which contains the incisors. The suture line (when visible) between the premaxilla and the palatine processes of the two maxillae is called the *incisive suture,* and runs from the incisive foramen to separate the premaxilla portion of the hard palate adjacent to the incisors from the more posterior portion of the palate.

### (4) Maxillary Sinus

The maxillary sinuses within the maxillae are one pair of four sinuses that surround the nasal passages. The other three are the frontal, ethmoid, and sphenoid sinuses located within those respective bones. The maxillary sinus functions to (a) lighten the skull, (b) give resonance to the voice, (c) warm the air we breathe, and (d) moisten the nasal cavity.

This large, four-sided, pyramid-shaped cavity is located within the body of each maxilla, right and left (Fig. 1.5). The average size of the maxillary sinus in an adult is 25 mm transversely, 30 mm anteroposteriorly, and 30 mm vertically, with an average capacity of 15 ml (range: 9.5–20 ml) (1), or about 1 tablespoon.

The sinus cavity floor extends inferiorly into the base or top of the alveolar process where many projections of the apical ends of the molar roots and sometimes premolar roots are found. The most intimate relationship between the teeth and sinus is seen in Figure 1.9. Only *very* thin bone lies between the floor of the sinus and the apices of the roots of the maxillary molars. Rarely, no bone separates the root apices from the sinus. There is always soft tissue, made up of the periodontal ligament on the tooth root and the sinus mucous membrane lining the sinus cavity, between the cementum of the root and the space of the cavity. Sometimes when a dentist extracts a molar and the root breaks off, he is unjustly accused of pushing the root into the sinus. It may have been located in the maxillary sinus prior to the extraction. The other three walls of the sinus are orbital, facial, and infratemporal (posterolateral).

The maxillary sinus is a significant structure because of the close relationship it has to the oral cavity. An infection in either place can spread to the other. Pain caused by a maxillary sinus infection can be mistaken for pain originating in any one or all of the molars or premolars on that side. The nerve and blood supply to the upper teeth travels just beneath the membrane lining of the sinus or through bony canals in the walls of the sinus (Fig. 1.26). Unfortunately, healthy teeth are sometimes extracted in a futile attempt to alleviate pain that was caused by a maxillary sinus infection.

The maxillary sinus is lined with ciliated columnar epithelium similar to that found in the respiratory tract. The mucous film it secretes moves spirally and superiorly (against gravity) across the membrane to the opening located on the anterosuperior portion of the sinus (Fig. 1.5), where it drains into the middle nasal fossa. Without humans' upright posture, this opening for drainage would be on the floor, not the roof, and humans would have fewer sinus problems. Many people can get pain relief by placing their head in a prone position for several minutes to permit more rapid drainage of the maxillary sinuses.

The blood, lymph, and nerve supply to the maxillary sinus are the same that supply the upper posterior teeth (see Chapter 1, Sections V and VI).

## Mandible

The single, horseshoe-shaped mandible is the largest and strongest bone of the skull (Figs. 1.4, 1.7, and 1.12). Generally, speaking, it is bilaterally symmetrical. It bears the mandibular teeth, and is attached only by ligaments and muscles to the relatively immovable bones of the skull. The craniomandibular joints just in front of the ear are movable articulations—the only visible movable articulations in the head (Fig. 1.4). The mandible is the only bone of the skull that can move. The rest of the bones move only when the whole head is moved and then they move in unison. The insertion ends of all chewing muscles attach to the relatively movable mandible.

The mandible has three parts: one horizontal *body* and two vertical *rami* (singular, ramus) (Figs. 1.4 and 1.12). The bulky, curved horizontal body and the flat-

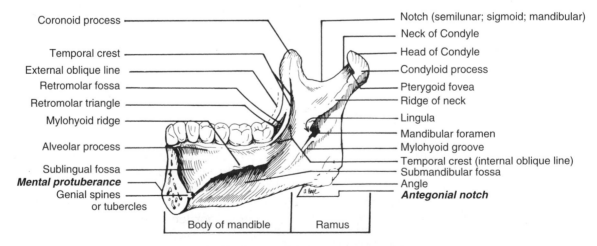

**Figure 1.12.** Medial surface of the mandible. Notice the major divisions of the body of the mandible and the ramus. The alveolar process extends superiorly from the apical ends of the tooth roots to the alveolar ridge crest that surrounds the cervical portion of each tooth (Fig. 1.10). Study each landmark and try to find it on an actual mandible as you read the text and study this illustration. You will be able to feel the angle externally and the anterior border of the ramus easily. The mylohyoid ridge beneath the mucosa can be felt by gently pressing laterally with a finger beneath your tongue.

tened vertical ramus join at the *angle of the mandible* on either side. The *angle* of the mandible is located where the inferior border of the body joins the posterior border of the ramus. The landmarks of the mandible will be discussed according to their location: external surface of the body, then ramus, then the internal surface.

### (1) Body (Lateral Surface)

The human *chin* consists of the two *mental tubercles* and the mental *protuberance* (Fig. 1.7). No other mammal has a chin. *Mental tubercles* lie on either side of the symphysis near the inferior border of the mandible. The *symphysis* (not evident on the adult mandible) is the line of fusion of the right and left sides at the midline where the two halves of the mandible fuse (join together) during the first year after birth. The centered *mental protuberance* is 10 mm above but between the two mental tubercles, and is on the midline. This protuberance and the tubercles are more prominent on men than on women.

As in the maxillae, an alveolar process supports the teeth (Fig. 1.7). Alveolar *eminences* are elevations over tooth roots on the facial side. The vertical elevations overlying the roots of the canines are called the *canine eminences.*

The *mental foramen* on each side lies near the apex (root end) of the second premolar (Fig. 1.7). On dental radiographs it looks dark, similar to the lesion formed by a periapical abscess (i.e., an infection that destroys bone around the end [apex] of the tooth root), especially when it is superimposed over the premolar root apex. The nerves and vessels that exit the mandible through the mental foramen traverse a canal within bone and then travel outward, upward, and posteriorly exiting the bone. Place a flexible probe carefully into this canal to confirm this direction. The mental foramen transmits vessels and nerves (see the mental nerve exiting the mental foramen in Fig. 1.27) and has been shown to be located at practically the same level on most humans (13–15 mm superior to the inferior border of the mandible).

In a study of 40 skulls (2), the mental foramen was found to be:

Under the apex of the first premolar—never

Between the apices of the first and second premolars—40%

Directly under the second premolar—42.5%

Distal to the apex of the second premolar—17.5%

The lateral surface of the angle is where the insertion of the masseter muscle attaches. Just posterior to this is the attachment of the stylomandibular ligament.

An e*xternal oblique* ridge (Fig. 1.4) extends from each mental tubercle (canine region) to the anterior border of the ramus. The nearly horizontal ledge or zone in the molar region between the external oblique ridge and alveolar process is named the *buccal shelf.* This is the location of the long buccal nerve.

### (2) Ramus (Lateral Surface)

There are two processes on the upper end of each ramus:

*(a) Coronoid Process*

This process is the more anterior process, roundly pointed on the upper border and flat on the lateral and medial surfaces (Fig. 1.4). The tendon from all of the fibers of the wide, flat, fan-shaped temporalis muscle has its insertion on this process and onto the anterior border of the ramus.

*(b) Condyloid Process or Mandibular Condyle*

This process is composed of a condyle head, and a neck to which the head is attached (Fig. 1.4). The mandibular condyle is about the size and shape of a large date pit with the greater dimension mediolaterally (Fig. 1.16). From the side, it looks like a round knob. From the posterior aspect, it is wide and narrow mediolaterally with a narrow neck. The upper surface of the mandibular condyle is strongly convex anteroposteriorly, and mildly convex mediolaterally.

The head of the condyle fits into and functions beneath the articular (glenoid) fossa of the temporal bone of the cranium (is part of mandibular fossa in Fig. 1.6) with a disc in between the condyle and temporal bone. "CMJ" stands for the bones that make up this joint: the craniomandibular joint. This term is preferable to the previously used term: temporomandibular joint (TMJ).

A portion of one of the important muscles of mastication, the lateral pterygoid, attaches to the front of the neck of the condyloid process.

The *sigmoid notch* or mandibular notch or semilunar notch (Fig. 1.4), is between the coronoid process and the condyloid process.

### (3) Medial Surface of Mandible

The *genial tubercles or spines* are on either side of the midline on the medial surface of the mandible. Two large muscles (genioglossus [seen in Fig. 1.10] and geniohyoid) attach to the genial spines (Fig. 1.20) and the elevated and roughened bone near them.

The *mylohyoid ridge* or *mylohyoid line* (Fig. 1.12) is the rough irregular bone ridge running downward and forward from the molar region to the genial tubercles. The mylohyoid muscle forming part of the floor of the mouth attaches here. This ridge separates two shallow depressions or fossae above and below. The *sublingual fossa* is just above and lateral to the genial tubercles on each side. The sublingual salivary gland rests against this fossa. The *submandibular* fossa, where the large submandibular gland rests, is below the mylohyoid ridge in the premolar and molar regions.

The *temporal crest* (Fig. 1.12) is a ridge extending downward from the tip of the coronoid process, continuing inward onto the medial surface of the ramus, and terminating near the third molar. This crest is where the tendon of the temporalis muscle attaches. The *internal oblique line* is the inferior one-fourth of the temporal crest. It is really a radiographic, rather than an anatomic, term, since it appears on radiographs as a short, curved line somewhat inferior to the image of the external oblique line. IT IS NOT SYNONYMOUS WITH THE MYLOHYOID RIDGE as incorrectly stated in some radiographic textbooks.

The *retromolar fossa* (Fig. 1.12) is a roughened fossa distal to the last molar and located between the temporal crest (lowest portion) and the external oblique line. The *retromolar triangle* is in the lowest most anterior, or only horizontal, portion of the retromolar fossa. The *buccinator crest* is a barely discernible ridge or line that divides the retromolar fossa from the retromolar triangle. The most posterior fibers of the buccinator muscle attach here. The buccinator muscle is the pouch-shaped muscle in our cheek (Fig. 1.10).

The *mandibular foramen* (Fig. 1.12) is a large opening located on the medial surface of the ramus below the sigmoid notch in the center of the ramus. It is the entrance into the mandibular canal which contains the inferior alveolar vessels and nerves. The *mandibular lingula* is a sharp ridge or projection of bone just anterior and slightly superior to the mandibular foramen. This is where the sphenomandibular ligament attaches to the mandible. The *mylohyoid groove* is a small groove running down and forward, below and anterior to the mandibular foramen, but posterior to the mylohyoid ridge. The mylohyoid nerve rests in this groove.

### c. Zygomatic Bone

The zygomatic bone (Fig. 1.4) (one on each side of the face) forms an arch along with the zygomatic process of the maxillae and zygomatic process of the temporal bones; the arch is often referred to as the cheek bone. This arch of bone serves as the origin for the powerful masseter muscle.

### d. Palatine Bone

The palatine bones mentioned earlier in the discussion about the hard palate, form the posterior one-forth of the hard palate (Fig. 1.8). They also project upward behind the maxillae, separated by a space from the pterygoid process of the sphenoid bone. This space is the *pterygopalatine space* which is the passageway of the major nerves from the brain and blood vessels from the heart to the jaws and muscles of mastication (in Fig. 1.5 the probe is in this space or canal).

### e. Vomer Bone

The vomer bone (Fig. 1.6) is a midline bone forming part of the nasal septum along with part of the ethmoid bone.

### f. Nasal Bones

The nasal bones form the lateral bridge of the nose (Fig. 1.7).

### g. Lachrimal Bones

The lachrimal bones, at the corner of each orbit, contain a depression for tear glands (Fig. 1.5).

### h. Inferior Turbinates

The inferior turbinates (nasal concha) are scrolled bones in the nasal cavity forming part of the maxillary sinus wall. These are best seen through the opening to the nasal passageway (piriform aperture) (Fig. 1.7). Along with other scrolled processes of the ethmoid bone, they increase the area of mucous membrane inside the nasal passageways to warm and moisten air that we breath. (See these scrolled bones bulging on both sides of the inside of the nasal cavity in Fig. 1.7.)

### i. Hyoid Bone

The hyoid bone is not a bone of the skull, but floats alone above the voice box (Fig. 2.10). Muscles extend superiorly from the hyoid bone to the mandible (suprahyoid muscles, e.g., geniohyoid), and inferiorly from the hyoid to the sternum (breast bone) and clavicle (common prefix is cleido). These muscles help to open and retrude the jaw. Another muscle that connects the breast bone (sternum) and collar bone (clavicle) to the mastoid process of the temporal bone is the sternocleidomastoid muscle (Fig. 2.10). This muscle can be felt at the junction of the anterior and lateral portions of the neck.

## LEARNING EXERCISES

*If you have an opportunity to examine a number of skulls, compare them for variations in bone form. Look at the following:*

Shape and height of the mandible.

Location of mental and mandibular foramina.

Thickness of the bone on the facial side of tooth roots (eminences).

Prominence of ridges and eminences on mandible (mylohyoid ridge, genial tubercles, lingula, mental protuberance). Usually these ridges are most noticeable on male skulls.

Relationship of the tooth root tips (apices) of maxillary anterior teeth to the floor of the nose.

Relationship of the apices of maxillary molars to maxillary sinuses.

See if you can find and identify all of the bony landmarks and fossae described in this chapter and shown in Figures 1.4, 1.7, and 1.12. Many of them are also shown in Figure 1.6.

Review the names of structures shown in Figure 1.6**A,** then cover them and name these structures as seen in Figure 1.6**B.** Do the same for Figures 1.3**A** and 1.3**B.**

## SECTION III: THE CRANIOMANDIBULAR JOINT (CMJ)

A joint, or articulation, is a connection between two separate parts of the skeleton.

### CRANIOMANDIBULAR JOINT

This joint is the articulation between the *mandible* and the two *temporal bones;* therefore, in the past it has been called the temporomandibular joint (TMJ). The mandibular articulation with the skull on each side is better termed the *craniomandibular articulation,* since it is the articulation between the movable mandible and the stationary cranium or skull (3). It is a bilateral articulation: the right and left sides work as a unit. It is the only visible free-moving articulation in the head; all others are sutures and are immovable (4). The coordinated movements of the right and left joints are complex and usually are controlled by reflexes. Within some limit or range, the great adaptability of the joints permit the freedom of movement of the mandible required during speech and mastication. One can learn, however, to move his mandible voluntarily into specific, well-defined positions or pathways (5–9). Both the maxillae and mandible carry teeth whose shape and position greatly influence the most closed portions of mandibular movements (3). Proper functioning of the craniomandibular joints has profound effect on the occlusal contacts of teeth which concern nearly all phases of dentistry.

## LEARNING EXERCISE

*Palpate the craniomandibular joint, and feel the movement of the mandibular condyle. In front of the ear: Put your index finger immediately in front of either ear and open and close your mouth. Then move your jaw to the right and left sides. You are feeling the movement of the outer pole (surface) of each mandibular condyle. In the ear opening: Put your little finger inside either ear, open and close your mouth, and pull your jaw back or posteriorly. You are feeling the upper and posterior portion of the mandibular condyle, especially when you close or retrude your mandible.*

# A. ANATOMY OF THE CRANIOMANDIBULAR JOINT

There are three articulating parts to each craniomandibular joint (Figs. 1.13 and 1.14): the mandibular condyle, the articular fossa and eminence (or tubercle) of the temporal bone, and the articular disc (interposed between the bony parts). These parts are enclosed by a *fibrous connective tissue capsule* (Fig. 1.15) (1, 4, 7).

## LEARNING EXERCISES

*Examine a skull and study how the mandibular condyle fits loosely into the articular fossa. The disc is not present in a prepared skull because the disc is not bone; for the same reason, the fibrous capsule is not present. With the posterior teeth in occlusion, there should be a visible space between the mandibular condyle and the articular fossa (normally occupied by the disc).*

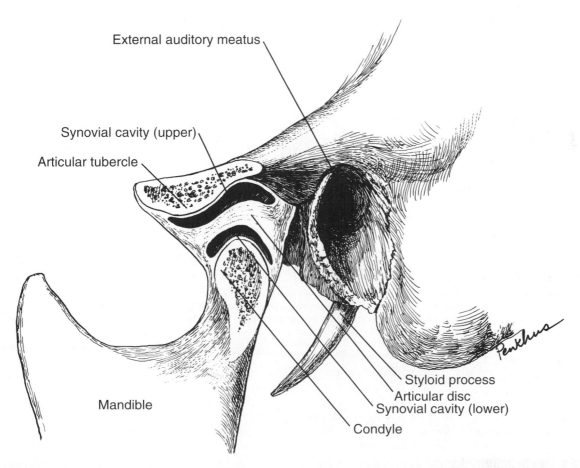

**Figure 1.13.** A sagittal section through the joint shown in Figure 1.17 reveals the condyle of the mandible, the articular fossa (the anterior part of the mandibular fossa identified in Figs. 1.6 and 1.14), and the disc. The articular eminence (tubercle) is a ridge extending mediolaterally just in front of the mandibular fossa. You will see this eminence if you examine the fossa of the undersurface of the skull. (Reproduced by permission from Clemente CD, ed. Gray's anatomy of the human body. 30th ed. Philadelphia: Lea & Febiger, 1985:340.)

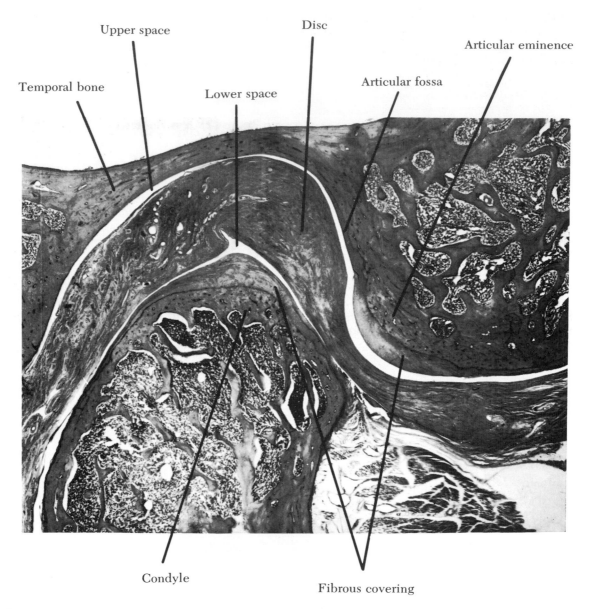

Upper space · Disc · Articular eminence · Temporal bone · Lower space · Articular fossa · Condyle · Fibrous covering

**Figure 1.14.** Photomicrograph of a human craniomandibular joint. The specimen was removed in a block of tissue, fixed in formalin, demineralized, embedded in celloidin, sectioned at a thickness of about 25 μm, and stained with hematoxylin and eosin. This is the joint seen from the lateral aspect. Anterior is toward the right of the picture; the white area across the top is the space of the brain case above the articular fossa. The condyle has a surface of compact bone, inside of which is the marrow cavity with bone trabeculae and bone marrow. The same kind of bone structure is seen in the articular eminence (*upper right*). Notice the difference in thickness of the fibrous covering on different parts of the articular fossa and mandibular condyle. The thicker regions are where the heaviest function occurs. (Courtesy of Professor Rudy Melfi.)

*Study Figures 1.6**A** and **B** to become familiar with the inferior view of the skull. The left half of the mandible has been removed, exposing the maxillary teeth, tuberosity, and articular fossa and eminence. Several of the structures and foramina mentioned previously are visible. Try to find as many of the named structures in Figure 1.6**A** on the photograph (Fig. 1.6**B**) as possible.*

## 1. MANDIBULAR CONDYLE

The mandibular condyle is a large, solid structure, about 10 mm thick antero-posteriorly and 20.4 mm wide mediolaterally (Figs. 1.6**A** and 1.6**B**). The outer tip or

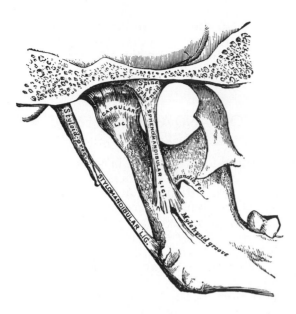

**Figure 1.15.** Medial aspect of the mandibular ramus and the craniomandibular joint. The fibrous capsule (capsular ligament) encloses the joint. Examine your prepared skull and locate the attachments of the stylomandibular and sphenomandibular ligaments. Most of these ligaments serve to prevent nonfunctional, damaging movements in the joint. (Reproduced by permission from Clemente CD, ed. Gray's anatomy of the human body. 30th ed. Philadelphia: Lea & Febiger, 1985:339.)

pole of the condyle is located about 15 mm beneath the skin in front of the ear (Fig. 1.16). Research by Drs. Woelfel and Igarashi on 25 men found the average depth on each side to be 15.0 mm; the range was 10.3 to 21.4 mm beneath skin. This is surprising since the outer pole of the condyle is readily palpated and its movements are visible (seemingly just beneath the skin) when eating. The articulating surface or functioning part of the condyle is located on the superior and anterior surfaces of the head of this condyloid process of the mandible (Fig. 1.13).

This surface of the condyle is covered or lined with a somewhat thickened a vascular layer of fibrous connective tissue, which may have a few cartilage cells. The fibrous connective tissue pad is particularly thick on top of the condyle over the region where most function occurs when the condyle is forward from its resting position (Fig. 1.14).

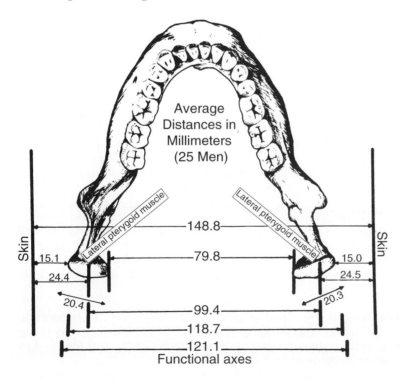

**Figure 1.16.** Summary of the information from a gnathologic cephalometric investigation in which metal markers were placed on the skin and some teeth prior to taking submental vertex cephalometric radiographs for analysis, tracing, and measuring. The location of the center of rotational opening of the mandible (the hinge axis) was found to pass through the center or near the center of the head of the condyle. The functional axes (controlling regions for all eccentric movement) were determined from pantographic recordings and the resultant articular settings and were found to be wider than the outer poles of the condyles. This means that lateral and protrusive excursions are controlled by ligaments and muscles, rather than by bone as previously reported. This research was conducted and supported by the Ohio State University College of Dentistry and Nihon University School of Dentistry in Tokyo.

All fibrous layers of the joint are avascular (also the disc), indicating that considerable force occurs on these surfaces of the joint. This avascular type of connective tissue is adapted to resist pressure. It lines the head of the condyle, the articulating surfaces of the articular eminence and fossa, and is found in the center portion of the disc (Fig. 1.14).

## 2. ARTICULAR FOSSA (NONFUNCTIONING PORTION) AND ARTICULAR EMINENCE (FUNCTIONING PORTION)

The *articular (glenoid) fossa* is the anterior three-fourths of the larger mandibular fossa (anterior to the petrotympanic fissure [Fig. 1.6]). This fossa is considered to be a nonfunctioning portion of the joint because, when the teeth are in tight occlusion, there is no tight contact between the head of the condyle, the disc, and the concave part of the articular fossa. The fossa is about 23 mm mediolaterally and extends 15 mm posteriorly from the eminence. The intracapsular surface is two to three times greater than on the mandibular condyle mainly because the anterior part of the capsule attaches 10 mm in front of the crest of the articulating eminence (10).

The *articular eminence* or transverse bony bar or ridge is located just anterior to and below the articular fossa (Fig. 1.6). Its surface is padded or lined by a thicker layer of fibrous connective tissue, more than the rest of the articular fossa, indicating that this is the functional portion of the joint when we are chewing food with the mandible in a protruded and/or lateral position. This thickened connective tissue lining is devoid of blood vessels and nerves (11). The thickest functional part of this lining is on the posterior inferior portion of the articular eminence. This is where the anterior-superior portion of the mandibular condyle rubs against it indirectly because the articular disc should always be interposed between the two functioning bony elements (Figs. 1.13 and 1.14). Confirm these surfaces of articulation on the skull.

## 3. ARTICULAR DISC

The disc (Figs. 1.13 and 1.14) is a tough oval pad of dense fibrous connective tissue located between (a) the mandibular condyle and (b) the articular fossa and articular eminence. The disc surfaces are very smooth.

It is thinner in the center than around the edges. It is thinner anteriorly and laterally and thicker medially and posteriorly. The disc acts as a buffer between the articular eminence of the temporal bone and the mandibular condyle. Rarely it may become perforated. The center of the disc has no blood supply (11), however, it is richly supplied elsewhere.

The upper contour of the disc is concavoconvex anteroposteriorly—concave anteriorly to fit under the articular eminence, and convex posteriorly, conforming to the shape of the articular fossa that it loosely rests against. The lower surface of the disc is concave in both directions, thus adapting to the upper surface of the mandibular condyle.

The disc forms a natural wedge anterior to the condyle head and a second wedge posterior to the condyle. Because of the extremely slippery surfaces, these two wedge portions help the disc move harmoniously with the condyle. When the wedge portions become flattened or the center of the disc thickens, the disc fails to move synchronously with the condyle, and popping (crepitus) occurs, which is quite annoying (Table 1.2).

Being elastically attached posteriorly, the disc moves with the head of the condyle in function, but only about half as far. It cushions all functional contacts between the articular eminence and the condyle when the jaw moves both laterally and forward in chewing.

**Table 1.2.** Prevalence of Crepitus During Maximum Opening*

|  | None % | Both Sides % | Right Side % | Left Side % | One Side (R or L) % |
|---|---|---|---|---|---|
| 594 Dental hygiene students | 52.0 | 13.3 | 18.2 | 16.8 | 35.0 |
| 505 Dental students | 72.0 | 4.2 | 15.9 | 7.9 | 23.8 |
| Percentage of all 1099 students | 61.2 | 9.1 | 17.1 | 12.7 | 29.8 |

*Determinations by Dr. Woelfel, 1970–1986. More than 20% of these professional students had or were undergoing orthodontic treatment.

The functions of the articular disc are (10, 12):

a. Partitioning the complex condylar movement into upper and lower functional components (12).

b. Lubricating with synovial fluid.

c. Stabilizing the condyle by filling the space between incongruous articulating surfaces (12).

d. Cushioning the loading of the joint at point of contact (shock-absorption).

e. Reducing physical wear and strain on joint surfaces.

f. Helping to regulate movements of the condyle because the anterior and posterior portions of the disc contain some proprioceptive nerve fibers that help determine the position of the mandible and some nerve fibers that mediate pain.

## 4. FIBROUS CAPSULE (SOMETIMES REFERRED TO AS THE CAPSULAR LIGAMENT)

The fibrous capsule is a sheet, sac, or tube of tissue that encloses the joint like a tube (Figs. 1.15 and 1.17). It is fairly thin, except laterally, where it forms the temporomandibular ligament seen as the lateral ligament in fig. 1.17 (13). The upper border of the capsule is attached to the temporal bone around the circumference of the articular fossa and the articular eminence. The lower border is attached around the neck of the condyloid process, thus enclosing the condyle completing the tube.

The *fibrous capsule* is composed of two layers:

### a. Inner Layer

The *inner layer* (synovial membrane), which lines the fibrous capsule and covers the bone to the borderline of the articulating surface and part of the mandibular neck. This is a thin layer of tissue that secretes a fluid, *synovia*, that lubricates the joint. The coefficient of friction of this fluid makes it three times as slippery as ice. The synovial fluid both lubricates and nourishes the joint surfaces, which lack a blood supply (fibrous covering of the articulating surfaces and center of the disc). In a normal joint space, there is only a small amount of fluid (1 or 2 drops). The synovial cavities are shown in Figure 1.13.

### b. Outer Layer

The *outer layer* is a somewhat thicker layer of fibrous tissue that is reinforced by accessory ligaments, which strengthen it. The anterior part of this fibrous capsule (*capsular ligament* [Fig. 1.17]) restricts posterior movement of the condyle of the mandible on wide openings as it becomes taut.

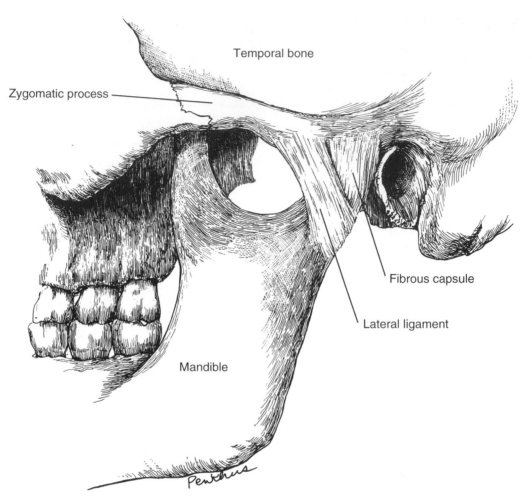

**Figure 1.17.** Lateral aspect of the mandible and part of the cranium. The craniomandibular joint is enclosed in the fibrous capsule, reinforced by the temporomandibular ligament (lateral ligament). (Reproduced by permission from Clemente CD, ed. Gray's anatomy of the human body. 30th ed. Philadelphia: Lea & Febiger, 1985:339.)

## 5. LIGAMENTS THAT SUPPORT THE JOINT AND LIMIT JOINT MOVEMENT

Ligaments are slightly elastic bands of tissue. They do not move the joint; muscles move the joint. They do support and confine the movement of the mandible to protect muscles from being stretched beyond their capabilities.

### a. Capsular Ligament

The capsular ligament was described above with the fibrous capsule.

### b. Temporomandibular Ligament or Craniomandibular Ligament

The *temporomandibular ligament* or craniomandibular ligament (the *lateral* portion of the fibrous capsule in Fig. 1.17) is the strong reinforcement of the lateral wall of the capsule. It is wide where it attaches to the zygomatic arch, then narrows as it drops obliquely down and backward to the side and back of the neck of the condyle. It keeps the condyle close to the fossa and helps to prevent lateral and posterior displacement of the mandible. It has no counterpart medially, and seemingly none is needed, since the right and left craniomandibular articulations work together as a unit. The temporomandibular ligament on the opposite side, by failing to stretch, prevents medial displacement on the side moving medially.

### c. Stylomandibular Ligament

The *stylomandibular ligament* (Fig. 1.15) is posterior to the joint and is separated from it, but it gives support to the mandible. It is relaxed when the mouth is closed but becomes tense on extreme protrusion of the mandible (13). It is attached above to the styloid process of the temporal bone and below to the posterior border and angle of the mandible and to the fascia of one of the muscles of the mastication, the medial pterygoid muscle.

### d. Sphenomandibular Ligament

The *sphenomandibular ligament* (Fig. 1.15) is medial to the joint. It gives some support to the mandible and may help limit maximum opening of the jaw. It is attached above to the *angular spine* of the sphenoid bone. Then it spreads out like a fan and attaches below to the lingula on the medial surface of the mandible near the mandibular foramen and to the lower border of the mylohyoid groove.

## 6. SUMMARY OF CAPSULE-TO-DISC AND OF DISC-TO-CONDYLE CONNECTIONS

Anteriorly, the disc and the capsule are fused. The disc is not attached to the skull. Posteriorly, the disc and the capsule are connected by an elastic bilaminar zone, a thick pad of loose elastic vascular connective tissue, which gives the disc freedom to move anteriorly, but limits it from excessive forward movement that could result in an anterior displacement of the disc (14).

Laterally and medially, the disc is tightly attached to the lateral and medial sides of the mandibular condyle, but not to the capsule. Therefore, the disc follows the movement of the condyle when the lateral pterygoid muscles move the mandible and disc forward or sideways.

## B. Development of the Craniomandibular Joint

### 1. IN INFANTS

The articular fossa, the articular eminence, and the condyle are rather flat. This flatness allows for a wide range of sliding motions in the craniomandibular joint. Also, they are at about the same level as the occlusal plane at birth with relatively no ramus height (Fig. 1.18).

### 2. DURING DEVELOPMENT

The articular fossa deepens, the articular eminence becomes prominent, the condyle becomes rounded, and the shape of the disc changes to conform to the change in shape of the fossa and condyle and the downward lengthening of the ramus.

### 3. GROWTH

The condyle contains cartilage beneath its surface, and the condyloid process and ramus lengthen until a person is 20–25 years old. This is one way the mandible grows in depth. As a result of growth in the condyle area, the body of the mandible is lowered from the skull, and the occlusal plane is about 1 inch below the level of the condyles in an adult.

### 4. MICROSCOPIC VIEW OF AN ADULT JOINT

Carefully examine the photomicrograph of a human craniomandibular joint seen in Figure 1.14. The condyle is in the position it would occupy when the teeth come

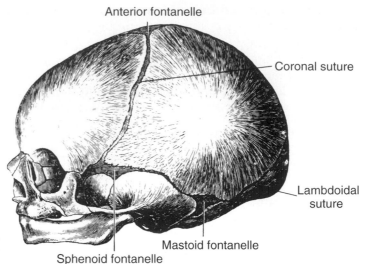

**Figure 1.18.** Skull at birth showing sphenoidal and mastoid fontanelles (membrane-covered openings between bones). Observe the small facial bones and the great difference in size between the facial and cranial vault bones in the neonatal skull. Notice that the mandibular condyle is barely higher than the crest of the mandibular ridge.

together as close as possible (are in maximum intercuspation), about 1 mm anterior to its most retruded position.

## LEARNING EXERCISES WITH SKULL

*Examine the space between the mandibular condyles and the articular fossae when the posterior teeth are in tight occlusion. Should this space exist? If so, what structure normally occupies this space?*

*Study a skull and see how the mandibular condyle fits into the mandibular fossa. The condyle, with the disc superimposed and attached medially and laterally, functions in the anterior part of this fossa. (The anterior part of the mandibular fossa is called the articular fossa.)*

# SECTION IV: MUSCLES OF CHEWING (MASTICATION)

## General Information on Muscles

The muscles of the body contribute 40–50% of the total body weight (15). Muscles produce the desired action by pulling or by shortening, never by pushing. Skeletal or voluntary muscles are made up of specialized tissue that contracts. Skeletal muscles are very active metabolically and therefore require a rich blood supply (15). There are two other kinds of muscles, cardiac and smooth, which we are unable to control or direct (involuntary muscles).

Muscle cells are small (10–40 microns [μm] in diameter), elongated contractile fibers, each enclosed in a delicate envelope of loose connective tissue. Many individual parallel muscle fibers make up a bundle, and various numbers of bundles comprise a muscle. The longest muscle fibers are 300 mm long. Each contractile unit can contract about 57% of its fully stretched length (16). The all-or-none law states that any single muscle fiber always contracts to its fullest extent (10). When a weak effort or contraction is required of the whole muscle, then only a few fibers contract (each to the fullest extent). Many fibers contracting produce greater power as needed. No single muscle acts alone to produce a movement or to maintain posture. Many muscles must work in perfect coordination to produce a steady, well-directed motion of a body part.

When a muscle becomes shorter as it moves a structure, the movement is called an *isotonic contraction*. When a muscle maintains its length as it contracts to stabilize a part, this movement is called *isometric contraction*. As you close your jaw until all teeth contact, the closing muscles work isotonically because they become shorter. If you maintain contact of all of your teeth but squeeze them together hard, these same muscles are contracting isometrically because they cannot shorten any more.

Some portions (a few or more individual muscles fibers) of all of our voluntary muscles are continually or alternately contracting during consciousness. This minimal amount of contraction needed to maintain posture is called tone or tonus, and the muscles involved are named "antigravity" muscles. As you read this, the muscles of mastication are probably in a state of minimal tonic contraction or balance with each other, with the neck muscles, and with gravity, enabling a comfortable, restful position for your mandible (teeth apart). This resting jaw position varies slightly according to whether you are sitting, lying on your back, or standing up, and depending on how tense or stressed you are.

Hopefully, this brief discussion will whet your appetite for seeking further knowledge. The reference list offers several choices.

## Muscular Functioning of the Craniomandibular Joint

**MUSCLES OF MASTICATION** move the mandible. There are four pairs of muscles (right and left): masseter, temporalis, medial pterygoid, and lateral pterygoid muscles. These muscles have the major control over all the movements of the mandible.

## A. Masseter Muscle

It is the most superficial, bulky, and powerful of the muscles of mastication (Figs. 1.19 and 1.20). It is quadrilateral in shape. Its average volume on 25 males was $30.4 \pm 4.1$ cm$^3$ which was 2.6 times larger than the medial pterygoid muscle (second largest one at $11.5 \pm 2.1$ cm$^3$) (17).

*Origin:* Zygomatic arch—inferior and medial surfaces of the zygomatic bone and the temporal process of zygomatic bone. From here it extends downward and posteriorly.

*Insertion:* Lateral surface of the ramus, angle, and lower border of mandible.

*Action:* Elevator closes jaw and applies great power in crushing food (6, 8, 9).

### LEARNING EXERCISE

*Feel contraction of the masseter by placing a finger on your cheek in the second molar region and then clenching your teeth several times. It will produce a noticeable bulge beneath your finger each time.*

## B. Temporalis Muscle

It is a fan-shaped, large, but flat muscle (Figs. 1.19 and 1.21).

*Origin:* Entire temporalis fossa (Fig. 1.4) (part of the frontal and parietal bones, squamous part of temporal, and greater wing of the sphenoid bones). From here its fibers are directed

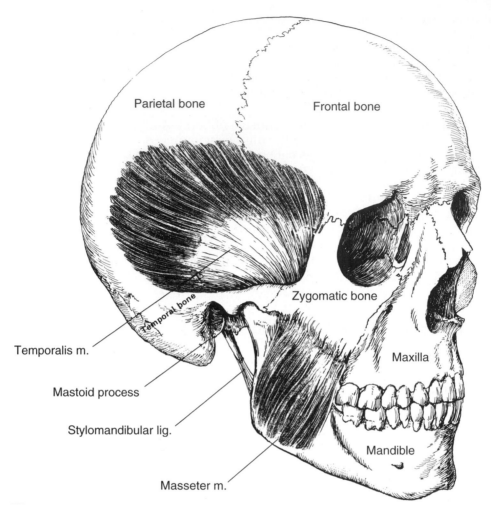

**Figure 1.19.** Masseter muscle below and fan-shaped temporalis muscle above. (Reproduced by permission from Clemente CD, ed. Gray's anatomy of the human body. 30th ed. Philadelphia: Lea & Febiger, 1985:450.)

downward (anterior part), and downward and anteriorly (posterior part), passing medial to the zygomatic arch.

*Insertion:* Coronoid process of the mandible, the anterior border of the ramus, and the temporal crest of the mandible (Fig. 1.12) via one common tendon (Fig. 1.21).

*Action:* Anterior vertical muscle fibers contract to act as an elevator to close the jaw especially when great power is not required (positioner) and the posterior, more horizontal fibers, retract or pull the jaw backward (6, 8, 9).

## LEARNING EXERCISE

*Feel contraction of the temporalis by placing several fingers above and in front of your ear while clenching your teeth several times. Feel the nearly horizontal fibers just above and behind your ears contract as you retrude or pull your mandible posteriorly (Figs. 1.19 and 1.21).*

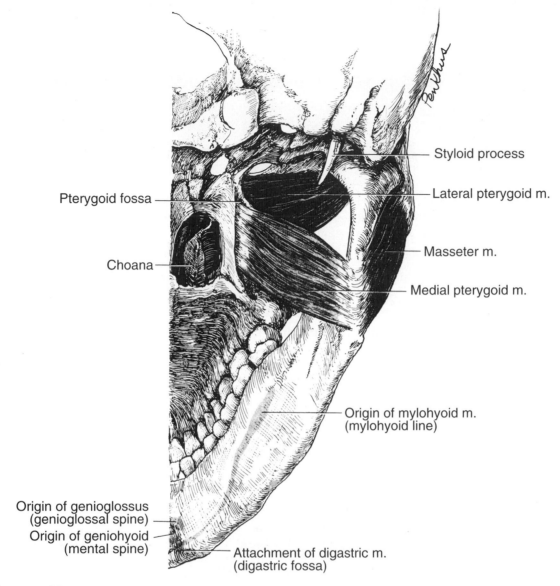

Styloid process

Lateral pterygoid m.

Pterygoid fossa

Masseter m.

Medial pterygoid m.

Choana

Origin of mylohyoid m.
(mylohyoid line)

Origin of genioglossus
(genioglossal spine)

Origin of geniohyoid
(mental spine)

Attachment of digastric m.
(digastric fossa)

**Figure 1.20.** The pterygoid and masseter muscles viewed from below. Note how the medial pterygoid and masseter muscles form a sling that, when contracted, act to close the teeth together and squeeze with considerable force. From this view, it is clear that the lateral pterygoid muscle has its origin (on the base of the cranium) more to the midline of the skull than its insertion, which is on the anterior portion of the head of the condyle and the articular disc. The insertion cannot be seen in this figure. If this muscle contracts only on the right side, the mandible shifts toward the left side. (Reproduced by permission from Clemente CD, ed. Gray's anatomy of the human body. 30th ed. Philadelphia: Lea & Febiger, 1985:452.)

## C. Medial Pterygoid Muscle

It is located medial to the ramus of the mandible much as the masseter is located on the lateral surface (Figs. 1.20 and 1.22).

*Origin:* Mainly from the medial surface of the lateral pterygoid plate and the pterygoid fossa between the medial and lateral plates (Figs. 1.6**A** and **B**) of the sphenoid bone. [Also from the pyramidal process of the palatine bone, with a few fibers to the maxillary tuberosity (3).] The fibers pass downward and laterally toward the angle of the mandible.

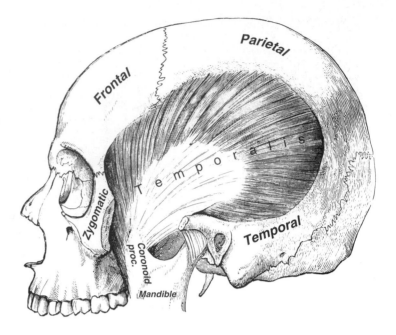

**Figure 1.21.** The zygomatic process of the temporal bone and temporal process of the zygomatic bones have been removed. Contraction of the anterior vertically oriented fibers of the temporal muscle act to close the jaw; contraction of the posteriorly placed horizontally oriented fibers act to pull the jaw back or to retract (retrude) the mandible (8). (Reproduced by permission from Clemente CD, ed. Gray's anatomy of the human body. 30th ed. Philadelphia: Lea & Febiger, 1985:449.)

*Insertion:* Medial surface of the mandible in a triangular region just above the angle and to the angle (Fig. 1.20).

*Direction from Origin to Insertion:* Downward, laterally, and backward.

*Action:* Elevator (closes jaw like the temporalis and masseter muscles). Although not as large or powerful, it is a synergist of (i.e., works together with) the masseter muscle in helping apply the power or great force on closures with the larger masseter muscle. Acting together, these two muscles form a sling on each side of the mandible.

## D. Lateral Pterygoid Muscle

Unlike the three other pairs of muscles that are primarily oriented vertically, this muscle has its fibers oriented horizontally (Figs. 1.20 and 1.22). The lateral pterygoid muscle is a short, thick, somewhat conical muscle located deep in the infratemporal fossa (behind the maxilla) and is the prime mover of the mandible except for closing the jaw.

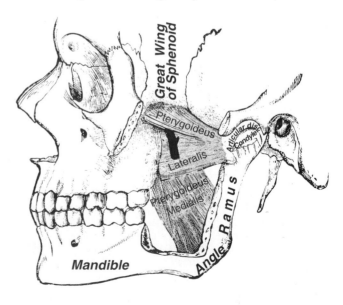

**Figure 1.22.** Removal of the zygomatic arch and the anterior part of the mandible reveals the medial and lateral pterygoid muscles. Contraction of the medial pterygoid muscle elevates (closes) the mandible. Simultaneous contraction of both lateral pterygoid muscles pulls the condyle and disc forward, which causes the mouth to open or protrude as in incising. Notice the horizontal orientation of the lateral pterygoid in direct contrast to the vertical direction of the fibers of the medial pterygoid muscle. (Reproduced by permission from Clemente CD, ed. Gray's anatomy of the human body. 30th ed. Philadelphia: Lea & Febiger, 1985:451.)

*Origin:* It has two heads. The smaller upper head is attached to the infratemporal surface on the great wing of the sphenoid bone; the larger lower head is attached to the lateral side of the lateral pterygoid plate on the sphenoid bone (Fig. 1.22).

*Insertion:* **Upper head:** front of the neck of the condyloid process and to the anteromedial surface of the capsular ligament penetrating the capsule and inserting into the disc. **Lower head:** roughened pterygoid fovea (Fig. 1.12) on the anterior surface of the neck of the condyle (Fig. 1.22). Minor forward contractions of the upper head work in concert with the stretching of the elastic band of retrodiscal tissues to prevent the disc from becoming displaced posteriorly (14).

*Direction from Origin to Insertion:* Posteriorly and laterally. The fibers from both heads travel in a virtually horizontally posterior direction toward the neck of the mandibular condyle. They travel laterally as well because their insertion in the mandible is lateral to their origin. Thus, when one muscle contracts, it pulls that condyle forward and inward (medially), causing the mandible to deviate from the contracting side toward the opposite side (see Fig. 1.16 for direction of action).

*Action:* (a) With both contracting simultaneously: opening the jaw. They do this by pulling the articular discs and the condyles forward down onto the articular eminences. In opening the jaw or depressing the mandible, the lateral pterygoids are assisted somewhat by the suprahyoid and infrahyoid muscles (for example, geniohyoid, digastric, and omohyoid muscles).

(b) With both lateral pterygoids contracting simultaneously: protruding the jaw. No other muscles are capable of doing this but can only assist in this action as stabilizers or by controlling the degree of jaw opening during the protrusion (5, 6, 8, 9, 18).

(c) Lateral movement of the mandible, which is produced by the unilateral contraction of one lateral pterygoid muscle. Contraction of the left lateral pterygoid muscle causes the mandible to move directly to the right side (lateral excursion) (8). Conversely, the contraction of the right lateral pterygoid muscle causes the mandible to move directly to the left side (left lateral excursion) (8). No other muscle is capable of moving the mandible sideways, although synergistic (in harmony with) unilateral contraction of the posterior fibers of the temporalis muscle occurs on the side toward which the jaw moves (8).

### LEARNING EXERCISE

*On a skull, imagine elastic bands passing from the origins to the insertions of the lateral pterygoid muscles, right and left. Since the origin on the base of the skull stays stationary, but the mandible can move, look at the direction of the mandible (forward and downward) if both elastic bands are contracted (shortened). Next, see what happens if only one band is shortened (contracted). The condyle of the mandible on that side will move closer to the pterygoid plate (medially) on that side so the teeth and the mandible together, will move toward the opposite side. Practice this until you understand why the jaw moves the way it does when one lateral pterygoid muscles works.*

## E. Other Muscles Affecting Mandibular Movement

The suprahyoid muscle group attaches above the hyoid bone to the mandible, while the infrahyoid muscle group attaches below the hyoid to the clavicle (collarbone) and sternum (breast bone) (Fig. 2.10).

The suprahyoid muscle group, the infrahyoid muscle group, and the posterior and deep muscles of the neck, as well as the overlying fascia and skin, all have a slight postural influence on the physiologic resting position of the mandible. To be effective in assisting mandibular movement (*opening and retruding*), the hyoid bone must be held firmly in place by the infrahyoid muscles while the suprahyoid muscles also contract. Other than this, the numerous facial muscles (Fig. 1.23), including the buccinator, *do not influence any movements of the mandible.*

## F. Other Factors Affecting Tooth Position or Movement

The temporomandibular ligament (lateral part of capsule), stylomandibular, and sphenomandibular ligaments provide the limits for protrusive, lateral, and opening movements originating from the craniomandibular joints (Figs. 1.15 and 1.17).

The cheeks (including muscles of facial expression shown in Fig. 1.23), the lips, and the tongue are thought to influence development, position, and shape of the dental arches (the maxillae and the mandible).

Fascia is connective tissue that forms sheets or bands between anatomic structures. Fascia attaches to bones and surrounds muscles, glands, vessels, nerves, and fat. Fascia is thought to limit movement of the mandible to some extent.

A person's posture, state of mind, stress, health, and physical and mental fatigue each have a decided effect on the resting posture of the mandible at any given time (19).

## G. Summary of Muscles That Move and Control the Mandible

There are five specifically different ways that we can voluntarily move our mandible. There are limitless combinations of these that occur throughout any 24 hours.

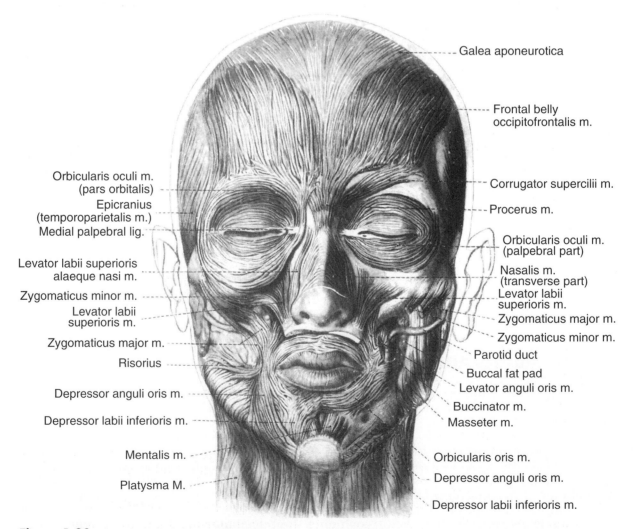

**Figure 1.23.** The muscles of facial expression (Reproduced by permission from Clemente CD, ed. Gray's anatomy of the human body. 30th ed. Philadelphia: Lea & Febiger, 1985:444.)

1. **ELEVATION** (closing the mouth) results from the bilateral contraction of three pairs of muscles:

   a. Right and left *temporalis* muscles (vertical fibers), which bring the mandible upward into position for crushing food. The temporalis muscles are primarily the positioning muscles, as they elevate the mandible upward until it is in position to have the real force applied by the other two pairs of closing muscles.

   b. Right and left *masseter* muscles and right and left *medial pterygoid* muscles which, acting together, apply the power on forceful jaw closures as in crushing food.

2. **DEPRESSION** (opening of mouth) results from the bilateral contraction of:

   Primarily both *lateral pterygoid* muscles but assisted by *suprahyoid* and *infrahyoid* muscles, primarily the anterior bellies of the digastric muscles (Fig. 1.20) and the omohyoid (*infrahyoid*) muscles which help fix or hold the hyoid bone.

3. **RETRACTION** (retruding the jaw) results from the bilateral contraction of the *posterior fibers of the temporalis* muscles assisted by the *suprahyoids:* the digastric muscles (anterior and posterior bellies).

4. **PROTRACTION** (or protrusion, protruding the jaw) results only from the simultaneous contraction of the right and left *lateral pterygoid* muscles.

5. **LATERAL EXCURSION** (move sideways) results from the contraction of *one lateral pterygoid* muscle on the opposite side (mandible is moved to the left by right lateral pterygoid muscle) (8). This can best be understood by manipulating a skull and looking at Figure 1.16.

   *Free movements* of the mandible are those in which teeth do not contact.

   *Contact movements* of the mandible occur when maxillary and mandibular teeth slide or glide over each other while maintaining contact (8, 20).

# SECTION V: THE NERVES OF THE ORAL CAVITY

## A. Twelve Cranial Nerves

There are 12 cranial nerves that are responsible for the following functions (1, 21, 23, 24–26):

| | | |
|---|---|---|
| I. | Olfactory: | Smell |
| II. | Optic: | Sight |
| III. | Oculomotor: | Orbital muscles for eye movement |
| IV. | Trochlear: | Orbital muscles for eye movement |
| V. | *Trigeminal: | Movement of the jaws and muscles of mastication; facial sensation, teeth and periodontal ligaments |
| VI. | Abducent: | Orbital muscles for eye movement |
| VII. | *Facial: | Motor to the muscles of facial expression, taste to anterior $2/3$ of tongue; taste |
| VIII. | Auditory/(Acoustic): | Sense of hearing, position and balance |
| IX. | *Glossopharyngeal: | Secretory to parotid gland, pharyngeal movements; sensory to pharynx and posterior $1/3$ of tongue, and taste to posterior $1/3$ of tongue |
| X. | Vagus: | Pharyngeal and laryngeal movements: digestive tract |
| XI. | Accessory: | Neck movements: sternocleidomastoid and trapezius |
| XII. | *Hypoglossal: | Tongue movement |

*Asterisked nerves are most important when discussing the function of the oral cavity and will be discussed in more detail. A detailed discussion of these nerves will include the major nerves to structures of the mouth including teeth, periodontal ligaments and alveolar processes, gingiva (gums), palate and floor of the mouth, muscles of mastication and facial expression, and tongue—muscular and sensory for taste.

There are several types of nerve fibers based on their function:

*Afferent (sensory)* fibers convey impulses from peripheral organs to the central nervous system. They supply the skin of the entire face, the mucous membrane of the oral and nasal cavities (except the pharynx and the base of the tongue), and the teeth and their supporting structures (i.e., periodontal ligament, the alveolar process, and gingiva).

*Efferent (motor)* fibers convey impulses from the central nervous system to the peripheral organs. They supply the four pairs of muscles of mastication, several other muscles in the region of the mouth (mylohyoid, anterior belly of the digastric, tensor veli palatini), and the tensor tympani in the ear.

*Secretory fibers* are specialized efferent nerve fibers which, upon stimulation, increase secretory activity of a salivary gland.

## B. Trigeminal Nerve (Fifth Cranial Nerve)

When discussing the function of the oral cavity, perhaps the most important nerve is the trigeminal (Figs. 1.24 and 1.25). The *trigeminal nerve* or fifth cranial nerve is the largest of the cranial nerves, and is the major sensory nerve of the face and scalp. It originates in the large semilunar or trigeminal ganglion within the skull, in a small depression above the carotid canal medial to the foramen ovale on the internal surface of the temporal bone (Fig. 1.3). It can be divided into three divisions:

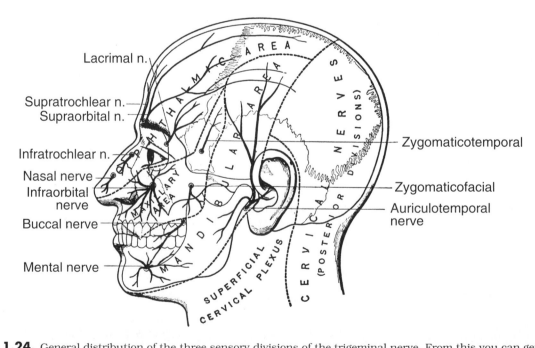

**Figure 1.24.** General distribution of the three sensory divisions of the trigeminal nerve. From this you can get a concept of the possible regions where pain might be referred when any one of these nerves becomes traumatized. (Reproduced by permission from Clemente CD, ed. Gray's anatomy of the human body. 30th ed. Philadelphia: Lea & Febiger, 1985:1164.)

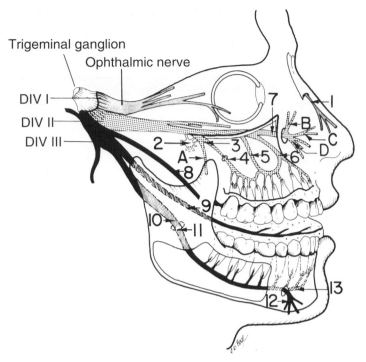

1. External nasal nerve
2. Pterygopalatine ganglion
3. Posterior superior
    Alveolar nerve
    A. Gingival branch
4. Alveolar canal
5. Middle superior alveolar nerve
6. Anterior superior alveolar nerve
7. Infraorbital nerve
    B. Palpebral branches
    C. Nasal branches
    D. Labial branches
8. Buccinator nerve
9. Lingual nerve
10. Inferior alveolar nerve
11. Mandibular foramen
12. Mental nerve
13. Incisive nerve

**Figure 1.25.** Distribution of the maxillary and mandibular divisions of the trigeminal nerve. Study these first. Then cover the names and test your knowledge by trying to identify each main branch. Note that the buccinator branch (*8*) of the mandibular (*III*) inferior division passes superficial to the ramus to the cheek, whereas the lingual (*9*) and inferior alveolar (*10*) branches pass medial to the ramus to the tongue, and enter the mandible through the mandibular foramen (*11*).

Division I    Ophthalmic Nerve (afferent [sensory] only) exits from the skull via superior orbital fissure (Fig. 1.3).

Division II   Maxillary Nerve (afferent [sensory] *only*) exits from the skull via *foramen rotundum* (Fig. 1.3).

Division III  Mandibular Nerve (afferent [sensory] *and* efferent [motor]) exits from the skull via *foramen ovale* (Figs. 1.3 and 1.6). The efferent fibers supply the muscles of mastication.

Each of the three divisions is further divided into branches and sub-branches. The branches of the *maxillary nerve* and the *mandibular nerve* are those that supply the region of and around the oral cavity (see Table 1.3). The maxillary and mandibular divisions of the trigeminal nerve supply afferent or sensory neurons that provide the brain with information about the position of the teeth and jaws. The interpretation of postural information by the brain is called *proprioception*. The periodontal ligament around each tooth is well supplied with proprioceptive (sense of position) neurons from the maxillary and mandibular divisions of the trigeminal nerve.

The craniomandibular joint has proprioceptive neurons in the capsule and disc that are innervated by the *auriculotemporal* branch of the mandibular division of the trigeminal nerve. Muscles and ligaments have proprioceptive nerve receptors as well as those around the teeth and in the lateral aspects of the joints.

Proprioceptive information, especially from the teeth (24, 25), to a great extent determines the subconscious, but well-coordinated, function of the two complex craniomandibular joints. Otherwise, we would experience many tooth interferences and frequent joint pain.

**Table 1.3.** Distribution of Branches of Trigeminal Nerve to the Teeth and Surrounding Structures*

Carefully study this comprehensive but simple table. Then, covering one column at a time, see how many nerves you can recall. These are the nerves any dental student, dental hygiene student, or graduate of either profession should be most familiar with. You should also be able to determine the location and source of each nerve.

| Teeth | Tooth Pulp | Gingiva | Periodontal Ligament and Alveolar Process | Hard Palate |
|---|---|---|---|---|
| **Maxillary Arch** | | | | |
| Anteriors | Anterior superior alveolar N. | Palatal—Nasopalatine N. Labial—Infraorbital and Anterior superior alveolar N. | Anterior superior alveolar N.† | Nasopalatine N. |
| Premolars | Middle superior alveolar N. | Palatal—Anterior palatine N. Buccal—Middle superior alevolar and Infraorbital N. | Middle superior alveolar N.† | Anterior palatine N. |
| Molars | Posterior superior alveolar N except MB root of first (supplied by middle superior alveolar N) | Palatal—Anterior palatine N. Buccal—Posterior superior alveolar N. | Posterior superior alveolar N. | Anterior palatine N. *SOFT PALATE* Middle and posterior palatine nerves |
| **Mandibular Arch** | | | | **Floor of Mouth** |
| Anteriors | Incisive branch of Inferior alveolar N. | Lingual—Lingual N. Labial—Mental N. | Incisive N. | Lingual N. |
| Premolars | Dental branch of Inferior alveolar N. | Lingual—Lingual N. Buccal—Mental N. | Dental branch of Inferior alveolar N. | Lingual N. |
| Molars | Dental branch of Inferior alveolar N. | Lingual—Lingual N. Buccal—Buccinator N. (Long buccal N.) | Dental branch of Inferior alevolar N. | Lingual N. |

*To follow the pathways and sources, refer to Figures 1.25 through 1.27.
†Also supply the maxillary sinus.

## 1. DIVISION I OF THE TRIGEMINAL NERVE: OPHTHALMIC NERVE

The *ophthalmic nerve* (Fig. 1.25) is about 25 mm long and exits from the skull by way of the superior orbital fissure (Fig. 1.3). It has three main branches: lacrimal, frontal (which divides into supraorbital and supratrochlear), and nasociliary. The ophthalmic nerve and its branches supply sensory innervation to the upper third of the face, i.e., the eyeball, the upper eyelid, the skin of the nose, the skin of the forehead, the skin of the scalp, part of the nasal mucosa and maxillary sinus, and the lacrimal glands (Fig. 1.24). THE OPHTHALMIC NERVE DOES NOT SUPPLY THE ORAL CAVITY.

## 2. DIVISION II OF THE TRIGEMINAL NERVE: MAXILLARY NERVE

The maxillary nerve exits from the skull through the foramen rotundum (Fig. 1.3) and has four principal branches:

Pterygopalatine

Posterior superior alveolar (terminal branch)

Infraorbital (terminal branch)

Zygomatic

It provides sensory innervation to the middle third of the face, including the palate and maxillary teeth (Figs. 1.24, 1.28).

### a. Pterygopalatine Nerve

This branch (Fig. 1.26) is closest to the origin of the *maxillary nerve*. It is given off in the *pterygopalatine fossa* and is attached to the pterygopalatine ganglion. The fibers of the pterygopalatine nerve pass through the ganglion and its two main branches (nasopalatine and palatine) are given off:

#### (1) Nasopalatine Nerve

This nerve passes diagonally downward and forward along the nasal septum to eventually pass through the *incisive canal* (Fig. 1.8) and exits to the palate through the *incisive foramen*. It goes to the anterior palatal mucosa, mucosa of the nasal septum, and palatal gingiva of the maxillary incisors and canines (Fig. 1.28). (The gingiva on the facial side of the mandible and maxillae in the premolar and molar regions is called the buccal gingiva. The gingiva on the facial side of the mandible and maxilla in the incisor regions is called the labial gingiva. The gingiva on the inside of the maxillary arch covering the alveolar process is called the palatal gingiva. This term should not be applied to the mucous membrane of the hard and soft palates. The mucous membrane in those areas is not gingiva; it is called palatal mucosa. The gingiva on the inside of the mandibular arch covering the alveolar process is called the lingual gingiva).

#### (2) Palatine Nerves

##### (a) Anterior Palatine Nerve (Greater Palatine Nerve)

After entering the oral cavity through the *greater palatine foramen* with the descending palatine artery (Fig. 1.8), this nerve (Fig.

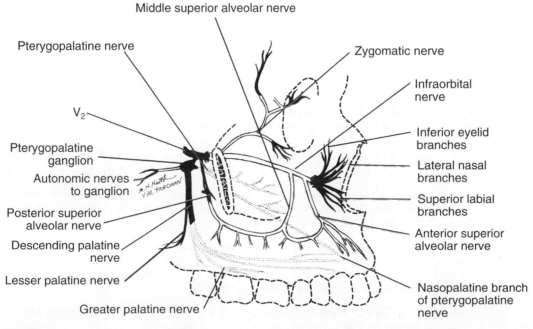

**Figure 1.26.** The branches of the maxillary nerve that supply the maxillary teeth and surrounding structures. (Reproduced by permission from Brand RW, Isselhard DE. Anatomy of oral structures. 2nd ed. St. Louis: C.V. Mosby, 1982.)

1.26) spreads anteriorly to supply the mucosa of the hard palate and the palatal gingiva of the premolars and molars (Fig. 1.28).

*(b) Middle and Posterior (Lesser) Palatine Nerves*

After entering the oral cavity through the *lesser palatine foramen* (Fig. 1.8), these nerves (Fig. 1.26) spread posteriorly to supply the tonsils and mucosa of the soft palate.

### b. Posterior Superior Alveolar Nerve

This first terminal branch of the maxillary division branches off within the pterygopalatine fossa and enters the body of the maxilla on the infratemporal surface via *alveolar* canals (Fig 1.25). Branches of the *posterior superior alveolar* (Fig. 1.25 and 1.26) nerve pass down through the wall of the maxillary sinus and supply:

1. The *pulp of the maxillary* molar teeth through the apical foramina, with the exception of the mesiobuccal root of the maxillary first molar (Fig. 1.28).

2. The buccal gingiva, periodontal ligament and the alveolar process of the maxillary molar teeth (Fig. 1.28).

3. The mucosa of the maxillary sinus and the cheek in part.

THE NERVE SUPPLY TO THE DECIDUOUS TEETH is precisely the same as that to the permanent teeth that will replace them. Consequently, no deciduous teeth are supplied by the posterior superior alveolar nerves, which supply only the permanent maxillary molars.

### c. Infraorbital Nerve

This is the second terminal branch of the *maxillary nerve.* It enters the orbit lodged in the infraorbital groove and then enters the infraorbital canal and passes out through the *infraorbital foramen* (Fig. 1.7) onto the face. It has several branches:

#### (1) Middle Superior Alveolar Nerve

(Comparison of description of the superior alveolar nerves indicates a great lack of uniformity in their distribution. Sometimes the middle superior alveolar is missing and the function is taken over by the anterior and posterior alveolar nerves.)

This branch (Figs. 1.25 and 1.26) arises from the *infraorbital nerve* while in the infraorbital groove, passes down through the lateral wall of the maxillary sinus, and supplies:

a. The *pulp of the maxillary premolars* through the apical foramina (earlier the deciduous molars), and the *pulp* in the *mesiobuccal root of the maxillary first* permanent molar (Fig. 1.28).

b. The buccal gingiva, periodontal ligament and the alveolar process in the maxillary premolar region (Fig. 1.28).

c. The mucosa of the maxillary sinus in part.

#### (2) Anterior Superior Alveolar Nerve

This branch (Figs. 1.25 and 1.26) arises from the *infraorbital nerve* while in the infraorbital canal and supplies:

a.  The *pulp of the maxillary incisors* and *canines* through their apical foramina (Fig. 1.26).

b.  The labial gingiva, periodontal ligament and the alveolar process in the maxillary incisor and canine region (Fig. 1.28).

c.  The mucosa of the maxillary sinus and of the nasal cavity.

### (3) Terminal Branches of the Infraorbital Nerve

After exiting from the infraorbital foramen, these branches (Fig. 1.25 Nos. 7B, 7C, and 7D) are:

a.  *Labial*—to skin and mucosa of upper lip, buccal gingiva of maxillary premolars, and maxillary labial gingiva.

b.  *Nasal*—to skin and mucosa of side of nose.

c.  *Palpebral*—to skin and mucosa of lower eyelid.

### d. Zygomatic Nerve

This nerve arises in the pterygopalatine fossa, enters the orbit via the inferior orbital fissure, and then divides into the *zygomaticotemporal* and *zygomaticofacial* nerves (the upper and lower branches, respectively, of the zygomatic nerve in Fig. 1.26). It supplies the bone and temporal region and the orbit.

## 3. DIVISION III OF THE TRIGEMINAL NERVE: MANDIBULAR NERVE

The mandibular nerve exits from the skull through the foramen ovale (Fig. 1.6), gives off the auriculotemporal and buccinator nerves, then passes through the infratemporal fossa (medial to and below the zygomatic arch). Then, within 12–15 mm, it divides into the inferior alveolar and lingual nerves (1, 29) (Fig. 1.25 Nos. 9 and 10).

The *mandibular nerve* is a mixed nerve; that is, it contains both afferent (sensory) and efferent (motor) fibers. It is the only efferent portion of the fifth nerve. These motor fibers supply the eight muscles of mastication. Sensory fibers innervate the lower third of the face, including the floor of the mouth, anterior of tongue (not taste), and mandibular teeth (Fig. 1.28).

### a. Efferent (Motor) Branches of the Mandibular Nerve

These nerves supply the muscles of mastication: the *masseteric nerve* to the masseter muscle as well as to the craniomandibular joint, the *posterior and anterior temporal nerve* to the temporalis muscle, the *medial pterygoid nerve* to the medial pterygoid muscle, and the *lateral pterygoid nerve* to the lateral pterygoid muscle.

Other efferent branches supply the mylohyoid muscle in the floor of mouth under tongue, the *anterior belly of digastric muscle* which helps retract the mandible (see Figs. 1.10 and 1.20), the *tensor veli palatini muscle* in the soft palate, and the tensor tympani muscle in the middle ear.

### b. Afferent (Sensory) Branches of the Mandibular Nerve

There are four divisions:

### (1) Buccinator Nerve (Long Buccal Nerve)

Buccinator nerve (long buccal nerve) (Fig. 1.25) comes off just below the foramen ovale, passes through the infratemporal fossa, between the two heads of the lateral pterygoid muscles, then down and forward emerging between the anterior border of the masseter and posterior border of the buccinator muscle to supply:

a. The *buccal gingiva in the area of the mandibular molars*, and sometimes second premolars (Fig. 1.28). The best place to anesthetize the buccinator nerve is inside the cheek by injecting or depositing the solution into the buccinator muscle.

b. The buccinator nerve also supplies the mucosa and skin of the cheek and corner of the mouth.

### (2) Lingual Nerve

Lingual nerve (Fig. 1.24) comes off the mandibular nerve about 15 mm below the oval foramen. Then it passes downward between the medial pterygoid muscles and ramus to the posterior part of the mylohyoid line resting closely beneath the mucous membrane near the last molar. This nerve supplies:

a. The *lingual gingiva of the entire mandibular arch* (Fig. 1.28).

b. The mucosa of the inner surface of the mandible and in the sublingual region (mucosa of floor of mouth).

c. The mucosa on the upper and lower surfaces of the body (anterior two-thirds) of the tongue (see Fig. 2.2). *This nerve supplies only general sensation:* touch, pain, pressure, temperature. It does not supply the sense of taste. *The sense of taste in this region is supplied by the facial nerve* (VII).

### (3) Inferior Alveolar Nerve

Inferior alveolar nerve (Figs. 1.25 and 1.27) is a large nerve coming off the mandibular nerve on the medial side of the lateral pterygoid muscle. It then descends between the sphenomandibular ligament and the ramus to the mandibular foramen where it gives off the mylohyoid nerve before it enters the mandible through the mandibular foramen (Fig. 1.12). The dental branches of this nerve supply the pulp of all the mandibular molar and premolar teeth through their apical foramina, the buccal gingiva, periodontal ligament and the alveolar process of mandibular molar and premolar teeth (Fig. 1.28).

The branches of the inferior alveolar nerve are the mylohyoid, mental, and incisive nerves.

#### (a) Mylohyoid Nerve

*Mylohyoid nerve* (efferent) comes off, pierces the sphenomandibular ligament. It then travels forward and down in the mylohyoid groove (Fig. 1.12), then into the digastric triangle where it supplies the mylohyoid muscle and the anterior belly of the digastric muscle (Fig. 1.10).

#### (b) Mental Nerve

This terminal branch (Figs. 1.25 and 1.27) exits from the body of the mandible via the *mental foramen* and supplies the facial gingiva of the mandibular incisors, canines, and premolars (Fig. 1.28), and the mucosa and skin of the lower lip.

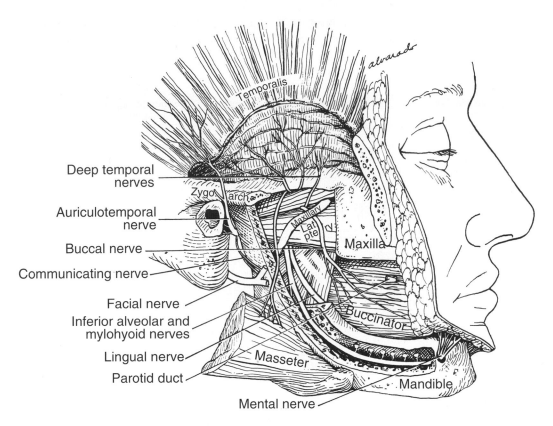

**Figure 1.27.** The external wall of the right mandible has been removed to expose the inferior alveolar nerve which gives off the many small branches to each mandibular tooth. (The teeth are not visible from this view.) This nerve continues within the mandible becoming the incisive branch of the inferior alveolar to the anterior teeth, but also gives off a mental branch which exits the mandible and supplies the lower lip on that side. The direction of the mental foramen canal from outside in, is downward, forward, and inward. This is the direction that local anesthetic solution must travel to penetrate the canal and successfully block the incisive nerve within the mandibular canal. (Reproduced by permission from Clemente CD, ed. Gray's anatomy of the human body. 30th ed. Philadelphia: Lea & Febiger, 1985:1166.)

*(c) Incisive Nerve*

This terminal branch (Fig. 1.25) continues forward within the body of the mandible in the mandibular canal and supplies the pulp of the mandibular incisor and canine teeth, the periodontal ligament, and the alveolar process of the incisors and canines (Fig. 1.28).

**(4) Auriculotemporal Nerve**

This nerve comes off the main trunk immediately below the base of the skull, turning backwards beneath the lateral pterygoid muscle to supply pain and proprioception fibers to the craniomandibular joint, also the outer ear, the skin of the lateral aspect of the skull and cheek, and the parotid gland (Fig. 2.10).

## C. Facial Nerve (Seventh Cranial Nerve)

The *facial nerve* is a mixed nerve (efferent and afferent).

The facial nerve enters the *internal acoustic meatus* (Fig. 1.3) and later exits from the skull through the *stylomastoid foramen* between styloid and mastoid processes (Fig. 1.6). It passes through the parotid gland. It divides into two terminal branches: temporofacial (side

## NERVES

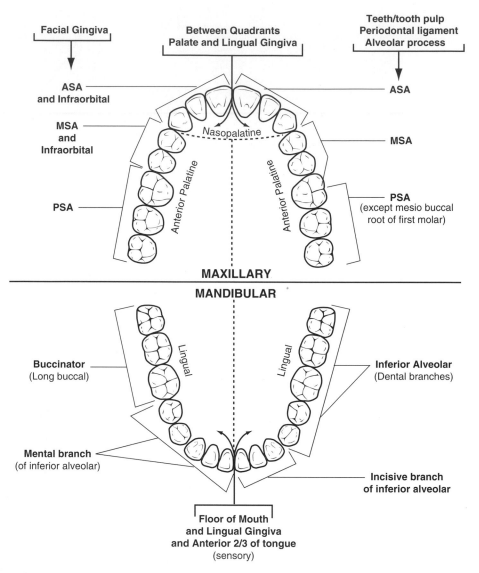

**Figure 1.28.** Distribution of nerves that innervate the tissues of the mouth. Nerves in the left column supply facial gingiva on the right and left side nerves to the teeth (etc.) in the right column supply the right and left side.

of forehead) and cervicofacial (lower side of face, orbicularis oris muscle, and chin), and supplies the following:

## 1. EFFERENT FIBERS

Efferent fibers innervate muscles of facial and visual expression of the face and the scalp, which are as follows (refer to Fig. 1.23):

Lips          Orbicularis oris (one) (no attachment in bone)

Cheek         Buccinator (Fig. 1.10)

| | |
|---|---|
| Upper Oral Group | Risorius |
| | Zygomaticus major |
| | Zygomaticus minor |
| | Levator labii superiorus |
| | Levator anguli oris alaeque nasi |
| | Levator anguli oris (caninus) |
| Lower Oral Group | Mentalis—one |
| | Depressor labii inferior |
| | Depressor anguli oris (triangularis) |
| Nose | Depressor septi nasi—one |
| | Dilator nares |
| | Nasalis |
| | Procerus |
| | Corrugator supercilii |
| Ears | Posterior auricular |
| | Superior auricular |
| | Anterior auricular |
| Scalp | Frontalis—one |
| | Occipitalis—one |

Other muscles supplied by the facial nerve include the posterior belly of the digastric muscle, platysma muscle (Fig. 1.10), stylohyoid muscle, and stapedius muscle (in middle ear cavity).

All of these muscles have little or no effect on moving the mandible. It has been said that it takes only six muscles to smile (the three levator pairs), yet 18 are active when one frowns. Perhaps we waste energy in frowning.

## 2. SECRETORY FIBERS OF THE FACIAL NERVE

These are efferent fibers ending in the pterygopalatine and submandibular ganglia that bring about secretions from two pairs of salivary glands: the sublingual glands located just under the mucosa in the floor of the mouth, and the submandibular glands located in the submandibular fossae.

## 3. AFFERENT FIBERS OF THE FACIAL NERVE

The *chorda tympani* branch comes off the facial nerve above the stylomastoid foramen (Fig. 1.6), courses through the tympanic cavity, eventually coming out of the skull by way of petrotympanic fissure, and joins with the lingual nerve (Fig. 1.25). It supplies the sense of *taste to the anterior two-thirds of the tongue* (the body and the tip of the tongue). The tip is where one best distinguishes sweet, salty, or alkaline substances, whereas the sides of the tongue are most sensitive to acid substances (27). There are only four primary tastes: sour (acid), sweet, salty, and bitter (27). Some authors add alkaline and metallic to the taste senses. The tip or anterior one-sixth of the tongue distinguishes sweet. Along the sides of the tongue, salt is detected anteriorly and sour is detected more posteriorly. There are approximately 9000 taste buds in the young adult, more in children, and fewer with advancing age (27).

## D. Glossopharyngeal Nerve (Ninth Cranial Nerve)

The glossopharyngeal nerve exits from the skull via the *jugular foramen* (Fig. 1.3) along with the vagus (tenth) and accessory (eleventh) nerves. It then passes down and forward, medial to the styloid process, to enter the tongue. It is a mixed nerve (efferent and afferent) and supplies parts of the tongue and pharynx.

1. *Efferent fibers*—The glossopharyngeal nerves' *efferent fibers* innervate the stylopharyngeus muscle of the pharynx.

2. Secretory fibers—Secretory fibers innervate the *parotid gland*, effecting secretion. This gland is located in front of each ear below the zygomatic arch.

3. The *afferent fibers* of this nerve supply the *sense of taste* to the posterior one-third of the tongue, general sensation of the same area and to the mucosa of the pharynx and tonsils (Fig. 2.2). [The circumvallate papillae area is particularly sensitive to bitter taste (27). Bitter sensations are noticed on the dorsal surface in the region of the circumvallate papillae. One text says there are other taste buds in the pillars of the fauces, hard and soft palate, epiglottis, and pharynx (28).] (See Fig. 2.2.)

## E. Hypoglossal Nerve (Twelfth Cranial Nerve)

The hypoglossal nerve exits from the skull through the *hypoglossal canal* just above the occipital condyles near the anterior border of the large foramen magnum (visible just inside the walls of the foramen magnum, which is seen on Fig. 1.6). It descends steeply, entering the oral cavity at the posterior border of the mylohyoid muscle.

This *efferent nerve* supplies the muscles that move the tongue. These are: genioglossus, styloglossus, hyoglossus, longitudinal, vertical, and transverse. If this nerve becomes damaged from injury or tumor, the tongue will deviate noticeably toward the affected side.

## Summary of Nerve Supply to the Tongue

### AFFERENT FIBERS

Lingual nerve (Division III of Fifth Nerve)—general sensation to the anterior two-thirds of the tongue (body of tongue).

Facial nerve (Seventh cranial nerve)—taste sensation to anterior two-thirds of tongue (body).

Glossopharyngeal nerve (Ninth cranial nerve)—responsible for taste and general sensation in the posterior one-third of the tongue (base of tongue).

### EFFERENT FIBERS

Hypoglossal nerve (Twelfth cranial nerve)—It supplies all of the muscles of the tongue.

## LEARNING EXERCISES

*Name the nerve supply for the deciduous incisors, canines, and molars.*

*Can you remember the names of the important foramina through which the maxillary and mandibular nerves exit from the skull?*

*Can you locate the regions referred to in this chapter on a dry skull?*

*Describe the region on your face where pain might be referred if the problem arose from the mandibular nerve. Do the same for the maxillary nerve.*

*Can you understand why the side of one's nose might feel cold after receiving a local anesthetic (injection) to block the maxillary nerve?*

*Which nerves pass just beneath the lining of the maxillary sinus and therefore might be affected by a sinus infection? How might a dentist determine whether the problem was due to an infected tooth or to an infection within the maxillary sinus that had some other origin?*

*Draw the tongue and label areas of innervation for general sensation, taste, and muscles.*

*Is the semilunar ganglion located within or outside of the cranial cavity?*

*How does the nerve supply to the deciduous teeth differ from that to the permanent teeth?*

*With a card, cover the names of nerves in Table 1.3 and see how many of them you can recall. In Figure 1.3, cover **A** and see how many of the structures and regions you are able to identify in **B**.*

*List all twelve cranial nerves.*

# SECTION VI: BLOOD VESSELS ASSOCIATED WITH THE ORAL CAVITY

Nerves and arteries tend to parallel one another, often passing through the same foramen and canals within bones after they meet. Vessels pass up from the heart and nerves come down from the brain.

## A. Arteries

Generally, arteries about the face and jaw run a more wiggly or corkscrew course than do veins.

Blood courses from the left ventricle of the heart through the aorta to the common carotid which ascends in the neck and divides into the **EXTERNAL CAROTID** (Figs. 1.29 and 1.30) which gives off the maxillary branches at the neck of the mandibular condyle, and the **INTERNAL CAROTID** (enters the skull; does not supply the mouth).

## LEARNING EXERCISE

*Feel the pulse of the external carotid, just in front of the sternocleidomastoid muscle.*

As the external carotid passes up the neck behind the angle of the mandible and up through the parotid gland where the maxillary artery branches off, the external carotid gives off the following branches that supply the area of the mouth:

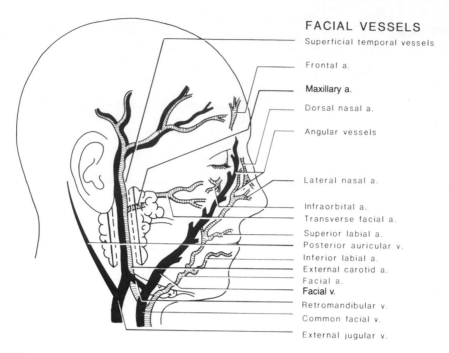

**FACIAL VESSELS**

Superficial temporal vessels

Frontal a.

**Maxillary a.**

Dorsal nasal a.

Angular vessels

Lateral nasal a.

Infraorbital a.
Transverse facial a.
Superior labial a.
Posterior auricular v.
Inferior labial a.
External carotid a.
Facial a.
Facial v.
Retromandibular v.
Common facial v.
External jugular v.

**Figure 1.29.** Facial vessels. The parotid gland is split apart to show the external carotid artery and vein, with the maxillary artery coming off and passing deep to this gland.

## 1. LINGUAL ARTERY

*Lingual artery* comes off near the hyoid bone, then enters the tongue deep to the hyoglossus muscle. As with the *lingual* nerve, this artery supplies the floor of the mouth, adjacent gingiva and the sublingual gland.

## 2. FACIAL ARTERY

*Facial artery* comes off just above or with the lingual artery. It then passes below the posterior belly of the digastric muscle and goes up and forward obliquely beneath

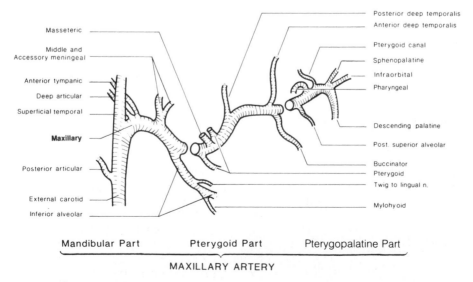

Masseteric

Middle and
Accessory meningeal

Anterior tympanic

Deep articular

Superficial temporal

**Maxillary**

Posterior articular

External carotid

Inferior alveolar

Posterior deep temporalis
Anterior deep temporalis

Pterygoid canal

Sphenopalatine

Infraorbital

Pharyngeal

Descending palatine

Post. superior alveolar

Buccinator
Pterygoid
Twig to lingual n.

Mylohyoid

Mandibular Part          Pterygoid Part          Pterygopalatine Part

MAXILLARY ARTERY

**Figure 1.30.** Maxillary artery and the branches of its three major portions.

the submandibular gland, then laterally around the lower border of the mandible. The facial artery and nerve pass through a notch on the inferior border of the mandible just anterior to the angle. This groove is called the *antegonial notch* (Fig. 1.12). It is an important landmark to become aware of so that you will be able to stop the flow of blood to the face in an emergency.

## *LEARNING EXERCISE*

*Try to find the facial artery at the antegonial notch with your finger or thumb. You may even feel pulsations of the facial artery if you are in the correct spot. From here it goes upward over the outer surface of the mandible.*

Branches of the facial artery are:

a. *Ascending palatine artery,* which comes off at the highest point of the first bend of the facial artery and then goes up along the superior pharyngeal constrictor and levator veli palatini muscles to supply the soft palate, the pharyngeal muscles, the mucosa of the pharynx, and the palatine tonsil.

b. *Submental artery,* which converges with the mylohyoid nerve and supplies the mylohyoid muscle, anterior belly of the digastric muscle, and lymph nodes in the submandibular triangle (Fig. 1.33).

c. *Inferior and superior labial arteries,* which supply the lips and the orbicularis oris muscle (Fig. 1.29).

d. *Lateral nasal and angular arteries,* which are the terminal branches of the facial arteries (Fig. 1.29).

There is considerable merging at the midline of the arteries from both sides of the face, rather than the more conventional system whereby an artery terminates with many small capillaries. This merging of small arteries from opposite sides is called an *end-to-end anastomosis.* One example is where the right and left superior and inferior labial arteries join at the midline. As one might guess, such an anastomosis can cause problems in arresting hemorrhage about the face.

## 3. MAXILLARY ARTERY

Maxillary artery (formerly called internal maxillary) is probably the *most important* to the dentist and dental hygienist. It arises from the external carotid within the parotid gland. The branches of this artery can be considered in three parts as shown in Figure 1.30. The mandibular and pterygopalatine parts (or first and third) are directly concerned with the blood supply to the mandibular and maxillary teeth respectively. The pterygoid (or middle) part supplies the four pairs of muscles of mastication (masseter, temporalis, medial, and lateral pterygoids). Study Figure 1.30 as you read about the branches of each part of the maxillary artery:

### a. Mandibular Part

**The mandibular part** (or first), part, has the seven branches. Of them, the anterior tympanic and middle meningeal help supply the craniomandibular joint; the accessory meningeal supplies the auditory tube and the semilunar ganglion. The branch of most dental interest is the INFERIOR ALVEOLAR artery, which, like the inferior alveolar nerve, enters the mandible through the *mandibular foramen,* supplying branches to the premolars and molars. It then divides into two branches: the mental artery, which exits from the mental foramen, and the incisive artery, which continues forward within the mandible to supply the anterior teeth (similar to the path of nerves in Fig. 1.27).

Refer to the Pathway of Blood From Heart to Tooth and Back to Heart (Fig. 1.32)

### b. Pterygoid Part

The **pterygoid part** is not involved directly with the teeth.

### c. Pterygopalatine Part

The **pterygopalatine part** of the maxillary artery gives off branches, two of which supply the maxillary teeth and the periodontal ligaments.

#### (1) Posterior Superior Alveolar Artery

The *posterior superior alveolar* artery enters into the maxillary sinus and like the posterior superior alveolar nerve supplies the maxillary molars.

#### (2) Infraorbital Artery

The *infraorbital* artery, like the infraorbital nerve, gives off the *middle superior alveolar* artery, which supplies the premolars, and just before it emerges from the infraorbital foramen, it gives off the *anterior superior alveolar* artery, which supplies the anterior teeth.

#### (3) Descending Palatine

The *descending palatine* branch of the maxillary artery supplies part of the nasal cavity, then descends through the pterygopalatine fossa and canal, emerging like the nerves from the *greater palatine foramen* (Fig. 1.6) to supply the mucosa of the hard and soft palate and the lingual gingiva. Its terminal part ascends through the *incisive canal* into the nasal cavity.

## 4. CRANIOMANDIBULAR JOINT

The **craniomandibular joint** is supplied with oxygenated blood from five sources: the ascending pharyngeal and superficial temporal branches of the external carotid (Fig. 1.29) and by the anterior tympanic, masseteric, and middle meningeal branches of the maxillary artery which also come off of the external carotid (Fig. 1.30).

## B. Veins

Veins (29, 30) tend to be straighter than arteries. In many instances, they travel almost the same course as arteries. There are no valves in any of the facial veins. Therefore, an infection in the face can go in either direction through veins. Drainage normally takes place through the vessels shown in Figure 1.31. All of these veins empty indirectly into the *internal jugular* vein via the *common facial* vein.

## 1. PTERYGOID PLEXUS

**Pterygoid plexus** is a plexus of veins medial to the upper part of the ramus of the mandible between the temporal and lateral pterygoid muscles or between the lateral and medial pterygoids (30). The pterygoid plexus receives blood from the area of the upper part of the face, the lips and muscles around the mouth, posterior part of

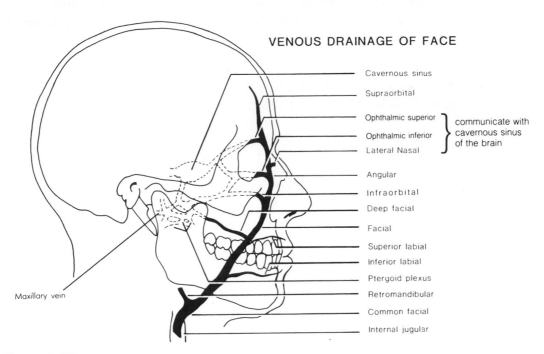

VENOUS DRAINAGE OF FACE

Cavernous sinus
Supraorbital
Ophthalmic superior ⎫
Ophthalmic inferior ⎬ communicate with cavernous sinus of the brain
Lateral Nasal ⎭
Angular
Infraorbital
Deep facial
Facial
Superior labial
Inferior labial
Ptergoid plexus
Retromandibular
Common facial
Internal jugular
Maxillary vein

**Figure 1.31.** Venous drainage of the face. The *dotted lines* represent deeper, less superficial vessels.

the nasal cavity, the palate, the maxillary alveolar process, and teeth. The pterygoid plexus empties into the maxillary vein (Fig. 1.31).

## 2. INFERIOR ALVEOLAR VEIN

The **inferior alveolar vein** drains the mandible and the mandibular teeth and empties into the pterygoid plexus of veins (not visible in Fig. 1.31).

## 3. DEEP FACIAL VEIN

The **deep facial vein** connects the pterygoid plexus with the facial vein.

## 4. LINGUAL VEINS

The **lingual veins** (not visible on Fig. 1.31) drain the tongue and empty into either the common facial or internal jugular vein.

## 5. FACIAL VEIN

The **facial vein** is formed by the angular and lateral nasal veins. It receives blood from the superior and inferior labial veins and from the muscles of mastication. The course of the facial vein closely parallels that of the facial artery but, of course, the blood flows in opposite directions.

## 6. RETROMANDIBULAR VEIN

The **retromandibular vein** is formed by the union of the superficial temporal and maxillary veins within the parotid gland. It drains the regions supplied by the maxillary and superficial temporal arteries. It drains into the facial vein.

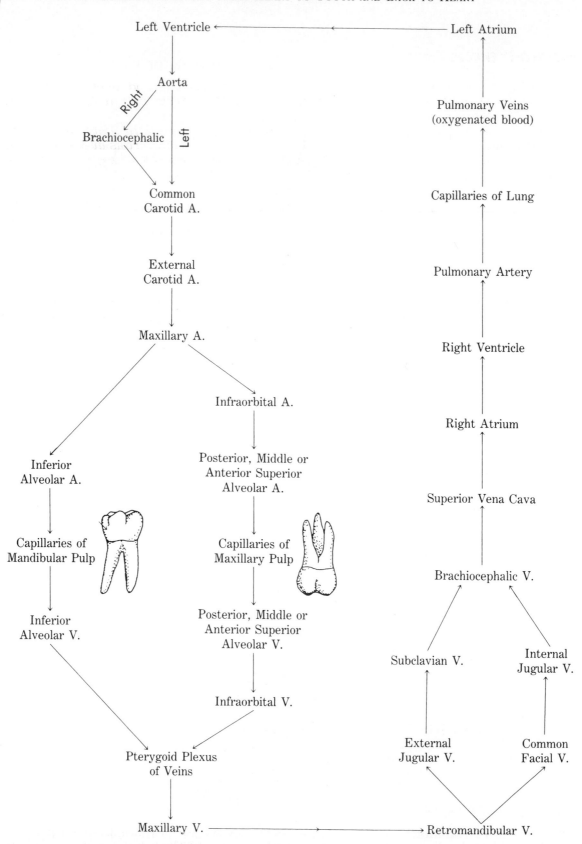

*(Think in terms of a drop of blood making this round trip.)

**Figure 1.32.** Pathway of blood from heart to tooth and back to heart. Become familiar with the similarities and differences in the blood flow to the maxillary and mandibular teeth.

### LEARNING EXERCISE

*Study Figure 1.32 to become familiar with the pathway that the blood takes from the heart in order to reach the maxillary or mandibular teeth. Practice naming these vessels after covering up their names.*

*Trace the route of a drop of blood from the heart to either a maxillary or mandibular tooth and then back to the heart as shown in Figure 1.32. Try to visualize this interesting round trip, which probably takes place every 10–15 seconds. The maxillary artery and its branches are most important to the dentist or dental hygienist.*

The dense venous plexus surrounding the maxillary artery helps protect it from becoming flattened when the masticatory muscles contract. During their contractions, however, the muscles drive blood from the veins (30). The *maxillary vein* drains the pterygoid plexus.

## C. Lymph

Lymph drainage (31) is somewhat more complex and is shown in Table 1.4 and Figure 1.33. In the arterial side of a capillary bed, blood pressure exceeds osmotic pressure and

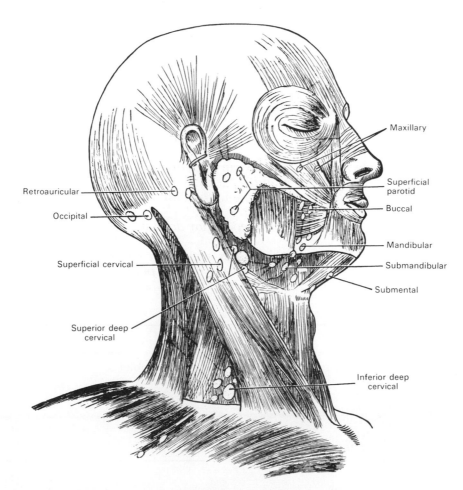

**Figure 1.33.** The lymph nodes palpated during a head and neck examination. Note that the superficial and deep cervical nodes are over the sternocleidomastoid muscle and below the angle of the mandible; the submental nodes are below the chin; the submandibular nodes are medial and inferior to the body of the mandible; the retroauricular and superficial parotid nodes are behind and in front of the ear; and the occipital nodes are near the base of the cranium over the occipital bone. (Reproduced by permission from Clemente CD, ed. Gray's anatomy of the human body. 30th ed. Philadelphia: Lea & Febiger, 1985:880.)

fluid escapes into the tissue spaces. On the venous side of each capillary bed, the blood pressure is lower and the osmotic pressure becomes higher, forcing 90% of the tissue fluid back into the venous capillary bed (32). The major bulk of the remaining 10% is the lymph which passes into the lumen of lymph capillaries, is then collected in the nodes, and returned to the blood vascular system (Table 1.4).

## 1. FUNCTIONS

The lymphatic system serves to collect tissue fluids that got outside the blood capillary bed and return them to the vascular system. During times of infection, trauma, or cancerous growth, abnormal amounts of fluids escape (with specialized cells to fight infection, etc.), resulting in swollen lymph glands.

### *LEARNING EXERCISES*

*Name two different pathways by which an infection might spread from a maxillary tooth to the neck.*

*Name two different pathways by which an infection might spread from a mandibular tooth to the neck.*

*What is unique about the arterial system of the face?*

*Why might application of finger pressure to block the facial artery on one side not stop a bleeding wound of the lip?*

*How does the blood supply to the deciduous teeth differ from that of the permanent dentition?*

*What are the terminal branches of the inferior alveolar artery?*

*How would the venous drainage of the temporomandibular joint differ from its arterial supply?*

*Of what artery is the middle superior alveolar a branch? What does the former artery supply?*

*Which teeth are supplied by the posterior superior alveolar artery?*

*What artery supplies blood to the mandibular canines and incisors?*

*If a patient is bleeding in the palate lingual to the first molars, what artery is producing the blood and of which artery is it a branch?*

*Where is the retromandibular vein located, what does it drain, and into what does it empty?*

*Where is the antegonial notch and what is its significance in the control of hemorrhage?*

*How might an infection spread directly to the brain if a pimple on the nose is squeezed?*

*Match the structures in Column A with the appropriate bone in Column B.*

| A | B |
|---|---|
| ___ a. Mental foramen | 1. Mandible |
| ___ b. Genial tubercles | 2. Maxilla |
| ___ c. Condylar process | |
| ___ d. Infraorbital foramen | |
| ___ e. Tuberosity | |
| ___ f. Lingula | |
| ___ g. Frontonasal process | |

*Identify the location of the following structures on your own head:*

a.  Submandibular fossa

b.  Mandibular condyle

c.  Coronoid process

**Table 1.4.** Lymphatic Drainage of Face and Jaws

**The following groups of nodes are associated with this area:**

A. Submental nodes (under chin) receive lymph from:
1. Chin
2. Tip of tongue
3. Anterior floor of mouth
4. Lower lip and mandibular incisors
B. Submandibular nodes (beneath angle of mandible) receive lymph from:
1. Submental nodes
2. Posterior floor of mouth
3. Tongue
4. Cheek, nose, upper lip
5. Vestibular gingiva of both jaws
6. Mucosa and gingiva of palate
7. All maxillary teeth, maxillary sinus, and mandibular teeth, except lower incisors
C. Parotid nodes (in front of ear over parotid gland) receive lymph from:
1. Scalp
2. Ear
3. Prominence of cheek
4. Eyelids
D. Deep cervical chain (on either side of neck) receives lymph from:
1. Mandible and lingual gingiva
2. Submandibular nodes
3. Parotid nodes
E. From here the lymph returns to the venous drainage of the cardiovascular system:

| On Left Side | On Right Side |
| --- | --- |
| Via the thoracic duct (which drains the lower body of both sides). The thoracic duct empties into the veins at the junction of the left subclavian and internal jugular veins. These two veins form the brachiocephalic (innominate) vein. | Via the right lymphatic duct (only 12.5 mm long), which in turn empties into the veins at junction of right subclavian and internal jugular veins. |

d. Lateral angle of the mandible

e. Medial angle of the mandible

f. Zygomatic arch

g. Palatine process

h. Head of the condyle

*Name the bones of the visceral cranium (that is, those that generally make up the face and NOT the neurocranium).*

# GLOSSARY

This glossary was added to this chapter to facilitate learning the vocabulary of dental anatomy. Since dental anatomy terms are often similar to common familiar words, the new terms are compared to familiar words wherever possible. Terms are placed alphabetically in categories that are related.

## Terms Related to Specific Bones of the Skull

**ethmoid:** cribriform; sieve-like

**maxillary:** refers to the bones (maxillae) supporting the upper arch of teeth

**mandibular:** refers to the bone (mandible) supporting the lower arch of teeth

**pterygo-:** [prefix] (compare the wing-like shape as a *ptero*dactyl flying dinosaur); pterygoid process of sphenoid bone has a notched wing-like appearance

**sphenoid:** bone at base of skull just anterior to temporal bone; its shape somewhat resembles a bat with its wings extended (1)

**temporal:** (compare the temples); pertaining to the lateral region of the head above the cheek bone, and above and in front of the ears

**vomer:** plow-shaped

## Anatomic Terms Related to Bones

**acoustic:** referring to sounds

**cervical:** related to the neck; like cervical vertebrae

**condyle:** an articular prominence of bones resembling a knuckle

**dura:** (compare *dura*ble); hard (not soft)

**glenoid:** socket-like

**lacrimal:** referring to the tears

**lamina:** (compare *lamina*ted wood); a thin layer

**lingula:** tongue shaped structure (cf. *lingu*al)

**malar:** referring to the cheek or cheek bone

**meatus:** a pathway or opening

**piriform:** pear-shaped

**palpebral:** referring to the eyelid

**septum:** a partition (compare *sep*aration)

**trochlea:** pulley-shaped

## Terms Related to the Junction Between Bones

**coronoid:** (compare coronation; where the crown fits or the shape of a crown); e.g., coronoid process of mandible is shaped like the point of a crown; e.g., coronoid suture is between the parietal and frontal bones

**lambdoid:** (compare lambda, the Greek letter which looks like this "λ", an upside down "V"); suture between the occipital and parietal bones in the shape of a lambda

**squamous:** (scale shape); suture between temporal and parietal bones that has a border in the shape of a fish scale

**suture line:** (compare sutures or stitches in surgery); lines of fibrous connective tissue that join two bones of the skull immovably together

**symphysis:** fibrocartilaginous joint where opposed bony surfaces are joined (a suture line may not be evident)

## Bumps and Depressions on the Bones and Teeth

### BUMPS (CONVEXITIES)

**eminence:** a prominence or projection

**process:** a prominence or projection of bone

**protuberance:** a prominence or swelling (of bone)

**ridge or line:** linear bump of bone or of enamel on a tooth

**tubercle:** a small eminence (spine) on a bone or of enamel on a tooth

### DEPRESSIONS (CONCAVITIES)

**alveolus:** socket for tooth within the alveolar process of the jaw bone that support the teeth

**cavity:** a hollow place or space within the body of bone (or within a tooth)

**fossa:** a hollow or depressed area

**fovea:** pit or depression, such as fovea palatini

**groove:** linear depression

**sinus:** air-filled cavity or space within cranial bones

## Opening (Holes) in Bones

**aperture:** an opening; compare a camera lens aperture

**foramen** (abbreviated **f.**): a hole through bone for passage of nerves and vessels; plural: foramina

**f. ovale:** an oval or egg shaped foramen (which is bigger than the round [rotundum] foramen)

**f. rotundum:** a round foramen; recall a building's rotunda or dome which is round

## Terms and Prefixes Related to a Relative Location or Surface of a Structure

**buccal:** related to the cheek; the long buccal nerve innervates the cheek; the *buccin*ator muscle is within the cheek; the *bucca*l surface of a tooth is the side toward the cheek (also called facial side because it is toward the face)

**cervix:** the neck portion

**facial:** toward the face

**infra:** (prefix) below

**inferior:** situated below

**retro:** (prefix) back, backward, or posterior

**sub:** (prefix) under or beneath

**superior or supra:** situated above

## Terms Related to Muscles

**anguli:** triangular area or *angle* of a structure

**auricular:** related to the ear

**depressor:** acts to depress or make lower

**insertion** of the muscles of mastication (place of attachment): place of attachment of muscles to the bone that moves like their attachment on the movable mandible

**labial:** related to the lips like the labial surface of a tooth

**lateral:** farther from the midline of the body

**levator:** acts to raise (cf. e*levator*)

**lingual:** related to the tongue; for example, the lingual nerve innervates the tongue, the lingual muscle is within the tongue, and the lingual surface of a tooth is the side toward the tongue.

**medial:** closer to the midline of the body

**mental:** referring to the chin; the mental foramen is the hole in the mandible where the mental nerve passes out of the mandible to the chin; the mentalis muscle inserts into the chin (1)

**mentalis:** related to the chin

**orbicularis:** round, compare an orbit

**origin:** (of muscles of mastication) are the source, beginning or fixed proximal end attachment of muscle as compared to insertion which is a muscle's more movable attachment or distal end (1)

**oris:** referring to the edge of the mouth; compare *oral*

**procerus:** long and slender

## Anatomic Terms Related to Nerves

**Afferent:** where "*a*" (as in *a*pproach) means sending impulses toward the brain (i.e., from an organ that receives sensory input) so the brain can "feel" it; therefore these impulses are sensory, related to the senses of feeling, touch, pain, taste, etc.

**Efferent:** where "*e*" (as in *e*xit) means sending an impulse from the brain, often to a muscle, to have that body part move in the intended direction; therefore these impulses are motor, leading to movement

**Ganglion:** a group of nerve cells bodies outside of the central nervous system

**Glossopharyngeal:** glosso (tongue) + pharyngeal (pharynx)

**Hypoglossal:** hypo (beneath; like a *hypo*dermic needle) + glossal (tongue)

**Ophthalmic:** related to the eye; compare *ophthalmo*logist, a physician who specializes in eyes

**Trigeminal:** *tri* refers to three parts, so the nerve would have three divisions

## Anatomic Terms Related to the Tongue

**circumvallate:** circum (around), vallate (valley or trench)

**filiform:** shaped like a thread or *fila*ment

**fungiform:** shaped like a *fungi* or mushroom

## Anatomic Terms Related to the Oral Cavity; Soft Tissues

**fornix:** referring to vault-like space

**frenum** (also frenulum; pl. frena): small fold of tissue that limits movement

**linea alba:** the white (alba) line (linea)

**mastication:** chewing food

**vestibule:** entrance to the mouth; like an anteroom, known as a vestibule in an old house

## References

1. Clemente CD, ed. Gray's anatomy of the human body. 30th Ed. Philadelphia: Lea & Febiger, 1985.
2. Roman-Ruiz LA. The mental foramen: a study of its positional relationship to the lower incisor and premolar teeth [Masters Thesis]. Columbus, OH: Ohio State University, College of Dentistry, 1970.
3. Sicher H, DuBrul EL. Oral anatomy. 7th ed. St. Louis: C.V. Mosby, 1975:174–209.
4. Edwards LF, Gaughran GRL. Concise anatomy. 3rd ed. New York: McGraw-Hill, 1971.
5. Hickey JC, Allison ML, Woelfel JB, et al. Mandibular movements in three dimensions. J Prosthet Dent 1963;13:72–92.

6. Hickey JC, Woelfel JB, et al. Influence of occlusal schemes on the muscular activity of edentulous patients. J Prosthet Dent 1963;13:444–451.
7. Woelfel JB, Hickey JC, Rinear L. Electromyographic evidence supporting the mandibular hinge axis theory. J Prosthet Dent 1957;7:361–367.
8. Woelfel JB, Hickey JC, Stacy RW. Electromyographic analysis of jaw movements. J Prosthet Dent 1960;10:688–697.
9. Woelfel JB, Hickey JC, Allison ML. Effect of posterior tooth form on jaw and denture movement. J Prosthet Dent 1962;12:922–939.
10. Sharry JJ. Complete denture prosthodontics. New York: McGraw-Hill, 1962:45–86.
11. Melfi RC. Permar's oral embryology and microscopic anatomy. 8th ed. Philadelphia: Lea & Febiger, 1988:247–257.
12. Ricketts RM. Abnormal function of the temporomandibular joint. Am J Orthod 1955;41:425, 435–441.
13. Burch JG. Activity of the accessory ligaments of the temporomandibular joint. J Prosthet Dent 1970;24:621–628.
14. Turell J, Ruiz HG. Normal and abnormal findings in temporomandibular joints in autopsy specimens. J Craniomandibular Disorders: Facial and Oral Pain 1987;1:257–275.
15. Osborn JW, ed., with Armstrong WG, Speirs RL. Anatomy, biochemistry and physiology. Oxford: Blackwell Scientific Publications, 1982:324–343.
16. Haines RW. On muscles of full and of short action. J Anat 1934;69:20–24.
17. Gionhaku N, Lowe AA. Relationship between jaw muscle volume and craniofacial form. J Dent Res 1989;68:805–809.
18. Montgomery RL. Head and neck anatomy with clinical correlations. New York: McGraw-Hill, 1981:202–214.
19. Winter CM, Woelfel JB, Igarashi T. Five-year changes in the edentulous mandible as determined on oblique cephalometric radiographs. J Dent Res 1974;53(6):1455–1467.
20. Kraus B, Jordan R, Abrams L. Dental anatomy and occlusion. Baltimore: Williams & Wilkins, 1969:203–222.
21. Basmajian JV. Grant's medical method of anatomy. 9th ed. Baltimore: Williams & Wilkins, 1975.
22. Edward LF, Gaughran GRL. Concise anatomy. 3rd ed. New York: McGraw-Hill, 1971.
23. Sicher H, DuBrul EL. Oral anatomy. 6th ed. St. Louis: C.V. Mosby, 1975:344–378.
24. Crum RJ, Loiselle RJ. Oral perception and proprioception. A review of the literature and its significance to prosthodontics. J Prosthet Dent 1972;28:215–230.
25. Jerge CR. Organization and function of the trigeminal mesencephalic nucleus. J Neurophysiol 1963;26:379–392.
26. Renner RP. An introduction to dental anatomy and esthetics. Chicago: Quintessence Publishing, 1985:162.
27. Jenkins GN. The physiology of the mouth. 3rd ed. Revised reprint. Oxford: Blackwell Scientific Publications, 1970:310–328.
28. Osborn JW, ed. Anatomy, biochemistry and physiology. Oxford: Blackwell Scientific Publications, 1982:542.
29. Edwards LF, Gaughran GRL. Concise anatomy. 3rd ed. New York: McGraw-Hill, 1971.
30. Sicher H, DuBrul EL. Oral anatomy. 7th ed. St. Louis: C.V. Mosby, 1980:351–376.
31. Montgomery RL. Head anatomy with clinical correlations. New York: McGraw-Hill, 1981:75–82.
32. Paff GH. Anatomy of the head and neck. Philadelphia: W.B. Saunders, 1973.
33. Osborn JR, ed. Dental anatomy and embryology. Oxford: Blackwell Scientific Publications, 1981:133.
34. Palmer RS. Elephants. World Book Encyclopedia 1979;6:178C.
35. Brant, D. Beavers. World Book Encyclopedia 1979;2;147.
36. Melfi RC. Permar's oral embryology and microscopic anatomy. 8th ed. Philadelphia: Lea & Febiger, 1988.
37. Osborn JW, ed. Dental anatomy and embryology. Oxford: Blackwell Scientific Publications, 1981.
38. Montgomery RL. Head and neck anatomy with clinical correlations. New York: McGraw-Hill, 1981.
39. Brand W, Isselhard B. Anatomy of orofacial structures. 5th ed. St. Louis: C.V. Mosby, 1994.
40. Francis CC. Introduction to human anatomy. 6th ed. St. Louis: C.V. Mosby, 1973.
41. Osborn JW, ed. Anatomy, biochemistry and physiology. Oxford: Blackwell Scientific Publications, 1982.
42. Zoo Books: Elephants. Wildlife Education Ltd. San Diego: Frye & Smith, 1980:14.

## General References

Reed GM, Sheppard VF. Basic structures of the head and neck. Philadelphia: W.B. Saunders, 1976.

Fehrenbach MJ, Herring SW. Illustrated anatomy of the head and neck. Philadelphia: W.B. Saunders, 1996.

Ash MM. Wheeler's dental anatomy, physiology and occlusion. 7th ed. Philadelphia: W.B. Saunders, 1993.

Dorland's illustrated medical dictionary. 27th ed. Philadelphia: W.B. Saunders, 1985.

# Oral Examination: Normal Anatomy of the Oral Cavity

*While following Chapter 2, examine a partner (using infection control procedures) and iden-tify each of the structures listed below. (The order of structures on this list is the same as that encountered within the chapter.)*

I.  Intraoral

    A.  Lips

    __  1.  Vermilion zone, mucocutaneous junction, wet line

    __  2.  Upper lip

        __  a.  tubercle

        __  b.  philtrum

        __  c.  nasolabial fold

    __  3.  Continue:

        __  a.  Commissure

        __  b.  Commissural papule

        __  c.  Labiomental groove

    B.  Vestibule (and cheeks) with labial mucosa

    __  1.  Fornix

__  2.  Labial frenum

__  3.  Buccal frenum

C.  Cheeks with buccal mucosa

__  1.  Linea alba

__  2.  Parotid papilla (drains Stensen's duct, see if saliva drains by gently milking the cheek from posterior toward the duct)

__  3.  Fordyce spots

D.  Teeth—maxillary and mandibular

How many in each arch? Maxillary __      Mandibular __

__  Maxillary tuberosity

__  Retromolar pad

E.  Gingiva

What is the color? __

Is it stippled? __

__  1.  Gingival margin

__  2.  Interdental papilla

__  3.  Free Gingiva

__  4.  Free gingival groove

__  5.  Gingival sulcus (not visible)

__  6.  Junctional epithelium (not visible)

__  7.  Attached gingiva

__  8.  Keratinized gingiva (describes character of both free and attached gingiva)

__  9.  Mucogingival junction

__  10. Alveolar mucosa

F.  Tongue

1.  Dorsum (top) with papillae that have taste buds

__  Filiform papilla

__  Fungiform papilla

__  Foliate papilla

__  Circumvallate papilla (difficult to see; way back)

__  Foramen cecum and terminal sulcus (probably not visible)

2.  Ventral (underneath) surface

__  Lingual frenum

__  Plica fimbriata

G.  Floor of mouth

__  1.  Sublingual folds (plica sublingualis) and sublingual caruncles (draining Wharton's duct; try to milk out saliva with your finger pressing gently from posterior to anterior)

__  2.  Alveolingual sulcus

__ 3. Are the following present?

__ Mandibular torus

__ Buccal exostosis

H. Roof of mouth

1. Hard palate

__ a. Incisive papilla

__ b. Palatine raphe

__ c. Rugae

__ d. Torus palatinus

2. Soft palate

__ a. Vibrating line (have partner say Ah, ah, ah)

__ b. Uvula

__ c. Fovea palatinae

I. Fauces

1. Arches

__ Glossopalatine arch

__ Pharyngopalatine arch

__ Palatine tonsils (if present)

2. Fauces

3. Pterygomandibular fold (an important landmark for future injections)

II. Structures to palpate extraorally

A. Muscles

__ 1. Masseter

__ 2. Medial pterygoid

__ 3. Temporalis

__ Anterior fibers (closing mandible)

__ Posterior fibers (retracting mandible)

__ 4. Lateral pterygoid (palpate intraorally)

B. Craniomandibular Joint (palpate during movements)

__ Lateral surface

__ Posterior surface

Pressure Spots to Palpate the Muscles of Mastication and Craniomandibular Joint:

#1: Lateral to craniomandibular joint

#2: Posterior to craniomandibular joint

#3: Masseter (origin)

#4: Masseter (insertion)

#5: Temporalis (anterior fibers that close mandible)

**Sequence and Sites For Palpation**

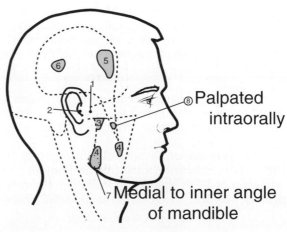

⑧Palpated intraorally

Medial to inner angle of mandible

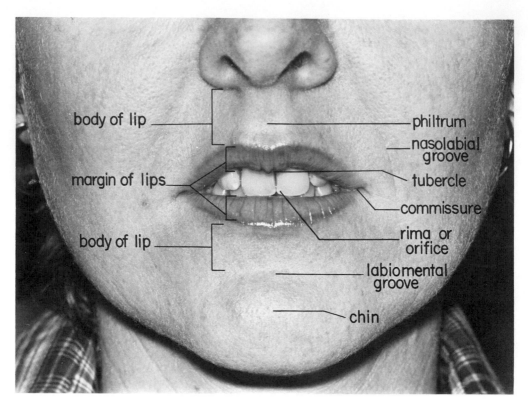

**Figure 2.1.** Surface anatomy of structures in the lower half of the face. The margin of the lip is sometimes called the vermilion border. The wet-dry line does not show because the margins were moistened by the tongue in order to photograph well.

#6: Temporalis (posterior fibers that retract mandible)

#7: Medial pterygoid

#8: Lateral pterygoid (palpated intraorally)

## SECTION I. INTRAORAL EXAMINATION

During the periodic oral, head, and neck cancer screening examination, the dental professional should evaluate all oral and surrounding structures for evidence of pathology. This examination begins with an assessment of the patient's general health, and then proceeds to an assessment *of extraoral* structures of the head and neck, and an *intraoral* examination that includes an evaluation of structures from the lips to the throat.

Soft tissue structures cover the bones of the skull and are supplied by the nerves and blood vessels discussed in Chapter 1. As you study this material and examine the mouth, attempt to recall these underlying bones, nerves, and vessels.

The *oral cavity* is bounded anteriorly by the lips, laterally by the cheeks, superiorly by the palate, and inferiorly by the floor of the mouth. The oral cavity can be divided into the *oral vestibule,* or space between the teeth (with alveolar arches) and lips, and the oral cavity proper, beyond the teeth and alveolar processes.

**LEARNING EXERCISE**

*Look into someone's mouth as you read this description and locate each structure mentioned. Use a tongue depressor or a mouth mirror to retract the lips and cheeks. The mouth mirror is useful for reflecting light into remote areas and for holding the tongue or cheek out of the way during your examination. Use the form provided at the beginning of the chapter to check off each structure as you find it.*

### UPON LOOKING INTO THE ORAL CAVITY, YOU SHOULD BE ABLE TO SEE:

1. Lips (entrance) with commissure (corner of the mouth)
2. Vestibule
3. Cheeks
4. Teeth
5. Gingiva (gums)
6. Tongue
7. Floor of Mouth
8. Roof of Mouth
   a. Hard palate and rugae
   b. Soft palate and fovea palatini
9. Fauces (posterior extent of oral cavity)
   a. Glossopalatine arch (anterior pillar)
   b. Pharyngopalatine arch (posterior pillar)

## Oral Mucous Membrane (Oral Mucosa)

A *mucous membrane* lines any body cavity that opens to the outside of the body. The *oral mucous membrane* lines the oral cavity. It is made up of two layers: stratified surface epithelium, and the underlying connective tissue. It resembles the skin on the outside of the body, except that it is more delicate in structure and is moist. It is most sturdy in the areas where it is subjected to the most wear. Look at the roof the mouth and the gingiva. This toughened layer is called the *keratin* layer, and, as wear occurs, it is replaced by underlying cells. Its appearance in these areas of greater wear is grayish, rather than red, compared to the floor of the mouth and cheeks where tissue is more protected. The mucosa beneath the tongue has no keratin layer, and this lining mucosa is so thin that the blood vessels located in the underlying connective tissue can easily be seen giving it a reddish or bluish color.

## A. Examine the Lips Visually Using Fig. 2.1 as a Guide

The lips are the two fleshy borders of the mouth (an upper and a lower) which join at the commissure. The upper lip is bounded by the cheeks (laterally) at the *nasolabial* groove, and by the nose (superiorly). The lower lip is also bounded laterally by the cheeks, and inferiorly by the chin at the *labiomental* groove. The orbicularis oris muscle is the muscle surrounding the opening between the lips that permits us to close the lips around a straw.

The lips are important in the head and neck exam because changes here may be caused by exposure to the sun which could lead to skin cancer.

1. Vermilion border (or zone)—the red border of the lips, representing a transitional zone where the lips merge into mucous membrane. It is the area where females often place lipstick. It is bounded in the mouth by the wet line where labial mucosa begins, and externally by the mucocutaneous junction.

    a. *Mucocutaneous junction* or margin of the lips—junction between skin of the face and vermilion border of the lips.

    b. *Wet line* (or wet-dry line)—the junction or division between the inner (more smooth and moist) and outer red portion of the lips, which is usually dry. The wet line is located in the red zone, only 10 mm back from the skin. The lips are redder in younger persons than in older persons. In some individuals, the lip color is reddish brown due to the presence of brown melanin pigment.

2. *Examine the Upper Lip* (and surrounding skin): (Fig. 2.1)

    a. *Tubercle*—the small rounded nodule of tissue in the center of the lowest part of the upper lip.

    b. *Philtrum*—the depression running from the tubercle to the nostrils.

    c. *Nasolabial groove*—the groove running diagonally downward on each side of the nostril toward the corner of the lip.

3. *Continue to examine the lips:*

    a. *Commissure*—the corner of the mouth where the upper and lower lips meets (right and left sides).

    b. *Commissural papule*—an elevation of mucous membrane immediately inside the mouth, usually 4–6 mm posterior to the commissure (not visible in Fig. 2.1).

    c. *Labiomental groove*—the horizontal groove between the lower lip and the chin.

## B. Examine the Vestibule and Cheeks and Identify Its Parts and Landmarks Using Fig. 2.2 as a Guide

The arch or vault-shaped space between the cheek or lip on one side, and the teeth and gingiva of the maxilla or mandible on the other side, is called a *vestibule* (maxillary or mandibular). It is covered with pinkish labial and deeper colored alveolar mucosa, and is rich in blood vessels (can you name the vessel to this area?) and minor salivary glands. The tip of your tongue can reach into each vestibule to assist in cleaning the facial surfaces of the teeth.

1. The *vestibular fornix* is the depth (mandible) or height (maxillae) of the vestibule. This is where food may collect in patients with nerve damage to the cheek.

2. The *labial frenum* (plural: frena) is the thin sheet of tissue that attaches the center of the lip (upper and lower) to the mucosa covering the jaw between the central incisors.

3. The *buccal frenum*, in the area of the premolars (maxillary and mandibular), loosely attaches the cheek to the mucosa of the jaw. These frena may be seen by pulling the lower lip and cheek out and down, and upper lip and cheek out and up. Our facial muscles move the buccal frena forward and backward and upward and downward in eating to help place our food back over the chewing surfaces of our teeth prior to swallowing. They also can dislodge complete dentures if the denture is designed improperly.

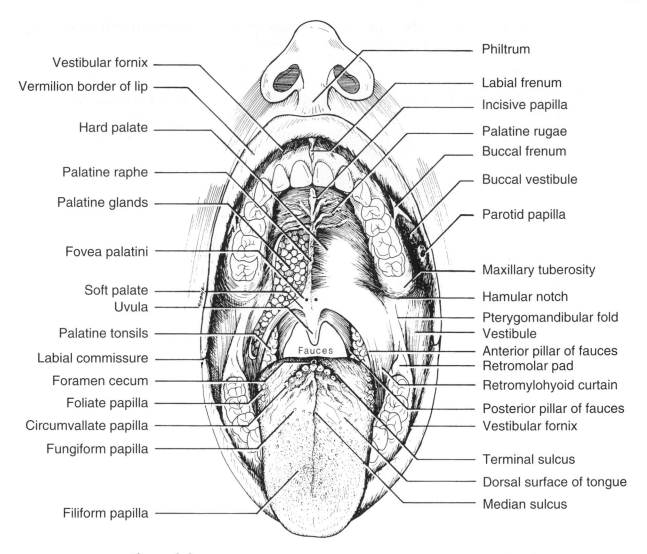

Vestibular fornix

Vermilion border of lip

Hard palate

Palatine raphe

Palatine glands

Fovea palatini

Soft palate
Uvula

Palatine tonsils

Labial commissure

Foramen cecum

Foliate papilla

Circumvallate papilla

Fungiform papilla

Filiform papilla

Philtrum

Labial frenum

Incisive papilla

Palatine rugae

Buccal frenum

Buccal vestibule

Parotid papilla

Maxillary tuberosity

Hamular notch

Pterygomandibular fold
Vestibule

Anterior pillar of fauces
Retromolar pad

Retromylohyoid curtain

Posterior pillar of fauces

Vestibular fornix

Terminal sulcus

Dorsal surface of tongue

Median sulcus

Fauces

**Figure 2.2.** Structures in the oral cavity. (Drawn by Amelia A. Boye.)

## C. Examine the Cheeks

The *buccal mucosa* lining of the inside of the cheeks is shiny, and in spots it is rough.

1.  Often there is a horizontal white line running posteriorly on each side at the level where the upper and lower teeth come together. This is called the *linea alba buccalis* ("linea" means line, "alba" means white). It may extend from the commissural area anteriorly to the pterygomandibular raphe posteriorly. This area is often irritated by trauma from biting the cheek.

2.  The *parotid papilla* (Fig. 2.2) is a rounded elevation of tissue next to the first and second molars at or just above the occlusal *plane.* Survey of parotid papilla location: [In 1971 and 1972, Dr. Woelfel and Dr. Igarashi supervised 331 dental students as they recorded the position of the right and left parotid papilla on each other. Of 662 parotid papillae, 78% were located between the maxillary first and second molar or by the second molar. Only 22% were by the first molar. In height, 87% of these same papillae were located level with (34%) or above the level (53%) of the occlusal plane. Only 13% were found below the level of the occlusal plane. The widest variation in location among these dental students was on two men, one having his parotid papilla

on each side 11 mm above the occlusal plane; the other man with his 8 mm below the level of the occlusal plane. In a similar study of 407 adults (258 Caucasian, 11 black, 9 Hispanic) with 293 men and 114 women, the parotid papilla averaged 3.3 mm above the occlusal plane (right 3.0, left 3.5 mm) (2).] These papillae cover the duct openings (*Stensen's duct*) from the parotid gland. The large quadrilateral-shaped parotid glands are located in front of each ear and produce 23–33% of our saliva (serous type) (1). They are also the glands affected during mumps.

3. *Fordyce's spots* are small, yellowish, irregular areas and may be conspicuous inside the lips or buccal mucosa, especially inside the cheeks just posterior to the corner of the mouth. They are produced by the presence of sebaceous glands—glands of a type otherwise found only in the skin on the outside of the body. Their presence here is often said to be the result of fusion of the upper and lower parts of the cheek during embryonic development. Such glands have also been found, however, on other parts of the oral mucosa.

## D. Identify the Teeth—Count Them

A full complement of adult teeth is 32 (16 upper and 16 lower). There are two *dental arches* (curved rows of teeth): maxillary or upper and mandibular or lower (Fig. 1.2).

### 1. NUMBER OF TEETH

The total number of teeth depends on the age of the individual, the stage of development of the teeth, and the number of teeth lost by disease, accident, or removed for orthodontic treatment.

The complete *primary dentition* (baby teeth) consists of 20 teeth (Fig. 1.1). Children between $2^1/_2$ and $5^3/_4$ years of age will usually have 20 teeth (all primary dentition).

From approximately $5^3/_4$ to 12 years of age, a *mixed dentition* with some primary and some permanent teeth is present. The mixed dentition of a 6-year-old would have 24 teeth, and by 12 years of age there would be 28 teeth.

The complete permanent or secondary dentition consists of 32 teeth, including the four third molars, which come in during the late teens. Immediately posterior to the maxillary last molar is a firm tissue bulge of the alveolar ridge named the *maxillary tuberosity* (Fig. 2.2). A similar, less prominent, pear-shaped elevation of movable tissue distal to the mandibular last molar is the *retromolar pad* (Fig. 2.2) ("retro" means behind or distal to the last molar). When a person has fully erupted third molars, the maxillary tuberosities and retromolar pads are small because these teeth occupy these regions.

## E. Periodontium and Gingiva

The periodontium is defined as the supporting tissues of the teeth and includes surrounding alveolar bone (already discussed), the gingiva, periodontal ligament, and the outer layer of the tooth roots (cementum) (Fig. 1.11).

The gingiva is that part of the masticatory (keratinized) oral mucous membrane that covers the alveolar process of the jaws and surrounds the cervical portions of the teeth (Fig. 2.3). Therefore, the gingiva is the part of the periodontium that is evaluated in the oral examination.

**EXAMINE THE GINGIVA AND IDENTIFY THE ZONES USING FIG. 2.3 AS A GUIDE.**

The *gingiva* is that part of the masticatory (keratinized) tissue that surrounds the cervical part of teeth. It is firmly attached to the teeth and to their surrounding bone. The gingiva

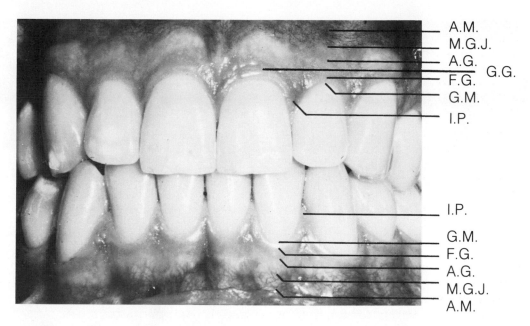

A.M.
M.G.J.
A.G.
G.G.
F.G.
G.M.
I.P.

I.P.

G.M.
F.G.
A.G.
M.G.J.
A.M.

**Figure 2.3.** Clinical components of the gingiva. *G.M.*, gingival margins; *F.G.*, free gingiva; *I.P.*, interdental papilla; *G.G.*, gingival groove; *A.G.*, attached gingiva; *M.G.J.*, mucogingival junction; *A.M.*, alveolar mucosa. Note that the interdental papillae should, but do not completely, fill the interproximal spaces between the mandibular incisors. The tissues are otherwise healthy. (Courtesy of Lewis J. Claman, D.D.S., M.S.)

is stippled (Fig. 2.4) and coral pink in persons with light pigmentation. In persons with dark coloring of the hair and skin, and in those of Mediterranean origin, the gingiva may be brown or spotted with brown (melanin pigmentation) (Fig. 2.5).

## ZONES OF GINGIVA (FIG. 2.3 SHOWS MOST OF THESE STRUCTURES)

1. *Gingival margin* is the occlusal (incisal) border at which the gingiva meets the tooth.

2. *Interdental (interproximal) papilla* is that portion of the gingiva that fills the interproximal space. The interdental gingiva (papilla) between the facial and lingual papillae conforms to the shape of the contact area.

3. *Free gingiva (marginal gingiva)* is the collar of tissue that is not attached to the tooth or alveolar bone. It surrounds the root of each tooth from the gingival margin to form the collar of space or gingival crevice or sulcus (where dental floss can fit).

4. *Attached gingiva* is a band or zone of gray to light or coral pink of keratinized masticatory mucosa that is firmly bound down to the underlying bone. It is present between the free gingiva and the more movable alveolar mucosa. The amount or height of attached gingiva varies from 3 to 12 mm.

5. *Free gingival groove* (Fig. 2.3) separates free gingiva from attached gingiva. It is present in about one-third of adults.

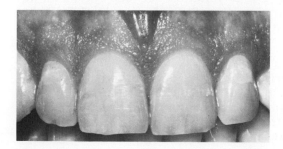

**Figure 2.4.** Healthy gingiva, close up. Note the ideal contours. The stippled (orange peel) surface texture is usually most noticeable on the maxillary labial attached gingiva.

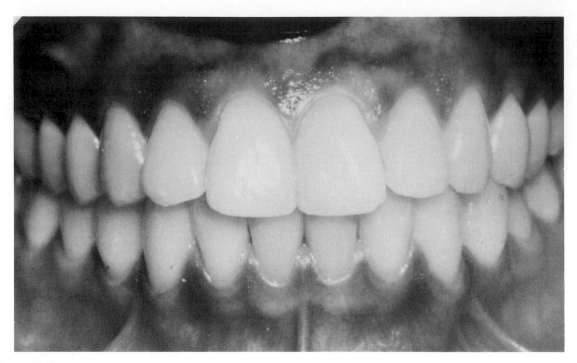

**Figure 2.5.** Healthy teeth, gingiva, and mouth with several streaks and patches of melanin pigmentation in the attached gingiva. It is especially evident over the maxillary incisors and mesial to the mandibular canines. This pigmentation may occur up to the mucogingival junction. It is a common occurrence in people with darkly colored and Negroid skin, Asians, people from India, and people of Mediterranean origins (Italians, Arabs, Yemenites, Turks, and some Jewish people). (Courtesy of Lewis J. Claman, D.D.S., M.S.)

6. *Gingival sulcus* (Fig. 2.6) is *not seen visually* but can be evaluated with a probe. It is a space or potential space between the tooth surface and the narrow unattached cervical margin of gingiva called free gingiva. It is lined with the sulcular epithelium. It extends from the free gingival margin to the junctional epithelium (histologically) and averages 0.69 mm in depth (3).

7. *Junctional or attached epithelium* (epithelial attachment *not visible* during the oral exam) begins at the most apical portion of the gingival sulcus and is a band that attaches the gingiva to the tooth (Fig. 1.11). It is about 1 mm in height (3); then there is a 1–1.5 mm connective tissue attachment to the root above the osseous crest of bone. It is usually recommended that the margins of crowns and inlays be kept 3 mm from the bony osseous crest.

8. *Keratinized gingiva* is the term used to describe masticatory mucosa that occurs between the gingival margin and the mucogingival junction (line). It includes both the free and the attached gingiva and is widest on the facial (vestibular) aspect of maxillary anterior teeth and the lingual aspect of mandibular molars. It is narrowest on the facial aspect of mandibular premolars (4).

9. *Mucogingival junction (line)* is a scalloped line or junction between the facial attached gingiva and the redder alveolar mucosa (Fig. 2.3). The hard palate, however, has firm keratinized tissue for almost the entire surface (Fig. 2.2). The mucogingival line is therefore present on maxillary and mandibular facial aspects and mandibular lingual aspects.

10. *Alveolar mucosa* is movable mucosa, dark pink to red, due to increased vascularity and more delicate nonkeratinized tissue just apical to the mucogingival junction (Fig. 2.3). It is found in three places: maxillary and mandibular facial and mandibular lingual aspects, not on the palate. Alveolar mucosa is more delicate and less firmly attached to the underlying bone than the attached gingiva

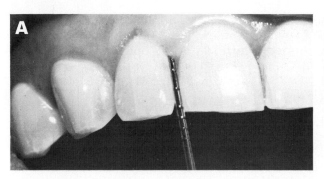
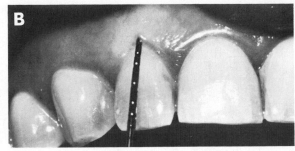

**Figure 2.6.** Periodontal probe in place in the gingival sulcus. **A.** Interproximal probing. **B.** Facial probing. In health, the area probed is the gingiva sulcus. If periodontal disease is present, it is called a pocket.

and is more displaceable as well, because of the underlying vessels and connective tissue. Palpate these two zones and you will feel the difference in firmness.

Ideal, healthy gingiva varies in appearance from individual to individual and in different areas of the same mouth. It is usually pink (or pigmented), with thin margins that are just coronal to the cementoenamel junction. The *papillae* are pointed and fill the interproximal spaces between teeth. The contours around each tooth are escalloped and follow a parabolic form. Clinically, the gingival sulcus varies in probing depth from less than 1 mm to 3 mm and should not bleed when probed (Fig. 2.6). The periodontal probe usually penetrates into the junctional epithelium, hence the difference between clinical and histologic depths (5).

[In a survey by Dr. Woelfel, 267 dental hygiene students measured their gingival sulcus depth with a calibrated periodontal probe. The average gingival sulcus depths for mandibular first molars midbuccal were: $1.5 \pm 0.5$ mm; midlingual: $1.7 \pm 0.6$ mm; mesiolingual and distolingual: $2.5 \pm 0.5$ mm. These measurements indicate that the gingival sulcus is usually deeper interproximally. Similar measurements made on the mesiofacial aspect of mandibular canines ($1.9 \pm 0.8$ mm), maxillary canines (1.8 mm), maxillary first premolars ($1.9 \pm 0.7$ mm), and maxillary first molars ($2.1 \pm 0.7$ mm) indicate sulci slightly deeper on posterior teeth than those on anterior teeth.]

In health, the gingiva functions in providing support, protection, and aesthetics. The gingiva somewhat supports the tooth because the junctional epithelium attaches to the tooth by the gingival fibers that insert into the tooth root covering (cementum), and the attached gingiva that is connected down to supporting bone. The gingiva protects underlying tissues because it has keratinized epithelium covering dense connective tissue on the oral aspect. It is resistant to bacterial, chemical, thermal, and mechanical irritants. Moreover, the attached gingiva helps prevent the spread of inflammation to deeper periodontal tissues. Healthy gingiva, with ideal contours, in turn is somewhat protected by ideally positioned natural teeth or well-contoured restorations. The protection it provides prevents injury from food deflected onto the gingival margins or impacted into the interdental space but doesn't prevent the formation on teeth of bacterial plaque, a bacterial layer that contributes to tooth decay and periodontal disease.

An imperfect area of protective function of the gingiva is the sulcular lining (epithelium) of the marginal gingiva and junctional epithelium, including the interdental papillae. This lining is not keratinized and is, therefore, permeable to bacterial products. It is a weak barrier to bacterial irritants.

## F. Examine the Tongue

Examine the tongue by wrapping it in a damp 4" × 4" gauze square and *gently* pulling it first to one side, then the other. Use Fig. 2.2 as a guide for the top of the tongue.

The tongue is a broad, flat organ composed of muscle fibers and glands. It rests in the floor of the mouth within the curvature of the body of the mandible. The tongue changes its shape with each functional movement. The anterior two-thirds is the body, and the posterior one-third is the tongue base or root.

## 1. DORSUM OF THE TONGUE

The *dorsum* (dorsal or superior surface) of the tongue (Fig. 2.2) is the principle organ of taste, and is invaluable during speech and during mastication and deglutition (swallowing). The *dorsum* of the tongue is grayish-red and is rough. It is covered by two kinds of papillae: *filiform papillae,* which are the most numerous, fine, and hair-like, covering the anterior two-thirds of the dorsal surface arranged in lines somewhat parallel to the terminal sulcus (6). There are also the larger, more sparse, scattered, and shorter *fungiform papillae* (Fig. 11.26**B**) that are easy to identify because of their round mushroom shape and deep red color. Fungiform papillae are more concentrated near the tip of the tongue (6).

*Foliate papillae* are large, red, leaf-like projections found on the lateral surfaces of the tongue in the posterior one-third. They contain some taste buds. The *circumvallate papillae* are 8 to 12 large, flat, mushroom-shaped papillae that form a V-shaped row on the dorsum near the posterior third of the tongue. Their walls contain numerous taste buds. These are sometimes difficult to see if the patient cannot extend his or her tongue sufficiently. The *foramen cecum* is a small circular opening immediately posterior to the V formed by the circumvallate papilla. It is the remains of the thyroglossal duct from which the thyroid gland developed. The *terminal sulcus* is a shallow groove running laterally and forward on either side of the foramen cecum and posterior to the circumvallate papillae. It is usually necessary to hold the tongue firmly with gauze and pull it forward in order to see the circumvallate papilla and its neighboring structures because of their extremely posterior location. The smoother posterior third of the dorsum contains numerous muciparous glands and lymph follicles referred to as the *lingual tonsil* (not visible on Fig. 2.2).

## 2. VENTRAL SURFACE OF THE TONGUE

The *ventral* or undersurface of the tongue is shiny and blood vessels are visible. Refer to Fig. 2.7.

The *lingual frenum* (fre´num) is a thin sheet of tissue that attaches the center of the undersurface of the tongue to the floor of the mouth. Raise your tongue and watch how this cord-like structure limits the amount of tongue movement. [Measurements on 333 casts by Dr. Woelfel indicated the frenum attachment to be 8.03 + 1.5 mm below the gingival sulcus of the mandibular central incisors; range 5.4–11 mm. Assuming an average length mandibular central incisor (8.8 mm), the lingual frenum attaches about 17 mm below the incisal edge of these teeth.] In a person who is tongue-tied, the lingual frenum is firmly attached perhaps only 3 or 4 mm below the gingival margins of the central incisors and may cause periodontal problems.

*Plica fimbriata* (fimbriated folds) are delicate folds of mucous membrane on each side of the frenum on the ventral surface of the tongue. The free edge of this fold may have a series of fringe-like processes. These are very delicate and often difficult to see unless gently moved by the tongue blade or mirror. In some animals, these fringes of tissue serve to keep the teeth clean.

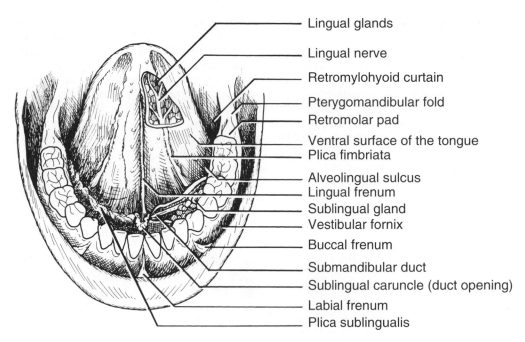

Lingual glands
Lingual nerve
Retromylohyoid curtain
Pterygomandibular fold
Retromolar pad
Ventral surface of the tongue
Plica fimbriata
Alveolingual sulcus
Lingual frenum
Sublingual gland
Vestibular fornix
Buccal frenum
Submandibular duct
Sublingual caruncle (duct opening)
Labial frenum
Plica sublingualis

**Figure 2.7.** Structures of the under surface of the tongue (ventral surface) and floor of the mouth. Note that the submandibular duct from the submandibular gland to the floor of the mouth is also known as Wharton's duct.

## G. Examine the Floor of the Mouth

Examine the floor of the mouth by having the patient raise the tongue. Refer to Fig. 2.7.

### 1. VENTRAL OF THE TONGUE

The ventral or undersurface of the tongue and the floor of the mouth are shiny, and some large blood vessels may be seen near the surface.

On the floor, the overlying *sublingual folds,* called the *plica sublingualis* (pli´ka sub lĭng guàl ĭs), extend anteriorly on each side of the floor of the mouth from the first molar to the *lingual frenum* where the broad underside of the tongue is attached to the floor of the mouth. Along these folds are openings of ducts from underlying sublingual salivary glands located in this region. The sublingual glands secrete purely mucous (ropy type) saliva, producing only 5–8% of our saliva (1).

In the center line at the junction between the right and left sublingual folds on either side of the sublingual frenum, is a pair of bulges called *sublingual caruncles,* each with an opening from ducts of salivary glands (Wharton's ducts). Wharton's ducts drain the larger, more posteriorly located submandibular glands, which produce about two-thirds of our saliva (1). Their secretions are primarily serous (two-thirds serous cells, one-third mucous cells (7)). If you gently move your finger from posterior to anterior over the sublingual folds, saliva should come out of the caruncles.

A person normally secretes over a pint of saliva during 24 hours (300 ml between meals, 300 ml while eating, and only 20 ml while sleeping) based on averages from 600 people (1).

### 2. ALVEOLINGUAL SULCUS

*Alveolingual sulcus* is a valley-shaped space between the tongue and mandibular alveolar bone. You can gently place your finger in this broad sulcus.

## 3. MANDIBULAR TORUS

*Mandibular torus* (plural *tori*) may be present (Fig. 2.8). It is a bulbous protuberance of bone beneath a thin mucous membrane covering on the lingual side of the mandible often found in the premolar region opposite the mental foramen. Mandibular tori are probably transmitted as a genetic trait, and are not uncommon. They usually cause no problems, but may be irritated (by being in the way) when lower impressions are made. After several or all lower teeth have been lost and removable dentures are to be made, mandibular tori must be surgically excised. A similar torus may also occur in the middle of the palate (called a *torus palatinus*).

*Exostosis* is a general term used to describe a hyperplastic bony growth projecting outward from the bone surface, such as a torus palatinus, or mandibular torus, but can also be used to describe bony ridges which may form on the buccal surface of the mandible or maxillae.

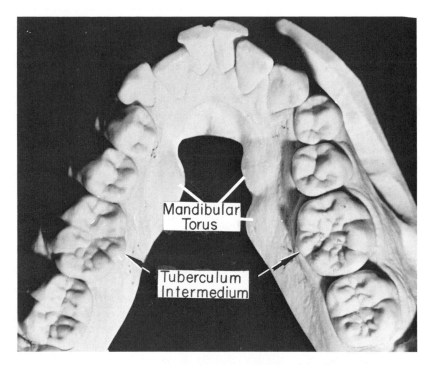

A

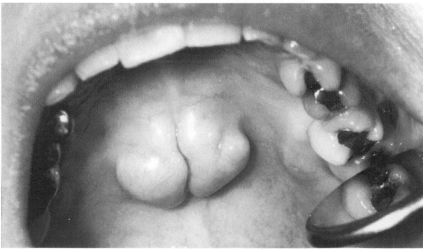

**Figure 2.8. A**. Dental stone cast of permanent mandibular dentition. Notice the three mandibular tori (large bulbous elevations of bone) on each side and the mandibular first molars, which have six, instead of the usual five, cusps. The anterior teeth are somewhat crowded. The mandibular first premolars each have two lingual cusps. Notice that the second premolars are widest lingually. **B**. A maxillary torus palatinus.

B

*Retromylohyoid curtain* (Fig. 2.2) is a zone of mucous membrane in the floor of the mouth between the anterior pillar of the fauces and the pterygomandibular fold. It is an important limiting structure in forming the lingual flange (edge) of a mandibular complete denture.

## H. Evaluate the Roof of the Mouth with a Good Light and Mouth Mirror

The *hard palate* is the firm anterior part of the roof of the mouth, ending opposite the third molars and immediately anterior to the fovea palatine (Fig. 2.2).

The *soft palate* is the posterior movable part of the roof of the mouth.

The *vibrating line* is the junction between the hard and soft palate.

### 1. HARD PALATE (FIG. 2.9)

The color is grayish red to coral pink.

#### a. Incisive (Nasopalatine) Papilla

*Incisive (nasopalatine) papilla* is the small rounded elevation of tissue on the midline just behind or lingual to the central incisors. There is a relatively constant 8.5-mm distance from the facial surface of the maxillary central incisors and the center of the incisive papilla. [On 326 casts measured by Dr. Woelfel, the average distance was 8.4 mm with a range of 5.5 to 12 mm.] This papilla is over the incisive foramen where the nasopalatine nerve passes to innervate the anterior hard palate.

#### b. Palatine Raphe

*Palatine raphe* (pronounced rā´fē) is the slightly elevated center line running anteroposteriorly in the hard palate. The median suture attachment or place of union between right and left maxillae is immediately under the mucosa along this line. The mucosa is firm over the raphe because it is firmly attached to the underlying periosteum and bone without intervening fat or gland cells. The sides of the hard palate are less hard than the palatine raphe because there is fat or

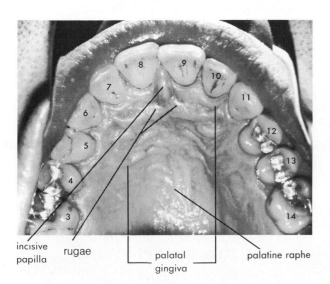

incisive papilla  rugae  palatal gingiva  palatine raphe

**Figure 2.9.** The hard palate is bordered by the maxillary dental arch. The teeth in the picture are, on either side of the arch, the central incisor, lateral incisor, canine, first premolar, second premolar, and first molar. The posterior parts of the arch and the soft palate are not in the picture. The palatine rugae are prominent, as is the incisive papilla (the enlargement between the right and left central incisors). The palatine raphe is seen, but is not conspicuous in this subject. In some mouths, this raphe is more ridge-like, extending anteroposteriorly in the center of the hard palate, and is readily distinguished. Notice the correct universal number on each tooth.

salivary gland tissue beneath the surface tissue. There are over 350 palatine glands in the posterior third of the hard palate (6). They secrete thick mucinous saliva.

### c. Palatine Rugae

*Palatine rugae* (Fig. 2.9) are more distinct in young persons than in other persons. They are a series of elevations, or wrinkles, running from side to side, like branches on a tree, on the anterior portion of the palate behind the maxillary anterior teeth from a common stem or trunk, the palatine raphe. [Among casts from 939 hygiene students, rugae trees had 3, 4, or 5 branches on each side in 87% of the students. The first main branch was aligned lingual to the canine in 72%. The rugae were well elevated in 85% of the students and flattened in only 14%.]

A longitudinal study on 20 females and 21 males, from age 4 to 22 years, indicated a slight but steady growth of the rugae during this period (average: 1.4–2.3 mm). Rugae growth occurred earlier in females, but the males had more branches (8).

Rugae function in two important ways: in tactilely sensing objects or food position and in aiding the tongue's proper placement for the production of certain speech sounds (9).

## 2. STRUCTURES OF THE SOFT PALATE

The soft palate (Fig. 2.2) is found posterior to the hard palate, and separates the mouth from the nasal passage. It is sometimes redder than the hard palate because of its somewhat increased vascularity. Its anterior border extends between the right and left third molars.

### a. Vibrating Line

Unlike the hard palate, there is no bone beneath the surface of the soft palate. (Say ah, ah, ah, and look.) The soft palate moves or vibrates. The hinged place, or the place where you observe the beginning of the soft palate, is the *vibrating line.*

### b. Uvula

*Uvula* (both u's are pronounced like the u in use) is a small fleshy structure hanging from the center of the posterior border of the soft palate.

### c. Fovea Palatini

*Fovea palatini* (fō´ve ah pāl´ ah tin ē) are a pair of pits in the soft palate located on either side of the center line near but posterior to the vibrating line. They are openings of ducts of minor palatine mucous glands (9).

## 3. FUNCTIONS OF THE SOFT PALATE (9)

### a. Swallowing

The nasal pharynx is closed off from the oral pharynx to prevent regurgitation of food into the nasal cavity.

### b. Blowing or Producing Explosive Consonants (Like B and P)

The soft palate is raised to seal the oral cavity from the nasal cavity.

## I. Examine the Fauces and Palatine Arches

Examine the fauces and palatine arches (Fig. 2.2) by having the patient open and say "ahhh. . . . ". You may have to *gently* push the tongue down with a tongue depressor. *BE CAREFUL,* patients may gag.

### 1. ARCHES OR PILLARS

The arches on either side of the uvula are the anterior and posterior palatine pillars or arches that descend from the soft palate. The anterior pillar is also named the *glossopalatine arch* and the posterior pillar is named the *pharyngopalatine arch* after the muscles beneath them. They are composed of an aggregation of lymphoid tissue beneath the mucous membrane. The *palatine tonsils* are located between the anterior and posterior pillars. They may become enlarged and inflamed during infections of the respiratory system. Patients may have had these surgically removed.

### 2. FAUCES

The opening between the free borders of the soft palate, the right and left posterior pillars, and the base of the tongue is called the *fauces.* It is the posterior boundary of the oral cavity. Behind the soft palate is the *oropharynx,* which leads to the esophagus.

### 3. PTERYGOMANDIBULAR FOLD

Laterally on each side is a curtain of tissue that appears to connect the mandible and the maxilla. This is the *pterygomandibular fold.* This is easy to see when the mouth is opened wide, as this action stretches this fold, extending from the retromolar pad on the mandible to the maxillary tuberosity.

### LEARNING EXERCISE ON ORAL ANATOMIC LANDMARK

*Test your newly acquired knowledge now by matching the landmarks with their description.*

**QUIZ ON ORAL ANATOMIC LANDMARKS**

Place appropriate letter or letters on line on left.

___ 1. Dorsum of tongue

___ 2. Hard palate

___ 3. Pharynx

___ 4. Elevated midline of hard palate

___ 5. Stensen's duct

___ 6. Alveolar mucosa

___ 7. Fordyce's spots

___ 8. Melanin

___ 9. Gingiva between teeth numbers 11 and 12 or 19 and 20

___10. Enlargement between teeth numbers 8 and 9 on the palatal side

___11. Vibrating line

a. Mouth

b. Dark pigment on attached gingiva

c. Anteriorly in floor of mouth where the plica sublingualis meet

d. Underside of tongue

e. Has rugae

f. Top side of tongue

g. Sebaceous glands on inside of cheek

h. Interdental papillae

i. Opens on inside of cheek near maxillary first molar

j. Palatine raphe

k. Attaches lip to mucosa covering jaw (upper and lower)

(continued)

___12. Wharton's duct openings

___13. Labial frenum

___14. Ventral surface of tongue

___15. Oral cavity

___16. Retromolar pad

___17. Maxillary tuberosity

___18. Filiform papillae

___19. Torus mandibularis

___20. Attached gingiva

___21. Alveolar mucosa

___22. Mandibular first molar

___23. Clinical crown

___24. Parotid gland

___25. Philtrum

___26. Commissure

___27. Fauces

___28. Nasolabial groove

___29. Labiomental groove

___30. Sublingual gland

___31. Submandibular gland

___32. Anatomic crown

___33. Anatomic root

___34. Clinical root

___35. Fovea palatini

___36. Diastema

___37. Plica sublingualis

___38. Uvula

___39. Plica fimbriata

___40. Foliate papilla

___41. Circumvallate papillae

___42. Alveololingual sulcus

___43. Deglutition

___44. Palatine tonsils

___45. Retromylohyoid curtain

___46. Mandibular torus

___47. Fungiform papillae

l.  Behind soft palate

m.  Incisive papilla

n.  Lines floor of vestibule

o.  Found between hard and soft palate

p.  Ridge of bone lingual to mandibular premolars

q.  Elevation of tissue distal to mandibular second molar

r.  Elevation of tissue distal to maxillary second molar

s.  Junction of hard and soft palate

t.  Tightly attached—pink color

u.  Loosely attached—reddish color

v.  Five major cusps

w.  Exposed to mouth

x.  Firm, covered by gingiva, has rugae

y.  Covered with enamel

z.  Hairlike papillae covering two thirds of dorsum of tongue

aa.  Crown of tooth exposed to saliva

bb.  Mucous salivary glands beneath anterior third of tongue

cc.  Large serous salivary gland beneath posterior third of tongue

dd.  At corners of mouth where lips join

ee.  Diagonal grooves from nostrils to corner of mouth

ff.  Horizontal depression below lower lip

gg.  Vertical depression on upper lip

hh.  Opening from oral cavity to pharynx

ii.  Serous salivary gland just in front of ear

jj.  Covered with cementum

kk.  That part of tooth embedded in the jaw

ll.  Space between two adjacent teeth

mm.  Act of swallowing

nn.  Fold in floor of mouth beneath tongue

oo.  Slight fold on each side of ventral surface of tongue

pp.  Hangs downward in center of soft palate

qq.  On lateral surfaces of posterior third of tongue

rr.  Space between mandibular teeth and tongue

ss.  8 to 12 circular papillae arranged in a V shape

tt.  Pocket of mucous membrane between anterior pillar and pterygomandibular fold

uu.  Located between anterior and posterior fold

vv.  Bulbous protuberance on inner side of mandible in premolar region

ww.  Sparce round mushroom-shaped papillae on dorsum of tongue

(See Answer Key at end of this chapter.)

## SECTION II. LOCATION OF STRUCTURES THAT CAN BE PALPATED EXTRAORALLY

### LEARNING EXERCISE

*While reading this section, palpate on a partner (this can also be done on yourself, looking in a mirror) the locations indicated to identify the structures as they are discussed. Use the figure on page 67 and figure 2.10.*

## A. Muscles of Mastication

Muscles of the head and neck can be palpated to identify pain or tenderness that could be related to problems in the craniomandibular joint or imbalance in the occlusion. For this reason, it is important to be able to locate these muscles extraorally.

Each muscle pair can be palpated bilaterally with the middle finger of each hand while using the index and fourth finger to palpate surrounding structures.

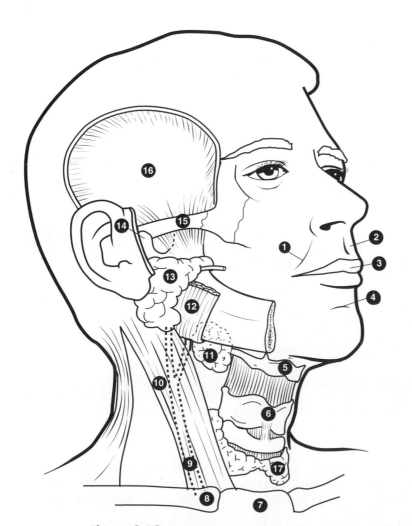

1. Nasolabial groove
2. Philtrum
3. Tubercle (upper lip)
4. Labiomental groove
5. Hyoid bone
6. Larygeal Prominence (Adam's apple)
7. Sternum
8. Clavicle
9. Carotid artery (dotted lines)
10. Sterno-cleidomastoid muscle
11. Submandibular gland
12. Masseter muscle
13. Parotid gland
14. Head of condyle
15. Zygomatic process
16. Temporalis muscle
17. Thyroid gland

**Figure 2.10.** Structures described in the first two chapters that relate to oral function.

## 1. MASSETER

Feel the body of the masseter by palpating the bulge over the angle of the mandible when your partner clenches; move your finger down toward the angle of the mandible to feel the insertion, and up toward the zygomatic arch (inferior border of the zygomatic process) to feel the origin.

## 2. MEDIAL PTERYGOID

Feel the bulge when your partner clenches while palpating the medial surface of the angle of the mandible at the insertion. It may help to have your partner lean the head forward as you palpate inward and upward.

## 3. TEMPORALIS

### a. Anterior Portion

Palpate just above a line between the eyebrow and superior border of the ear; feel the bulge when your partner clenches.

### b. Posterior Portion

Palpate this part of the temporalis just above and distal to the superior border of the ear. Since this muscle is involved in retruding the mandible, see if you can feel a bulge when the partner retrudes (pulls back) the mandible.

## 4. LATERAL PTERYGOID (INTRAORAL PALPATION)

The lateral pterygoid can only be palpated intraorally.

Feel this muscle by placing your index finger in the vestibule behind the maxillary tuberosity. (Use a skull to see how to reach the lateral plate of the pterygoid process of the sphenoid bone.) With your partner's mouth *slightly* open, and mandible moved slightly toward the side being palpated, slide your finger back toward the lateral pterygoid plate for the origin of the lateral pterygoid muscle. The anterior border of the coronoid process is the location of part of the insertion of this muscle. (Note: This may be uncomfortable to a patient even if the muscle is not sore.)

## B. Craniomandibular Joint

Palpate the lateral aspect of the joint by pressing directly over the joint just anterior to the external opening of the ear and below and posterior to the zygomatic arch. Feel the head of the condyle move as your partner opens and closes the mandible, and as your partner slides the mandible from side to side. You should feel the most movement over the right condyle when opening and moving the mandible to the left, and feel the most movement over the left condyle when moving to the right. Can you demonstrate this on a skull?

Palpate the dorsal or posterior surface of the joint by placing your little finger into the external auditory meatus (ear canal opening) and press anteriorly forward. Feel the condyle when your partner opens, closes and moves the mandible laterally from side to side.

## ANSWER KEY FOR ANATOMIC LANDMARKS FROM EARLIER IN THIS CHAPTER

1-f, 2-x, 3-l, 4-j, 5-i, 6-n, 7-g, 8-b, 9-h, 10-m, 11-s, 12-c, 13-k, 14-d, 15-a, 16-q, 17-r, 18-z, 19-p or vv, 20-t, 21-u, 22-v, 23-aa, 24-ii, 25-gg, 26-dd, 27-hh, 28-ee, 29-ff, 30-bb, 31-cc, 32-y, 33-jj, 34-kk, 35-o, 36-ll, 37-nn, 38-pp, 39-oo, 40-qq, 41-ss, .42-rr, 43-mm, 44-uu, 45-tt, 46-vv or p, 47-ww

## References

1. Jenkins GN. The physiology of the mouth. 3rd ed. Revised reprint. Oxford: Blackwell Scientific, 1970:310–328.
2. Foley PF, Latta GH. A study of the position of the parotid papillae relative to the occlusal plane. J Prosthet Dent 1985;53:124–126.
3. Gargiulo A, Wentz F, Orban B. Dimensions and relationships of the dentogingival junction in humans. J Periodontol 1961;32:261.
4. Lang N, Loe H. The relationship between the width of keratinized gingiva and gingival health. J Periodontol 1972;43:623.
5. Polson A, Caton J, Yeaple R, Zander H. Histological determination of probe tip penetration into gingival sulcus of humans using an electronic pressure-sensitive probe. J Clin Periodontol 1980;7:479.
6. Osborn JW, Armstrong WG, Speirs RL, eds. Anatomy, biochemistry and physiology. Oxford: Blackwell Scientific, 1982:535.
7. Brand RW, Isselhard DE. Anatomy of orofacial structures. 5th ed. St. Louis: C.V. Mosby, 1994.
8. Simmons JD, Moore RN, Errickson LC. A longitudinal study of anteroposterior growth changes in the palatine rugae. J Dent Res 1987;66:1512–1515.
9. Renner RP. An introduction to dental anatomy and esthetics. Chicago: Quintessence Publishing, 1985.

## Other General References

Clemente CD, ed. Gray's anatomy of the human body. 30th ed. Philadelphia: Lea & Febiger, 1985.
DuBrul EL. Sicher's oral anatomy. St. Louis: C.V. Mosby, 1980.
Beck EW. Mosby's atlas of functional human anatomy. St. Louis: C.V. Mosby, 1982.
Dunn MJ, Shapiro CZ. Dental anatomy/head and neck anatomy. Baltimore: Williams & Wilkins, 1975.
Montgomery RL. Head and neck anatomy with clinical correlations. New York: McGraw-Hill, 1981:236–240.

# 3

# Basic Terminology for Understanding Tooth Morphology

Prior to reading this chapter, be sure to master the tooth terms used to identify teeth in Chapter 1, Section I.

When we enter into any new field of study, it is necessary to learn at once the particular language of that field. Without an adequate vocabulary, we can neither understand nor make ourselves understood. Definitions and explanations of terms used in descriptive tooth morphology are the basic foundation for understanding subject matter in subsequent chapters. You must learn a few basics, similar to learning the multiplication tables. You will soon become nearly as familiar with these dental terms as you are with your name, and you will continue to use many of them throughout your professional dental career.

## SECTION I. TOOTH IDENTIFICATION SYSTEMS

The making and storage of accurate dental records is an important task in any dental practice. To do so expeditiously, it is necessary to adopt a type of code or numbering system for teeth. Otherwise, one must write for each tooth being charted something like, "maxillary right second molar mesio-occlusodistal amalgam restoration with a buccal extension" (11 words or 81 letters). Simplified by using the Universal Numbering System (Figure 3.1), this same information would be "2MODBA" (only six symbols). As can be seen in Table 3.1, this same tooth by the Palmer Notation System would be 7⌋ or, using the International System, 17. The MODBA describing the type of cavity and restoration is used with all three systems and is fully described in Chapter 12.

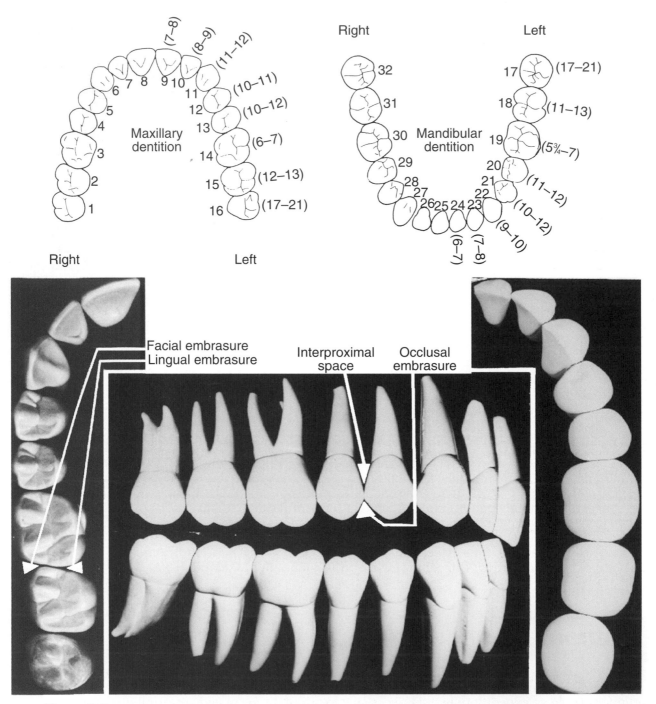

**Figure 3.1.** A drawing and photographs of the occlusal, incisal, and facial surfaces of the maxillary and mandibular adult dentitions. The numbers in parentheses give the usual emergence time into the mouth. The numerals 1 to 32 inside the arches give the Universal Numbering Code commonly used for record keeping. The photographs below are of large plastic tooth models and give an indication of the location of contact points between adjacent teeth. The quadrant of teeth on the *left* are the occlusal and incisal surfaces of the permanent maxillary dentition; on the *right* are the mandibular dentition. Also shown are embrasure spaces.

**Table 3.1.** Various Tooth Identification Systems

| | Tooth | Universal | | Palmer Notation | | International (F.D.I.) | |
|---|---|---|---|---|---|---|---|
| | | Right | Left | Right | Left | Right | Left |
| **Deciduous Dentition — Maxillary Teeth** | Central incisor | E | F | A⌐ | ⌐A | 51 | 61 |
| | Lateral incisor | D | G | B⌐ | ⌐B | 52 | 62 |
| | Canine | C | H | C⌐ | ⌐C | 53 | 63 |
| | First molar | B | I | D⌐ | ⌐D | 54 | 64 |
| | Second molar | A | J | E⌐ | ⌐E | 55 | 65 |
| **Deciduous Dentition — Mandibular Teeth** | Central incisor | P | O | A⌐ | ⌐A | 81 | 71 |
| | Lateral incisor | Q | N | B⌐ | ⌐B | 82 | 72 |
| | Canine | R | M | C⌐ | ⌐C | 83 | 73 |
| | First molar | S | L | D⌐ | ⌐D | 84 | 74 |
| | Second molar | T | K | E⌐ | ⌐E | 85 | 75 |
| **Permanent Dentition — Maxillary Teeth** | Central incisor | 8 | 9 | 1⌐ | ⌐1 | 11 | 21 |
| | Lateral incisor | 7 | 10 | 2⌐ | ⌐2 | 12 | 22 |
| | Canine | 6 | 11 | 3⌐ | ⌐3 | 13 | 23 |
| | First premolar | 5 | 12 | 4⌐ | ⌐4 | 14 | 24 |
| | Second premolar | 4 | 13 | 5⌐ | ⌐5 | 15 | 25 |
| | First molar | 3 | 14 | 6⌐ | ⌐6 | 16 | 26 |
| | Second molar | 2 | 15 | 7⌐ | ⌐7 | 17 | 27 |
| | Third molar | 1 | 16 | 8⌐ | ⌐8 | 18 | 28 |
| **Permanent Dentition — Mandibular Teeth** | Central incisor | 25 | 24 | 1⌐ | ⌐1 | 41 | 31 |
| | Lateral incisor | 26 | 23 | 2⌐ | ⌐2 | 42 | 32 |
| | Canine | 27 | 22 | 3⌐ | ⌐3 | 43 | 33 |
| | First premolar | 28 | 21 | 4⌐ | ⌐4 | 44 | 34 |
| | Second premolar | 29 | 20 | 5⌐ | ⌐5 | 45 | 35 |
| | First molar | 30 | 19 | 6⌐ | ⌐6 | 46 | 36 |
| | Second molar | 31 | 18 | 7⌐ | ⌐7 | 47 | 37 |
| | Third molar | 32 | 17 | 8⌐ | ⌐8 | 48 | 38 |

The *Universal Numbering System,* first suggested by Parreidt in 1882, was officially adopted by the American Dental Association in 1975. It is accepted by third party providers and is endorsed by the American Society of Forensic Odontology. Basically, it uses numbers 1 through 32 for the permanent dentition starting with 1 for the maxillary right third molar, going around the arch to the upper left third molar as 16; dropping down on the same side, the left mandibular third molar becomes 17, and then the numbers increase clockwise around the lower arch to 32, which is the lower right third molar. For the deciduous dentition, letters of the alphabet are used from A through T. A is the maxillary right second molar, sequentially through the alphabet to J for the upper left second molar, then dropping down on the same side to K for the mandibular left second molar, and then clockwise around the lower arch to T for the lower right second molar.

The *Palmer Notation System* utilizes simple brackets to represent the four quadrants of the dentition as if you are facing the patient: ⌐ is upper right, ⌐ is upper left, ⌐ is lower right, and ⌐ is lower left. The permanent teeth are numbered from 1 to 8 on each side from the midline, so 1 is a central incisor, 3 is a canine, and 8 is a third molar. The number is placed within the bracket; so, for example, lower left central incisor, lower left second premolar, and upper right canine would be shown as ⌐1, ⌐5, and 3⌐, respectively. On deciduous teeth, the same four brackets are used, but letters of the alphabet A through E represent the primary teeth, central incisors becoming A, lateral incisors B, canines C, etc. If you are confused, refer to Table 3.1.

The *International Numbering System* (Federation Dentaire Internationale) uses two digits for each tooth, permanent or primary. The first digit always denotes the dentition, arch, and side, and the second digit denotes the tooth (1 to 8 for permanent and 1 to 5 for deciduous teeth from the midline posteriorly). The first digit of the two digits used in this system is designated as follows:

1   Permanent dentition, maxillary, right side.

2   Permanent dentition, maxillary, left side.

3   Permanent dentition, mandibular, left side.

4   Permanent dentition, mandibular, right side.

5   Deciduous dentition, maxillary, right side.

6   Deciduous dentition, maxillary, left side.

7   Deciduous dentition, mandibular, left side.

8   Deciduous dentition, mandibular, right side.

Thus, with the FDI system, numbers 11 through 48 represent permanent teeth (maxillary right central incisor, and mandibular right third molar), and numbers 51 through 85 represent deciduous teeth (maxillary right central incisor and mandibular right second molar). All of the tooth numbers are shown in Table 3.1. You will find it easy to become familiar with any system by first learning (memorizing) the number of letters for key teeth, possibly the central incisors, canines, and first molars.

**NOTE: Unless otherwise stated, the Universal System is used throughout this text.**

## SECTION II. TRAIT CATEGORIES HELPFUL IN DESCRIBING TOOTH SIMILARITIES AND DIFFERENCES

A trait is distinguishing characteristic, quality, peculiarity, or attribute.

### A. Set Traits

*Set traits* (dentition traits) distinguish teeth in the primary (deciduous) from secondary (permanent) dentition.

### B. Arch Traits

*Arch traits* distinguish maxillary from mandibular teeth.

### C. Class Traits

*Class traits* distinguish the four categories (or classes) of teeth described in the introduction: namely incisors, canines, premolars, and molars. Examples of class traits: *incisors* have crowns compressed labiolingually for efficient cutting; *canines* have single pointed cusps for piercing food; *premolars* have two or three cusps for shearing and grinding; *molars* have three to five somewhat flattened cusps, ideally suited for grinding food morsels.

## D. Type Traits

*Type traits* differentiate teeth within one class (such as differences between central and lateral incisors, or between first and second premolars, or between first, second, and third molars).

# SECTION III. TERMINOLOGY USED TO DESCRIBE THE PARTS OF AN INDIVIDUAL TOOTH

## A. Tissues of a Tooth

### 1. FOUR TISSUES OF A TOOTH

#### a. Enamel

*Enamel* (mostly inorganic, calcified) is the hard, white shiny surface of the *anatomic* crown. It develops from the enamel organ (from ectoderm).

*Composition:*  95% Calcium hydroxyapatite (inorganic calcified)

4% Water

1% Enamel matrix (organic matter)

#### b. Dentin

*Dentin* (mostly inorganic, calcified) is the hard yellowish tissue underlying the enamel and cementum making up the major bulk of the tooth. It develops from the dental papilla (from mesoderm).

*Composition:*  70% Calcium hydroxyapatite (inorganic calcified)

18% Organic matter (collagen fibers)

12% Water

#### c. Cementum

*Cementum* (mostly inorganic, calcified) is the dull yellow external surface of the *anatomic* root (covering the dentin). It develops from the dental sac (mesoderm).

*Composition:*  65% Calcium hydroxyapatite (inorganic calcified)

23% Organic matter (collagen fibers)

12% Water

#### d. Pulp

*Pulp* is the soft (not calcified) tissue in the pulp chamber (the cavity or space in the center of the crown and root). It develops from the dental papilla (mesoderm).

*Composition:*  Loose connective tissue

Fibroblasts, blood vessels, and nerves (collagen and reticulum)

Ground substance (water and long carbohydrate chains attached to protein backbones)

Undifferentiated mesenchymal cells that serve to replace injured or destroyed odontoblasts (a reparative function)

## 2. LOCATION OF THESE TISSUES (FIG. 3.2)

### a. Enamel

*Enamel* makes up the protective outer surface of the *anatomic crown.*

### b. Cementum

*Cementum* makes up the surface of the *anatomic root.* The cementum is very thin next to the cervical line (only 50–100 micrometers thick), no thicker than this page.

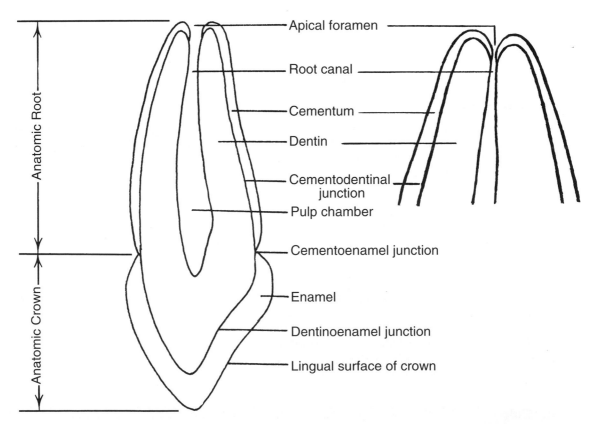

**Figure 3.2.** A maxillary anterior tooth sectioned longitudinally through the center to show the distribution of the tooth tissues and the shape of the pulp cavity (made up of pulp chamber and root canal). On the *right* is a close-up of the apical portion depicting the usual expected constriction of the root canal near the apical foramen. Note that the layer of cementum covering the root is proportionately much thinner on the actual tooth.

### c. Dentin

*Dentin* is found in the crown and the root making up the main bulk of each tooth, beneath the enamel and the cementum, and extending to the lining surrounding the pulp cavity. Dentin is not normally visible except on a dental radiograph, a sectioned tooth, or on a badly worn one.

### d. Pulp

*Pulp* is found in the center part of the tooth. The pulp cavity is surrounded by dentin except at a hole or holes near the root apex (apices or *apical foramen*). Like dentin, the pulp is normally not visible except on a dental radiograph, or sectioned tooth.

It has a coronal portion (*pulp chamber*) and a root portion (*pulp canal[s]*).

The functions of the dental pulp are:

1. Formative—dentin producing cells (odontoblasts) produce dentin throughout the life of a tooth. This is called *secondary dentin.*
2. Sensory—nerve endings permit the sense of pain from heat, cold, drilling, sweet, decay, trauma, or infection.
3. Nutritive—nutrient transport from blood stream to extensions of the pulp that reach into dentin. Blood in the tooth pulp passed through the heart six seconds previously.
4. Defensive or protective—responds to injury or decay by forming reparative dentin (by the odontoblasts).

## 3. JUNCTIONS OF TOOTH TISSUES (VISIBLE IN DIAGRAM IN FIG. 3.2)

### a. Cementoenamel Junction

The *cementoenamel junction* (cervical line) separates the enamel of the *anatomic* crown from the cementum of the *anatomic* root. This is also known as the cervical line. Refer to Table 3.4 for differences in the amount of curvature of these cervical lines when moving from anterior teeth to posterior teeth.

### b. Dentinoenamel Junction

*Dentinoenamel junction* is the inner surface of the enamel cap (only visible on a cross-section or when preparing a tooth for a restoration).

### c. Cementodentinal Junction

*Cementodentinal* (dentinocemental) junction is the inner surface of cementum lining the root (only visible on cross-section).

## B. Anatomic Versus Clinical Crown

## 1. ANATOMIC CROWN AND ROOT (CAN BE OBSERVED ON AN EXTRACTED TOOTH)

As stated earlier, the *anatomic crown* is the part of a tooth that has an enamel surface, (Figs. 3.2 and 3.5**B**) and the *anatomic root* is the part of a tooth that has a cementum surface. A *cervical line* separates the anatomic crown from anatomic root. This relationship does not change over a patient's lifetime.

## 2. CLINICAL CROWN AND ROOT (ONLY APPLIES WHEN THE TOOTH IS *IN THE MOUTH* AND AT LEAST PARTIALLY ERUPTED)

Clinically, the relationship of the gingival (gum) margin to the cervical line in a 25-year-old patient with healthy gingiva is as follows: The gingival margin approximately follows the curvature of the cervical line. However, it is not always at the level of the cervical line because of the eruption process or recession of the gingiva. In a 10-year-old with a healthy mouth, the gingival margin may cover some of the anatomic crown of the tooth enamel; in older persons who have had periodontal disease or periodontal therapy resulting in gingival recession, the gingiva may not cover all of the anatomic root (cementum).

### a. Clinical Crown

The *clinical crown* is the part of a tooth that is visible in the oral cavity. The clinical crown may be larger or smaller than the anatomic crown. It may include all of the anatomic crown and some of the anatomic root if there has been recession of the gingiva, or it may include only part of the anatomic crown if the cervical part of the crown is still covered by gingiva (especially on newly erupted teeth).

You will find an example of a *short clinical crown* if you look at the maxillary central incisors of a 9- or 10-year-old child—the cervical part of the anatomic crown will be covered by gingiva.

You probably will find an example of a *long clinical crown* if you look at the teeth of a 60-year-old person—the cervical cementum of the anatomic root will probably be exposed (as with tooth #11 in Fig. 3.10**B**).

### b. Clinical Root

The *clinical root* is that part of a tooth which is under the gingiva and is not exposed to the oral cavity. It may be longer than the anatomic root. On newly erupted teeth, any part of the crown not erupted is considered to be part of the clinical root. In an elderly person with considerable recession of the gingiva, the clinical root would be shorter than the anatomic root because the portion of the root that is exposed to saliva is considered to be a part of the clinical crown.

### *LEARNING EXERCISE*

*Examine the mouths of several persons of different ages to see if the cervical line is visible or hidden. As the individual grows older, the location of the margin of the gingiva may recede apically on the tooth because of periodontal disease or injury from the faulty use of oral hygiene aids. Of course, the location of the cervical line on the tooth remains the same, so the distinction between the anatomic crown and root does not change over a lifetime.*

## SECTION IV. TERMINOLOGY USED TO DISTINGUISH TOOTH SURFACES

### A. Terms That Identify Outer Surfaces of Anterior Versus Posterior Teeth

*Facial Surface*—the surface next to the face; the outer surface of a tooth in the mouth resting against or next to the cheeks or lips. Facial may be used to designate this portion of any tooth, anterior or posterior.

1. *Buccal surface* (pronounced like "buckle") meaning *cheek* is another name for the facial surface of the *posterior* teeth (next to the cheek). It is incorrect to use this term when speaking about the incisors or canines (see tooth #3 in Fig. 3.3).

2. *Labial surface* (meaning lip) is another name for the facial surface of *anterior* teeth (next to the lip). This term should not be used when referring to the premolars or the molars (see tooth #6 in Fig. 3.3).

## B. Terms That Differentiate Approximating Surfaces of Teeth

*Proximal surface* is the surface or side of a tooth that is next to an adjacent tooth (either the mesial or the distal surface). Proximal surfaces are generally not considered to be self-cleansing when compared to the facial, lingual, and occlusal surfaces which are more self-cleansing (see Fig. 3.3 labeled on third molar).

1. *Mesial surface* is the surface of the tooth nearest the midline of the dental arch, i.e., toward the plane between the right and left central incisors.

2. *Distal surface* is the surface of the tooth farthest from the midline of the dental arch.

Note: The *mesial* surface of all teeth approximate (face) the *distal* of the adjacent tooth except between the central incisors where *mesial* surface faces another mesial surface.

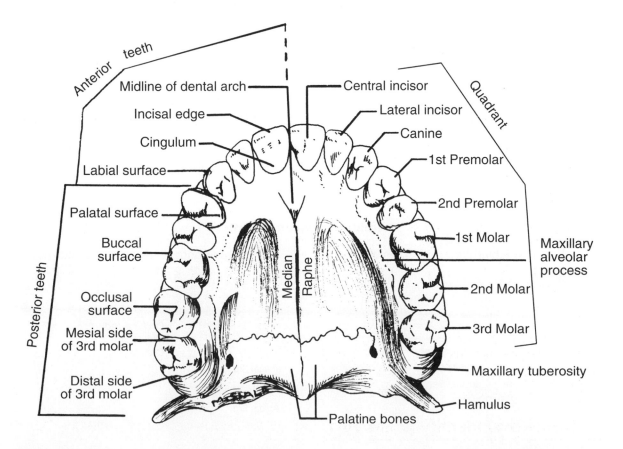

**Figure 3.3.** Maxillary dental arch and the bones of the hard palate. Remember that the labial surface of an anterior tooth and the buccal surface of a posterior tooth are both referred to as facial surfaces. Also, the mesial and distal sides or surfaces are correctly called proximal surfaces.

## C. Terms That Identify Inner or Medial Side Surfaces (Toward the Middle of the Mouth) of Maxillary Versus Mandibular Teeth

*Lingual surface* is the surface of maxillary and mandibular teeth nearest the tongue.

*Palatal surface* is the surface of maxillary teeth nearest the palate. This surface is more commonly called the lingual surface (labeled on tooth #5 in Fig. 3.3).

## D. Terms That Differentiate Biting Surfaces of Anterior Versus Posterior Teeth

*Occlusal surface* is the chewing surface of posterior teeth consisting of cusps, ridges, and grooves, and bounded anteroposteriorly by the marginal ridges and buccolingually by the cusp ridges. Incisors and canines do not have an occlusal surface (labeled on tooth #2 in Fig. 3.3).

*Incisal edge* is the cutting edge, ridge, or surface of anterior teeth (labeled on tooth #8 on Fig. 3.3).

## E. Points of Reference (General) Which Should Not Be Confused with Tooth Surface Terminology

*Medial*—toward the center line of the body.

*Lateral*—toward the sides of the body, i.e., toward the right or left (away from the midline).

## F. Divisions of the Crown of a Tooth (for Purposes of Description) (Fig. 3.4)

### 1. DIVISIONS CERVICO-OCCLUSALLY (CERVICOINCISALLY)

*Divisions cervico-occlusally (cervicoincisally)* are demonstrated by arbitrary lines drawn *horizontally* on the tooth crown to divide the crown into the following three parts:

Cervical third

Middle third

Occlusal (incisal) third

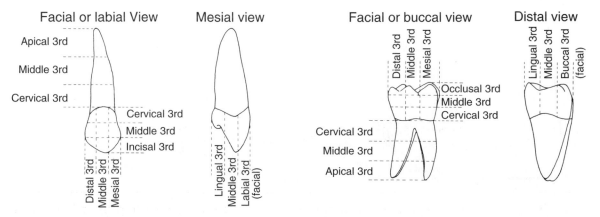

**Figure 3.4.** Diagram of a maxillary canine and a mandibular first molar to show the manner in which the parts of a tooth may be divided for purposes of description, location of anatomic landmarks, contact areas, and so forth.

## 2. DIVISIONS MESIODISTALLY

*Divisions mesiodistally* are demonstrated by similar equally spaced lines drawn *vertically* on the *facial or lingual surface* of the crown:

Mesial third

Middle third

Distal third

## 3. DIVISIONS FACIOLINGUALLY

*Divisions faciolingually* are demonstrated by lines drawn *vertically* on the *mesial or distal surface* of the crown:

Facial third (labial or buccal third)

Middle third

Lingual third

## G. Divisions of the Root of a Tooth

Mesiodistally and faciolingually, the divisions are exactly the same as for the crown.

Divisions cervicoapically are:

Cervical third

Middle third

Apical third

## H. Combined Terms

Combined terms (notice spelling) to denote the junction (area) where two surfaces meet (left column) or a dimension between the surfaces (right column). The "al" ending in the first term is changed to an "o" when combining these terms.

| | |
|---|---|
| Mesio-occlusal | Labiolingual |
| Mesioincisal | Buccolingual |
| Mesiolingual | Faciolingual |
| Mesiobuccal | Cervicoincisal |
| Distolingual | Cervico-occlusal |
| Disto-occlusal | |
| Distoincisal | |
| Distobuccal | |

# SECTION V. MORPHOLOGY OF THE TOOTH

## A. Morphology of an Anatomic Crown

To identify the following anatomic structures, reference will be made primarily to drawings of a canine (Fig. 3.5) and a premolar (Fig. 3.6). These drawings are being used as representative examples.

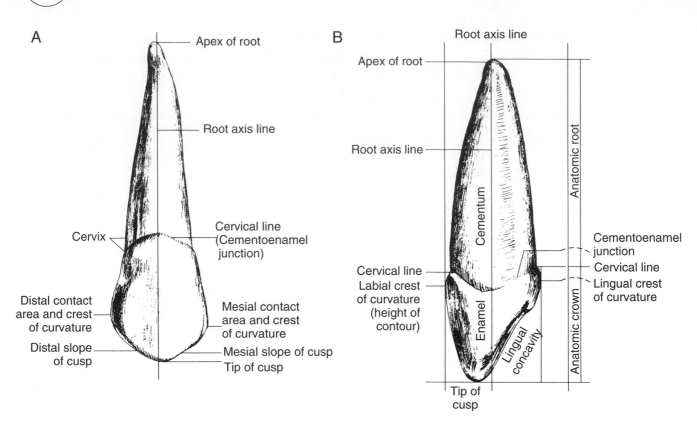

**Figure 3.5. A**. Labial surface of the maxillary right canine pictured in **B**. The root axis is determined by bisecting the root at the cervix. **B**. Mesial side of a maxillary right canine. The root axis line bisects the root in the cervical area. Customarily, other parts of the tooth are located or described relative to this line. In this case, for instance, the cusp tip is labial to the root axis line.

## 1. BUMPS AND RIDGES

### a. Cusp

*Cusp* (Figs. 3.5 and 3.6) is a point, or peak, on the chewing surface of molar and premolar teeth, and on the incisal edge of canines. *Cusp slopes* are the inclined surfaces or ridges that form an angle at the cusp tip when viewed from the facial or lingual aspect (Fig. 3.5**A**). These cusp slopes may also be called *cusp ridges* or *cusp arms* (Fig. 3.7).

### b. Cingulum

*Cingulum* (the c and g are pronounced as in *singular*) is the enlargement or bulge on the cervical third of the lingual surface of the crown on anterior teeth (incisors and canines). (See Fig. 3.5**B**.)

### c. Ridges—Longitudinal Convexities of Enamel

#### (1) Labial Ridge

The *labial ridge* (Fig. 3.5**A**) is a ridge running cervicoincisally in approximately the center of the labial surface of the canines (similar to the buccal ridge on premolars).

#### (2) Buccal (Cusp) Ridge

The *buccal (cusp) ridge* (Fig. 3.7) is a ridge running cervico-occlusally in approximately the center of the buccal surface of premo-

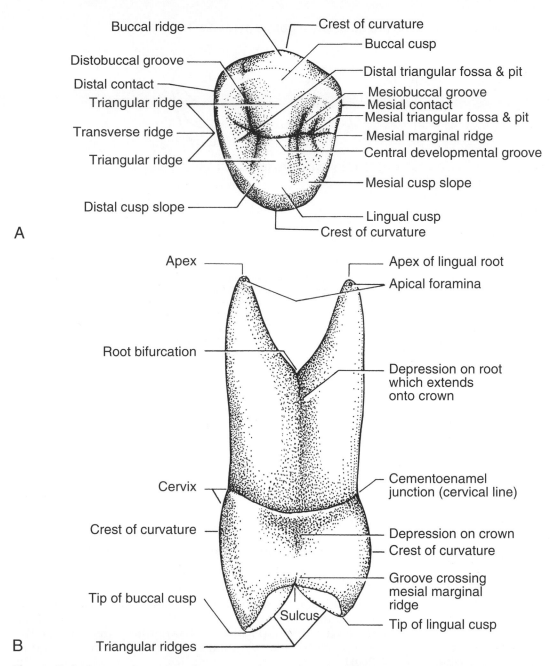

**Figure 3.6. A**. Maxillary right first premolar, occlusal surface. Notice proximal contact locations. **B**. Maxillary right first premolar, mesial surface. The sulcus is the occlusal depression between cusps (valley) that is seen on all posterior teeth. The space between the two roots is the furcal region, and the root area between the cervical line and root bifurcation is the root trunk.

lars, more pronounced on the first premolars than on the second premolars (Fig. 6.18).

### (3) Cervical Ridge

The *cervical ridge* (Fig. 7.30 Molar) is a ridge running mesiodistally on the cervical one-third of the buccal surface of the crown, found on all deciduous teeth but only on the permanent molars.

**All cusps are basically a gothic pyramid**

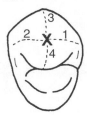

The cuspal gothic pyramid produces 4 ridges:

1. Mesial cusp ridge
2. Distal cusp ridge
3. Buccal cusp ridge (labial ridge on canines)
4. Triangular ridge on posterior teeth (lingual ridge on canines)

**Figure 3.7.** Buccal cusps and design with the four cusp ridges numbered *1–4* around the cusp tip (*X*) on a maxillary right first premolar. All cusps have four ridges. The facial ridge (*3*) is more prominent on some teeth than on others, particularly on maxillary canines and first premolars. Most triangular ridges incline toward the center of the tooth at a slope of approximately 45° (see Fig. 3.6**B**). The mesial and distal cusp ridges (*1* and *2*) form the triangular shape of the cusp when viewed from the facial (see Fig. 3.5**A**). (Courtesy of Dr. Richard W. Huffman and Dr. Ruth Paulson.)

### (4) *Marginal Ridge*

On incisor and canine teeth (Fig. 3.9**B**), a *marginal ridge* is located on the mesial and distal border of the lingual surface; on posterior teeth, it is located on the mesial and distal border of the occlusal surface (Fig. 3.6**A**).

### (5) *Oblique Ridge*

The *oblique ridge* is a ridge found only on maxillary molars that crosses the occlusal surface obliquely and is made up of the triangular ridges of the mesiolingual and the distobuccal cusps (Fig. 7.30).

### (6) *Triangular Ridge*

The *triangular ridge*, on the occlusal surface of posterior teeth, is the ridge from any cusp tip to the center of the occlusal surface (Fig. 3.6**A**). All posterior tooth cusps have a triangular ridge except the mesiolingual cusp on maxillary molars, which has two triangular ridges (Fig. 7.30**A**).

### (7) *Transverse Ridge*

The *transverse ridge* (Fig. 3.6**A**) is a ridge crossing the occlusal surface of most posterior teeth in a buccolingual direction and made up of connecting triangular ridges (e.g., between the mesiolingual and mesiobuccal or between the distolingual and distobuccal cusps on molars (see Fig. 7.11) or running between buccal and lingual cusps on premolars).

### d. Mamelon

*Mamelon* is one of three tubercles sometimes present on the incisal edge of an incisor tooth that has not been subjected to wear (attrition) (Fig. 4.1).

## 2. DEPRESSIONS AND GROOVES

### a. Sulcus

*Sulcus* is a broad depression or valley on the occlusal surfaces of posterior teeth, the inclines of which meet in a developmental groove and extend outward to the cusp tips (see Fig. 3.6**B**).

### b. Developmental Groove

The *developmental groove* is a sharply defined, narrow and linear depression, short or long, formed during tooth development and usually separating lobes or major portions of a tooth (Fig. 3.12). The major grooves are named according to their location (Fig. 3.6**A**). Grooves are important escape ways for cusps during lateral and protrusive jaw motions, and for food morsels during mastication. (Food squirts out toward the tongue and cheeks.)

A *fissure* is a narrow channel, cleft, ditch, or crevice, sometimes deep, formed at the depth of a developmental groove, caused or formed during the development of a tooth and extending inward toward the pulp from the groove (Fig. 12.1**A**). Decay (dental caries) often begins in a deep fissure (see Chapter 12).

### c. Supplemental Grooves

*Supplemental Grooves* are small, irregularly placed grooves, not at the junction of lobes or major portions of a tooth, found usually on occlusal surfaces. These can be named for the part of the tooth on which they are found (mesiobuccal supplemental groove, distolingual supplemental groove) (Figs. 3.6**A,** 3.8).

### d. Fossa

*Fossa* (plural, *fossae*) (Fig. 3.6**A**) is a depression, or hollow, found on the lingual surfaces of some anterior teeth (particularly maxillary incisors) and on the occlusal surfaces of all posterior teeth.

### e. Pits

*Pits* (Fig. 3.6**A**) often occur at the depth of a fossa where two or more grooves join. Like fissures at the depth of grooves, pits are areas where dental decay may begin.

Developmental grooves

Central developmental groove (**C**)

Fossa developmental grooves (**F**)

Supplemental grooves (**S**)

Marginal ridge groove (**M**)

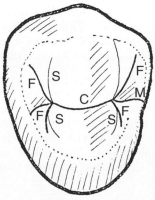

**Figure 3.8.** An occlusal surface of a maxillary right first premolar depicting various occlusal grooves. Some texts consider the fossa grooves as supplemental. Grooves are important escape ways for cusps in lateral and protrusive jaw motions, and for food morsels during mastication. (Courtesy of Dr. Richard W. Huffman and Dr. Ruth Paulson.) Refer to Figure 3.6**A** for the major developmental grooves.

## B. Anatomic Root Morphology Terms (External Anatomy)

### 1. ANATOMIC ROOT

The *anatomic root* is the part of a tooth that has a cementum surface (Fig. 3.5**B**).

### 2. APEX OF ROOT

The *apex of root* is the tip or peak at the end of the root (Fig. 3.5**B**).

### 3. CERVIX

The *cervix* is the part (neck) of the root (Fig. 3.5**A**) or crown (Fig. 3.6**B**) near the cementoenamel junction.

### 4. ROOT TRUNK

The *root trunk,* or *trunk base* (on multirooted teeth only), is the part of the root of a molar or two-rooted premolar near the cementoenamel junction. It is the part that is not furcated, i.e., not divided into two or more parts (Fig. 3.6**B**).

### 5. FURCATION

*Furcation* (Fig. 3.6**B**) is the place on multirooted teeth where the root trunk or root base divides into separate roots (bifurcation on two-rooted and trifurcation on three-rooted teeth).

### 6. FURCAL REGION OR ASPECT

The *furcal region or aspect* (Fig. 3.6**B**) is the region between two or more roots on a tooth (inter-radicular), apical to the place where the roots divide or separate from the root trunk.

### 7. DILACERATION

*Dilaceration* is an abnormal tooth that has both the crown and the root twisted (possibly severely) from the normal linear relationship (Fig. 11.20).

### LEARNING EXERCISE

*Views of many teeth are presented in Fig. 3.9**A**-**D** showing the location of cusps, ridges, fossae, and grooves for each type of tooth. This figure should be referred to often when learning this terminology and while reading Chapters 4 through 7.*

## C. Relative Size

Using a sample size of 4572 extracted teeth, the average dimensions of each type of tooth have been determined and serve as the basis for many statements made within this textbook. This data are presented in Table 3.2 and are useful for determining the tooth with the longest crown, the longest overall length, the shortest root, and so forth.

# CUSPS

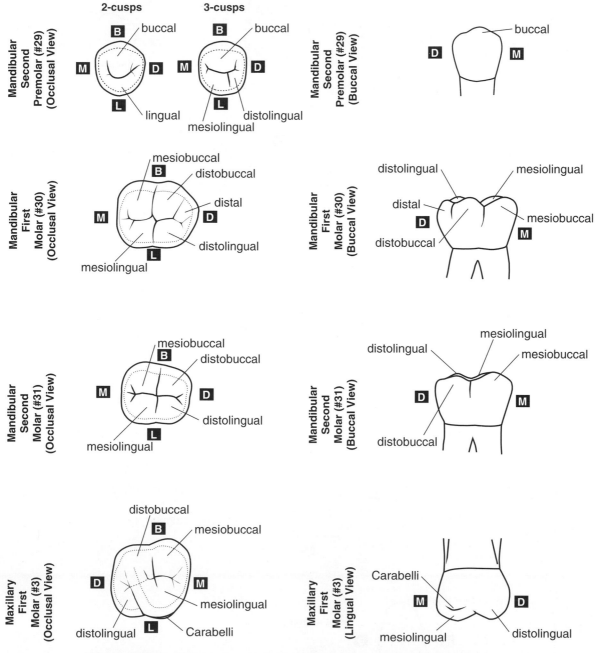

**Figure 3.9. A**. Major cusps on a variety of molars, premolars and incisors.

# RIDGES

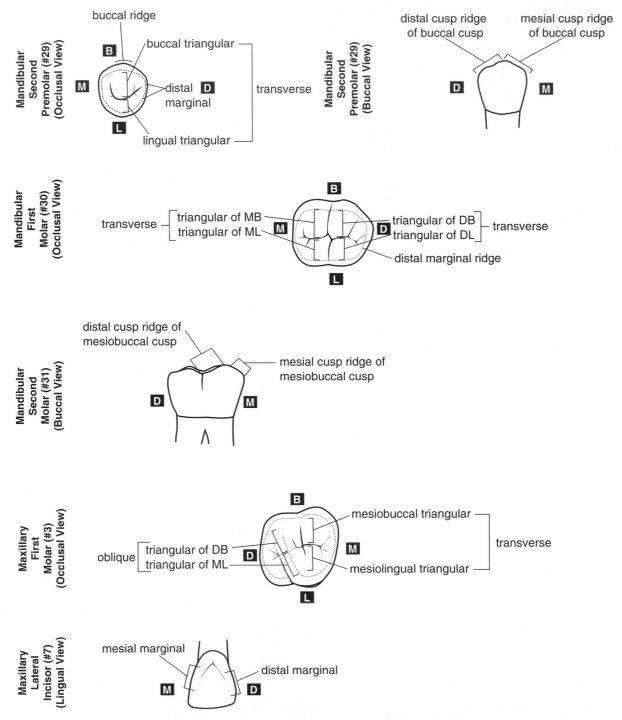

**Figure 3.9. B**. Examples of a variety of ridges on molars, premolars and incisors.

# FOSSAE AND PITS

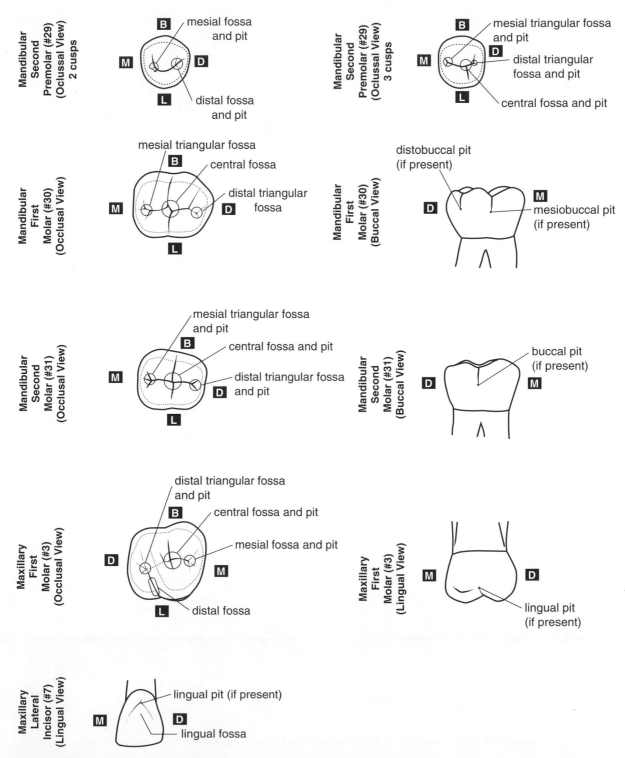

**Figure 3.9. C**. Examples of various fossae (often with associated pits) on molars, premolars, and incisors.

# GROOVES

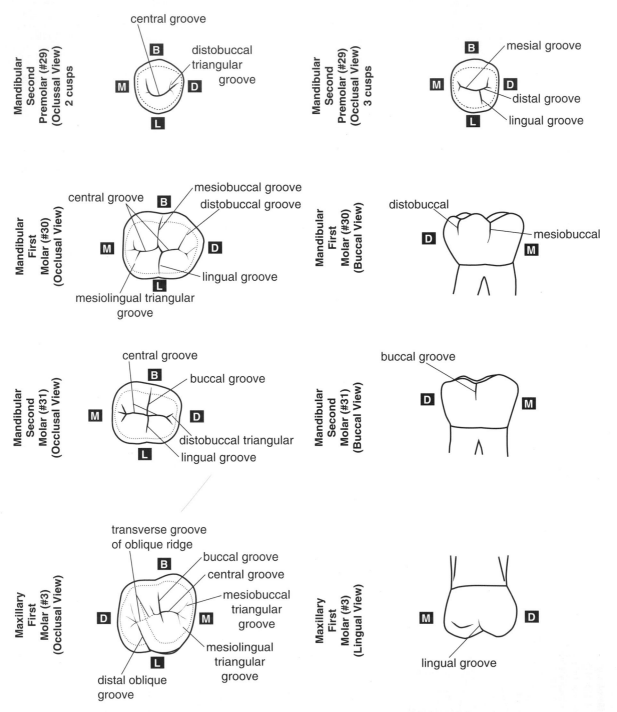

**Figure 3.9. D**. Examples of developmental grooves on molars and premolars.

**Table 3.2.** Average Measurements on 4572 Extracted Teeth from Ohio From a Study by Dr. Woelfel and His First-year Dental Hygiene Students at The Ohio State University College of Dentistry, 1974–1979. Size ranges are shown in tables in each chapter.

| Maxillary Teeth | Crown Length (mm) | | Root Length (mm) | Root to Crown Ratio | Overall Length (mm) | Crown Width M-D (mm) | Cervix Width M-D (mm) | Crown Width F-L (mm) | Cervix Width F-L (mm) | Mesial Cervical Curve (mm) | Distal Cervical Curve (mm) |
|---|---|---|---|---|---|---|---|---|---|---|---|
| Central incisor (398) | 11.2 | | 13.0 | 1.16 | 23.6 | 8.6 | 6.4 | 7.1 | 6.3 | 2.8 | 2.3 |
| Lateral incisor (295) | 9.8 | | 13.4 | 1.37 | 22.5 | 6.6 | 4.7 | 6.2 | 5.8 | 2.5 | 1.9 |
| Canine (321) | 10.6 | | 16.5 | 1.56 | 26.3 | 7.6 | 5.6 | 8.1 | 7.6 | 2.1 | 1.4 |
| First premolar (234) | 8.6 | | 13.4 | 1.56 | 21.5 | 7.1 | 4.8 | 9.2 | 8.2 | 1.1 | 0.7 |
| Second premolar (224) | 7.7 | | 14.0 | 1.82 | 21.2 | 6.6 | 4.7 | 9.0 | 8.1 | 0.9 | 0.6 |
| First molar (308) | 7.5 | MB 12.9 DB 12.2 L 13.7 | | 1.72 | 20.1 | 10.4 | 7.9 | 11.5 | 10.7 | 0.7 | 0.3 |
| Second molar (309) | 7.6 | MB 12.9 DB 12.1 L 13.5 | | 1.70 | 20.0 | 9.8 | 7.6 | 11.4 | 10.7 | 0.6 | 0.2 |
| Third molar (305) | 7.2 | MB 10.8 DB 10.1 L 11.2 | | 1.49 | 17.5 | 9.2 | 7.2 | 11.1 | 10.4 | 0.5 | 0.2 |
| Avg. 2392 Upper teeth | 8.77 | | 13.36 | 1.55 | 21.59 | 8.23 | 6.11 | 9.20 | 8.48 | 1.40 | 0.97 |

**Mandibular Teeth**

| Mandibular Teeth | Crown Length (mm) | | Root Length (mm) | Root to Crown Ratio | Overall Length (mm) | Crown Width M-D (mm) | Cervix Width M-D (mm) | Crown Width F-L (mm) | Cervix Width F-L (mm) | Mesial Cervical Curve (mm) | Distal Cervical Curve (mm) |
|---|---|---|---|---|---|---|---|---|---|---|---|
| Central incisor (226) | 8.8 | | 12.6 | 1.43 | 20.8 | 5.3 | 3.5 | 5.7 | 5.4 | 2.0 | 1.6 |
| Lateral incisor (234) | 9.4 | | 13.5 | 1.43 | 22.1 | 5.7 | 3.8 | 6.1 | 5.8 | 2.1 | 1.5 |
| Canine (316) | 11.0 | | 15.9 | 1.45 | 25.9 | 6.8 | 5.2 | 7.7 | 7.5 | 2.4 | 1.6 |
| First premolar (238) | 8.8 | | 14.4 | 1.64 | 22.4 | 7.0 | 4.8 | 7.7 | 7.0 | 0.9 | 0.6 |
| Second premolar (227) | 8.2 | | 14.7 | 1.80 | 22.1 | 7.1 | 5.0 | 8.2 | 7.3 | 0.8 | 0.5 |
| First molar (281) | 7.7 | M 14.0 D 13.0 | | 1.83 | 20.9 | 11.4 | 9.2 | 10.2 | 9.0 | 0.5 | 0.2 |
| Second molar (296) | 7.7 | M 13.9 D 13.0 | | 1.82 | 20.6 | 10.8 | 9.1 | 9.9 | 8.8 | 0.5 | 0.2 |
| Third molar (262) | 7.5 | M 11.8 D 10.8 | | 1.57 | 18.2 | 11.3 | 9.2 | 10.1 | 8.9 | 0.4 | 0.2 |
| Avg. 2180 Lower teeth | 8.62 | | 13.85 | 1.62 | 21.61 | 8.17 | 6.24 | 8.22 | 7.44 | 1.20 | 0.80 |

**Table 3.3.** Tooth Anatomy Trends from Anterior to Posterior Teeth

**Proximal Contacts (Proximal crest of curvature) viewed from the facial**

| | |
|---|---|
| **All teeth:** | Distal contacts are more cervical than mesial contacts except mandibular first premolars (where the mesial is more cervical) and mandibular central incisor (mesial and distal contacts are at the same level). |
| **All anterior teeth:** | Mesial contacts are in the incisal third (or for the maxillary canine, at the junction of the incisal and middle thirds). Contact areas become more cervical when moving from the midline (where they are almost at the incisal edge) to the distal of the canine. |
| **All posterior teeth:** | Mesial contacts are at or near the junction of the middle and occlusal thirds. Mesial and distal contact areas become more cervical toward the distal of the arch (accentuated by shorter crowns), but mesial and distal contacts are more nearly at the same level than for anterior teeth. |

**Contact Location viewed from the occlusal**
    **Anterior:** Tooth contacts are nearly centered faciolingually.
    **Posterior:** Contacts are larger than anterior contact areas and tend to be slightly buccal to the middle third buccolingually.

**Proximal Cervical Line (Cementoenamel junction) Curvatures**
    **All teeth:** Generally have greater proximal cervical line curvature on the mesial than the distal. Proximal cervical line curvatures are greater on the incisors and tend to get smaller when moving toward the last molar, where there may be no curvature at all.

**Facial and Lingual Crest of Curvatures**
    **All teeth** have the *facial* crest of curvature in the cervical third.
    **Anterior teeth** have the *lingual* crest of curvature in the cervical third (on the bulge of the cingulum).
    **Posterior teeth** have the *lingual* crest of curvature at or near the middle third of the crown.

# SECTION VI. TERMINOLOGY RELATED TO THE IDEAL ALIGNMENT OF TEETH IN THE DENTAL ARCHES

When viewed from the occlusal aspect, each dental arch is U-shaped (Fig. 3.1). The incisal edges and the buccal cusp tips follow a curved line around the outer edge of the dental arch; the lingual cusp tips of the posterior teeth follow a curved line nearly parallel to the buccal cusp tips. Between the buccal and lingual cusps is the *sulcular groove*, which runs anteroposteriorly the length of the posterior teeth.

*Curve of Spee* (Fig. 3.10) (anteroposterior curve of the curve occlusal plane)—When viewed from the buccal aspect, the cusp tips of posterior teeth follow a gradual concave curve anteroposteriorly. The curve of the maxillary arch is convex; that of the mandibular arch is concave.

*Curve of Wilson* (side-to-side curve) (Fig. 10.8)—When viewed from the anterior aspect with the mouth slightly open, the cusp tips of the posterior teeth follow a gradual curve from the left side to the right side. The curve of the maxillary arch is convex; that of the mandibular arch concave. Thus, the lingual cusps of the posterior teeth are aligned at a lower level than the buccal cusps on both sides and in both arches.

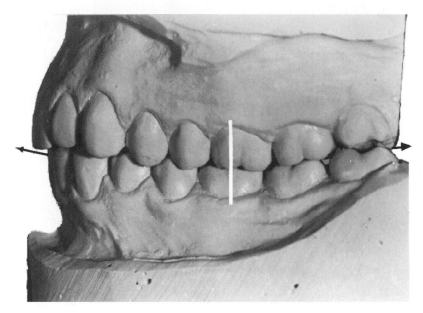

**Figure 3.10. A**. Dental stone casts fitting together in the maximum intercuspal position (centric occlusion). Notice that each tooth contacts two opposing teeth except the mandibular central incisor and the maxillary third molar. (Further information in Chapter 10.) The vertical white line marks the relationship of first molars in Class I occlusion; the mesiobuccal cusp of the maxillary first molar occludes in the mesial buccal groove of the mandibular first molar. The *curved arrows* denote the curve of Spee.

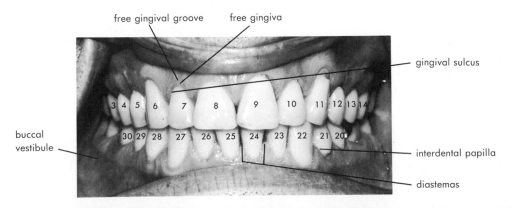

**Figure 3.10. B**. Maxillary and mandibular teeth of the permanent dentition are in centric occlusion; the labial surfaces of the anterior teeth and the buccal surfaces of the posterior teeth are seen. The gingiva surrounds the teeth and forms the interdental papillae between them. The mandibular vestibule is exposed. Notice how each tooth is in contact with the adjacent teeth, except between teeth numbers 24 and 25 and between teeth numbers 23 and 24. Spaces are called diastematas. Note how the maxillary arch overlaps the mandibular arch, and how the greater width of the maxillary central incisors causes each of them to overlap not only the mandibular central incisor, but also half of the mandibular lateral incisor. (See Chapter 10 on occlusion.) Notice the cervical abrasion on tooth number 11.

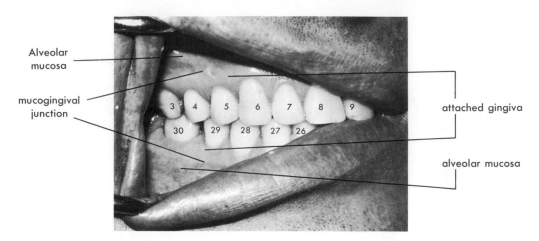

**Figure 3.10. C**. The subject is the same as in Figure 3.9**B,** but here the right cheek is drawn back. Notice the arrangement of the maxillary teeth relative to the mandibular teeth: each maxillary tooth overlaps two mandibular teeth. There is a clear line between the light-colored gingiva and the darker alveolar mucosa, the mucogingival junction. The attached gingiva is stippled above tooth number 7. Notice the metal restorations on teeth numbers 3 and 30.

## A. Crest of Curvature (Fig. 3.5)

The form of the curvature or convex bulges on teeth determines the direction of food as it is pushed cervically over the tooth surface during mastication. During chewing, these convexities divert food away from the collar of tissue (gingiva) that surrounds the neck of the tooth, and toward the buccal vestibule and toward the palate or tongue, thus preventing trauma to the gingiva. If teeth were flat in their middle and cervical thirds, much food would lodge and remain near the gingival margin and sulcus until removed by a toothpick or toothbrush or by dental floss.

The *crest of curvature* is the highest point of a curve or greatest convexity or bulge. The crest of curvature on the facial and lingual surfaces of the crown is where this greatest bulge would be touched by a tangent line drawn parallel to the root axis (Fig. 3.5**B**). The *location* of the crest of curvature on the facial and lingual surfaces of the crowns of teeth can be seen from the mesial and distal aspects, and are usually in one of two places:

1.  In the cervical third of the crown on:
    a.  Facial surfaces of all anterior and posterior teeth (maxillary and mandibular).
    b.  Lingual surfaces of all anterior teeth (maxillary and mandibular) on the cingulum.
2.  In the middle third of the crown on:
    a.  Lingual surface of maxillary and mandibular posterior teeth.
    b.  Lingual surface of all mandibular posterior teeth.

Refer to Table 3.4 for the changes in relative position of the facial and lingual crests of curvature when moving from anterior teeth to posterior teeth. The mesial and distal crest of curvatures (seen from the facial or lingual) are normally the same as contact areas (Fig. 3.5**A**).

## B. Contact Areas (Refer to Fig. 3.1)

*Contact areas* are the crests of curvature on the proximal surfaces of tooth crowns where a tooth touches the tooth adjacent to it in the same arch when the teeth are in proper alignment

**Table 3.4.** Chronology of the Human Dentition by Logan and Kronfeld (slightly modified by McCall and Schour)

| | Tooth | Hard Tissue Formation Begins | Crown Completed | Eruption | Root Completed |
|---|---|---|---|---|---|
| **Deciduous Dentition — Maxillary Teeth** | Central incisor | 4 mos. in utero | 4 mos. | 7½ mos. | 1½ yrs. |
| | Lateral incisor | 4½ mos. in utero | 5 mos. | 9 mos. | 2 yrs. |
| | Canine | 5 mos. in utero | 9 mos. | 18 mos. | 3¼ yrs. |
| | First molar | 5 mos. in utero | 6 mos. | 14 mos. | 2½ yrs. |
| | Second molar | 6 mos. in utero | 11 mos. | 24 mos. | 3 yrs. |
| **Deciduous Dentition — Mandibular Teeth** | Central incisor | 4½ mos. in utero | 3½ mos. | 6 mos. | 1½ yrs. |
| | Lateral incisor | 4½ mos. in utero | 4 mos. | 7 mos. | 1½ yrs. |
| | Canine | 5 mos. in utero | 9 mos. | 16 mos. | 3 yrs. |
| | First molar | 5 mos. in utero | 5½ mos. | 12 mos. | 2¼ yrs. |
| | Second molar | 6 mos. in utero | 10 mos. | 20 mos. | 3 yrs. |
| **Permanent Dentition — Maxillary Teeth** | Central incisor | 3–4 mos. | 4–5 yrs. | 7–8 yrs. | 10 yrs. |
| | Lateral incisor | 10–12 mos. | 4–5 yrs. | 8–9 yrs. | 11 yrs. |
| | Canine | 4–5 mos. | 6–7 yrs. | 11–12 yrs. | 13–15 yrs. |
| | First premolar | 1½–1¾ yrs. | 5–6 yrs. | 10–11 yrs. | 12–13 yrs. |
| | Second premolar | 2–2¼ yrs. | 6–7 yrs. | 10–12 yrs. | 12–14 yrs. |
| | First molar | birth | 2½–3 yrs. | 6–7 yrs. | 9–10 yrs. |
| | Second molar | 2½–3 yrs. | 7–8 yrs. | 12–15 yrs. | 14–16 yrs. |
| | Third molar | 7–9 yrs. | 12–16 yrs. | 17–21 yrs. | 18–25 yrs. |
| **Permanent Dentition — Mandibular Teeth** | Central incisor | 3–4 mos. | 4–5 yrs. | 6–7 yrs. | 9 yrs. |
| | Lateral incisor | 3–4 mos. | 4–5 yrs. | 7–8 yrs. | 10 yrs. |
| | Canine | 4–5 mos. | 6–7 yrs. | 9–10 yrs. | 12–14 yrs. |
| | First premolar | 1¾–2 yrs. | 5–6 yrs. | 10–12 yrs. | 12–13 yrs. |
| | Second premolar | 2¼–2½ yrs. | 6–7 yrs. | 11–12 yrs. | 13–14 yrs. |
| | First molar | birth | 2½–3 yrs. | 6–7 yrs. | 9–10 yrs. |
| | Second molar | 2½–3 yrs | 7–8 yrs. | 11–13 yrs. | 14–15 yrs. |
| | Third molar | 8–10 yrs. | 12–16 yrs. | 17–21 yrs. | 18–25 yrs. |

(also called *contact points*). Floss must pass through contact points to clean the spaces between teeth (their proximal surfaces).

On different teeth, contact areas characteristically may be in the incisal third, the middle third, or at the junction of the incisal or middle third. Contact points are never located more cervically than in the middle of tooth crowns.

The contact of each tooth with the adjacent teeth has important functions:

1. It stabilizes the tooth within its alveolus (bony tooth socket) which thereby stabilizes the dental arches (the combined anchorage of all teeth in both arches making positive contact with each other).

2. It helps prevent food impaction, which can lead to decay and periodontal problems.

3. It protects the interdental papillae of the gingiva by shunting food toward the buccal and lingual areas.

The contact areas on teeth are at first contact points. Then, as the teeth rub together in function, these points become somewhat flattened and are truly contact areas. It has been shown by careful measurements that, by age 40 in a healthy mouth with a complete dentition, 10 mm of enamel has been worn off the contact areas of the teeth in each arch. This averages 0.38 mm per contact area on each tooth, and certainly emphasizes the amount of proximal attrition that occurs. Therefore, we would expect contact areas on teeth of older people to be large and somewhat flattened.

Refer to Table 3.3 for the relative position of proximal contacts when moving from anterior teeth to posterior teeth.

***Diastema*** is a space between two adjacent teeth that do not contact each other (Fig. 3.10**B**).

When teeth contact, there are four continuous spaces that surround the contact area: an interproximal space gingivally, as well as a facial (buccal or labial), lingual and occlusal or incisal *embrasure:*

## 1. INTERPROXIMAL SPACE

The *interproximal space* is the triangular space between adjacent teeth cervical to their contact. The sides of the triangle are the proximal surfaces of the adjacent teeth, and the apex of the triangle is the area of contact of two teeth. This space is occupied in periodontally healthy persons by the *interdental papilla,* tissue which fills the base of the triangle. (See Figs. 3.1, 3.10**B** and **C.**) Sometimes this interproximal space is referred to as the *cervical embrasure* or the *gingival embrasure.*

## 2. EMBRASURES

An *embrasure* (see Fig. 3.1) is the V-shaped spillway space or triangular shaped space adjacent to the contact area on adjacent teeth, narrowest at contact and widening facially (buccal or labial embrasure), lingually (lingual embrasure), and occlusally (occlusal or incisal embrasure). As just stated, the fourth triangular space, cervical to the contact area is properly called the *interproximal space.*

The lingual embrasures are ordinarily larger than the facial embrasures, since most teeth are narrower on the lingual side than on the facial side and because their contact points are located in the facial third of the crowns. These contact area locations and the buccal and lingual embrasures are seen when the dental arch is examined from the occlusal view (Fig. 3.1).

The *occlusal* or *incisal embrasure* is usually shallow from the occlusal surface or incisal edge to the contact areas and is narrow faciolingually on anterior teeth but broad on posterior teeth. The occlusal embrasure is the area between and occlusal to the marginal ridges on two adjacent teeth (occlusal to their contact area). This is where we place the dental floss before passing it through the contact area to clean tooth surfaces in the interproximal space.

Embrasures act as spillways to direct food away from the gingiva. When the occlusal embrasure is incorrectly shaped in a dental restoration (amalgam, composite, or gold), food will readily lodge in the interproximal spaces and can be removed only with dental floss.

## C. Root Axis Line

The *root axis line* is an imaginary line on the facial and lingual surface that divides the root at the cervix into mesial and distal halves (Fig. 3.5**A**). On the mesial and distal surfaces, it divides the root at the cervix into facial and lingual halves (Fig. 3.5**B**).

## SECTION VII. IDEAL OCCLUSION: INTER (BETWEEN) ARCH RELATIONSHIPS OF TEETH

Ideal relationships between maxillary and mandibular teeth are discussed here. It is important to learn the concepts and relationships of ideal occlusion in order to identify malocclusions that could contribute to dental problems. *Occlusion* is contact of the chewing (masticating) and incising surfaces of opposing maxillary and mandibular teeth. To *occlude* means to *close,* as in shutting your mouth and clenching your teeth together forcibly. The importance of good occlusion cannot be overestimated. It is essential to both general and dental health and to a patient's comfort and ability to enjoy food and to effectively reduce it for consumption. In dentistry, the study of occlusion includes a study of the anatomy, physiology, and pathology of the teeth, bones, craniomandibular joints, and soft tissues of the oral cavity during function.

Understanding occlusion requires a knowledge of:

1. The arrangement of teeth within the dental arches (alignment, plane, rotation, and spaces) as discussed in this chapter, Section VI.

2. The relation of the mandibular dental arch of teeth to the maxillary dental arch (discussed in this Section).

3. The relation of the mandible to the maxilla (centric relation and eccentric relations) (discussed in Chapter 1, Section II, and in Chapter 10).

4. The craniomandibular joints and their complexities (discussed in Chapter 1, Section III).

5. The muscles, nerves, ligaments, and soft tissues that affect the position of the mandible (discussed in Chapter 1, Sections IV, V, and VI).

6. Abnormalities that may be detrimental to dental health (malaligned teeth, biting or bruxing habits, tongue thrust, mouth breathing, deflective tooth contacts, balancing side interferences, and improperly designed dental restorations).

## A. Ideal Tooth Relationships Between Arches (Interarch)

Ideal tooth relationships were described and classified in the early 1900s by Edward H. Angle. He classified ideal occlusion as Class I, and defined it based on the relationship between the maxillary and mandibular dental arches. When closed together the teeth are in *centric occlusion* (maximum intercuspation), as shown in Figure 3.10**A**. Centric occlusion is achieved on hand-held models when the maxillary teeth fit as tightly as possible against the mandibular teeth, i.e., are most stable (Fig. 3.10**A**). The following relationships are seen:

1. **Relationship of anterior teeth:**

   **THE MAXILLARY ANTERIOR TEETH overlap the mandibular teeth**

   a. *Horizontal overlap:* The incisal edges of maxillary anterior teeth are labial to the incisal edges of the mandibular teeth (Fig. 3.10**A**).

   b. *Vertical overlap:* The incisal edges of the maxillary anterior teeth extend below the incisal edges of the mandibular teeth (Figs. 3.10**A** and **B**).

2. **Relationship of posterior teeth:**

   **THE MAXILLARY POSTERIOR TEETH** are slightly buccal to the mandibular posterior teeth (Figs. 3.10**B** and **C**) so that:

    a. The buccal cusps and buccal surfaces of the maxillary teeth are buccal to those in the mandibular arch.

    b. The lingual cusps of maxillary teeth rest in occlusal fossae of the mandibular teeth.

    c. The buccal cusps of the mandibular teeth rest in the occlusal fossae of the maxillary teeth.

    d. The lingual cusps and lingual surfaces of the mandibular teeth are lingual to those in the maxillary arch.

3. **Relative Alignment**

**THE VERTICAL (LONG) AXIS MIDLINE OF EACH MAXILLARY TOOTH** is slightly distal to the vertical axis of the corresponding mandibular tooth (Figs. 3.10**A** and **B**) so that:

    a. The tip of the mesiobuccal cusp of the maxillary first molar is aligned directly over the mesiobuccal groove on the mandibular first molar (Fig. 3.10**A**). *This relationship of first molars (the first permanent teeth to erupt) is a key factor in the definition of Class I occlusion.*

    b. The distal surface of the maxillary first molar is posterior to the distal surface of the mandibular first molar (Fig. 3.10**A**).

4. **Opposing teeth**

**EACH TOOTH IN A DENTAL ARCH** occludes with two teeth in the opposing arch except the mandibular central incisor (which is narrower than the maxillary central incisor) and the maxillary last molar (Fig. 3.10).

To summarize, *normal occlusion* involves a Class I relationship between the maxillary and mandibular first molars in centric occlusion. Ideally, only the canines touch when the mandible moves to either side, without molar and premolar contacts. There should *not* be facets, bone loss, closed vertical dimension, crooked teeth, bruxing habits, loose teeth, or joint pain (2).

# SECTION VIII. DEVELOPMENTAL DATA

For the *deciduous* dentition, the crowns of all 20 teeth begin to calcify between 4 to 6 months *in utero* (Fig. 3.11) and on the average take 10 months for completion (range 6$^{1}/_{2}$ months for maxillary central incisor to 13 months crown calcification time for the canines and mandibular second molar). It is about 6 months later, on average, before the mandibular crowns emerge, and 9 months after crown completion before the maxillary teeth reach the oral cavity (range: 3$^{1}/_{2}$ months for mandibular central incisor to 13 months delay for the maxillary second molar). The deciduous roots are completed on average of 14 months after emergence for the mandibular dentition and 15 months after emergence for the maxillary teeth (range 8 months for the mandibular lateral incisor to 22 months later for the upper and lower canines). Only 3 years after the roots are complete, they begin to resorb as the permanent teeth begin their occlusal migration. All of this information is derived from Table 3.4.

Root formation for permanent and deciduous teeth begins immediately after the enamel on the crown is completely formed, and at this time the tooth starts its occlusal movement toward the oral cavity. This tooth movement is called *eruption*. In the process of eruption, the tooth crown emerges into the oral cavity. The eruptive movement continues after the incident of emergence, and eventually the tooth comes into occlusion with teeth in the oppo-

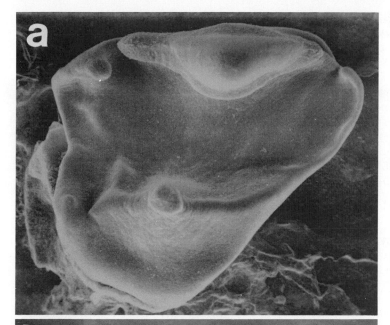

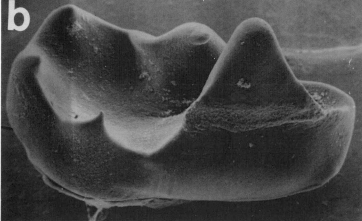

**Figure 3.11.** Developing human primary molars. **A.** Occlusal view of a 19-week in utero maxillary right first molar. Note the large, well-developed, mesiobuccal cusp, which is covered with a mineralized enamel cap and is the first formed and largest cusp of the trigon, the early molar form that has three cusps. The other cusps forming the trigon are the mesiolingual and distobuccal cusps, neither of which have started to mineralize. The distolingual cusp is barely discernible. Original magnification x36. **B.** Buccal view of a 20-week in utero mandibular right first molar. Note the strongly elevated mesiobuccal cusp that dominates the mesial portion of the tooth. The mesiolingual cusp is the second to differentiate and shows incipient mineralization. These two cusps make up the trigonid of the molar (in higher primates the third cusp, the paraconid, is lost). The distal half of the tooth is dominated by the talonid and its three surrounding cusps, the distobuccal, distolingual and distal cusps, which appear in that order. Original magnification x36. These two examples illustrate that the mesiobuccal cusp of both the maxillary and mandibular molars is the first to form and mineralize.

site arch. Even then it continues to erupt to compensate for wear (attrition) on its incisal or occlusal surface.

Each deciduous tooth is lost prior to being replaced by its succeeding permanent tooth. *Exfoliation* is the process of shedding the deciduous teeth usually caused by forces of the permanent teeth which will replace them. Sometimes severely diseased permanent teeth will become exfoliated if disease destroys the bony support of the teeth (alveolar bone).

On average for the permanent dentition, there is a 4-year span from completion of the crown calcification until the tooth emerges into the mouth, with a time range of from 2.7 years for the lower anterior teeth to 4.7 years for the lower posterior teeth.

In Table 3.4, the figures below *Eruption* indicate the approximate age of the individual at the time the tip of the tooth crown emerges through the oral mucosa into the mouth. There is a considerable normal range in emergence time for any given tooth (± 9 months).

The permanent dentition is also called the *succedaneous dentition* or that which succeeds the primary dentition. In the strict sense, succedaneous teeth would exclude the permanent molars because they have no predecessors or precursors as they erupt posterior to the deciduous molars. It has been estimated that a person 70 years of age will have spent

91% of this time chewing on permanent teeth (bridges, etc.) and only 6% of this time masticating with his or her deciduous dentition (1). The early years are important, and proper maintenance of the primary teeth will assure better tooth relationships and health long after the deciduous teeth have been shed.

In general, females' teeth emerge into the mouth a few months earlier than for males. Teeth of the same type usually come in the lower arch earlier than their maxillary counterparts. EXCEPTIONS include the permanent premolars. The roots on permanent teeth are not usually completely formed until about 2.5 years after the crowns have become visible in the mouth. In Table 3.4, the figures below *Root Completed* indicate the age of the individual at the time the root apex is completed. The tip of the root or apex is the last part to develop. On average, the root formation is completed 2.4 years after emergence, with an average time span range of from 2.3 years for the lower posterior teeth to 2.8 years for the lower anterior teeth.

Dental students and dental hygiene students should become quite familiar with the emergence dates in order to adequately and correctly inform worried parents and patients concerning the normal times at which teeth emerge. If the time is within 12–18 months (early or late) of the dates given in Table 3.4, there should be no real concern for permanent teeth. On the expected emergence times for deciduous teeth, a variation of 4–5 months (early or late) can be considered normal. Dental radiographs (x-ray films) are the best means for determining what is covered up or missing in a dentition when the expected teeth have not emerged, particularly when they are considerably overdue. Early emergence of teeth usually presents no problems other than a concern about instituting oral hygiene measures. An easy-to-understand sequence of tooth eruption or emergence is given in Table 9.1.

# SECTION IX. EVOLUTION OF TEETH AND LOBES

In terms of the evolution of the dentition, tooth crowns are said to have developed from *lobes* or primary centers (Fig. 3.12). For example, the mandibular first molar supposedly develops from five lobes: it has five cusps—three buccal and two lingual. Incisors develop from four lobes: three facial lobes that form three mamelons, and one lingual lobe forming the cingulum. Most canines and premolars develop from four (or five) lobes. The facial tooth surface develops from three lobes, usually evidenced by three subtle longitudinal ridges separated by two depressions. One lingual lobe forms the cingulum on canines and one (or two) lobes form the lingual cusps on premolars. All normal teeth show evidence of having developed from three or more lobes. Only some maxillary third molars have as few as three lobes. Peg-shaped maxillary lateral incisors and some supernumerary teeth have less than three lobes.

## LEARNING EXERCISE

For each of the following code letters and numbers (UNIVERSAL CODE), *write the complete tooth name:*

| DENTITION | ARCH | QUADRANT | TOOTH NAME |
|---|---|---|---|
| 28 | | | |
| 7 | | | |

16 _____

E _____

22 _____

3 _____

K _____

18 _____

R _____

Fill in the correct designation for the mandibular left lateral incisor according to the:

Universal Code_____

International Code (FDI)_____

Palmer Code _____

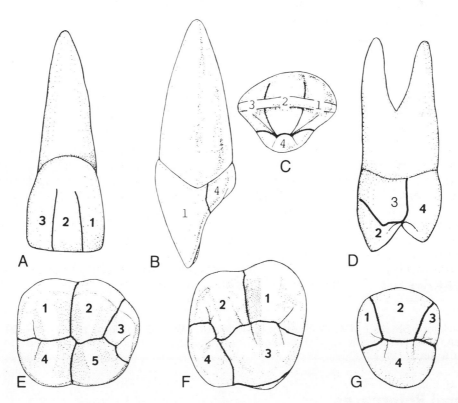

**Figure 3.12.** Lobes or primary anatomic divisions on teeth. **A.** Maxillary central incisor, like all anterior teeth has four lobes; the lingual lobe (4) beneath the cingulum is seen in the mesial view **B,** and incisal view **C. D** and **G.** Maxillary first premolar, mesial, and occlusal views. The divisions between the facial and lingual lobes are evidenced by the marginal ridge developmental grooves. **E.** Mandibular first molar with three buccal and two lingual lobes. **F.** Maxillary first molar with three large lobes and one small lobe. The Carabelli cusp, when present, is a part of the large mesiolingual lobe. On posterior teeth, major developmental grooves separate these divisions (Fig. 3.9**D**). Mamelons, when present, are an indication of the three labial lobes on incisors.

## THE TOOTH AND ITS SUPPORTING STRUCTURES

Sketch a tooth in cross-section and label the following structures:

1. Enamel
2. Dentin
3. Cementum
4. Pulp cavity
5. Pulp chamber
6. Pulp canal
7. Apical foramen
8. Dentinoenamel junction
9. Cementoenamel junction or cervical line
10. Cementodentinal junction
11. Periodontal ligament
12. Alveolar bone
13. Gingiva
14. Gingival sulcus

## RIDGES

Review your knowledge of occlusal morphology by naming the ridges (triangular, cusp, and marginal) on the premolar drawing in Fig. 3.13. There are 10, including the transverse ridge which is formed by two triangular ridges.

**Figure 3.13.** List ridges on Maxillary First or Second Premolar:

1. _____
2. _____
3. _____
4. _____
5. _____
6. _____
7. _____
8. _____
9. _____
10. Transverse

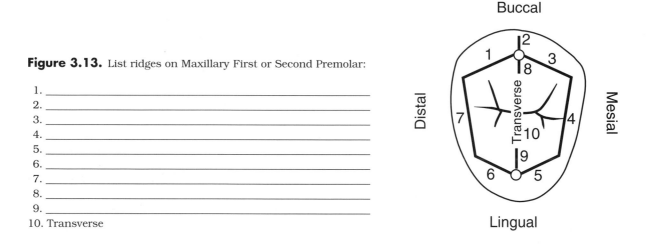

## References

1. Ramfjord SP, Ash MM. Occlusion. Philadelphia: W.B. Saunders, 1966:142–159.
2. Ash MM. Wheeler's dental anatomy, physiology, and occlusion. 6th ed. Philadelphia: W.B. Saunders, 1984.

## General References

Kraus B, Jordan R, Abrams L. Dental anatomy and occlusion. Baltimore: Williams & Wilkins, 1969.
Renner RP. An introduction to dental anatomy and esthetics. Chicago: Quintessence Publishing, 1985.

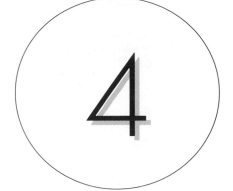

# Morphology of the Permanent Incisors

*As a suggestion for learning to describe and identify teeth, we suggest that you begin by placing a selection of all types of teeth in front of you. First, identify the incisors based on class traits. Second, identify the arch based on arch traits. Then third, identify the actual tooth (and the corresponding universal tooth number) based on type traits.*

*Using the maxillary right lateral incisor as a representative example for all incisors, refer to the Appendix, page 1, while reading Section I of this chapter. "Appendix" followed by a number and letter (e.g. Appendix 1a) is used within the text to denote reference to the page (number 1) and item (letter a) being referred to on that appendix page. The appendix pages are designed to be torn out to facilitate study and minimize page turns. Other appendix pages will be referred to throughout this chapter, also using the appendix page number and item letter.*

## SECTION I. GENERAL DESCRIPTION OF INCISORS

There are four maxillary incisors: two central incisors (first maxillary incisors: #8 and #9) and two lateral incisors (second maxillary incisors: #7 and #10). There are four mandibular incisors: two central incisors (first mandibular incisors: #24 and #25) and two lateral incisors (second mandibular incisors: #23 and #26).

The central incisors are located on either side of their respective arches (maxillary or mandibular) with their mesial surfaces next to one another at the midline, usually in contact.

(A space between these or other teeth is called a *diastema*.) Their distal surfaces contact the mesial surfaces of the lateral incisors. The lateral incisors are, therefore, just distal to the central incisors, with their mesial surfaces in contact with the distal surfaces of the adjacent central incisors and their distal surfaces contacting the canines. Did you know that the tusks on an elephant are maxillary central incisors (see Table 1.1)? They have the largest diastema in the world, large enough for the massive trunk between their central incisors. Two small diastemas between human mandibular incisors are shown in Figure 3.10**B.**

## A. Functions

The mandibular incisors function with the maxillary incisors in (a) cutting food (mandibular incisors are moving blades), (b) enabling articulate speech (consider the enunciation of a toothless person), and (c) helping to support the lip and maintain a good appearance (vanity). By our standards, a person lacking one or more incisors has an undesirable appearance. (Did you ever hear the song, "All I want for Christmas are my two front teeth"?) Their fourth function, by fitting the incisal edges of the mandibular incisors against the lingual surfaces of the maxillary incisors, is (d) to help guide the mandible posteriorly during the final phase of closing just before the posterior teeth contact.

## B. Morphology

In general, the morphology, or anatomy, of a tooth is described just as the morphology of a bone is described. Any tooth crown has five surfaces, i.e., four surfaces and a chewing or cutting surface or edge, depending on whether it is a posterior tooth (chewing in the back part of the mouth) or an anterior tooth (cutting in the front of the mouth). A tooth also has a number of characteristic grooves and ridges. In the study of tooth morphology, the grooves and ridges on the various surfaces are described and named. A knowledge of the character and location of these ridges, grooves, convexities, and concavities on teeth is invaluable in describing and identifying teeth in regard to *arch, type, class,* and *side* of the mouth.

When discussing traits, the external morphology of a tooth is customarily described from five aspects: (a) facial (i.e., labial or buccal), (b) lingual (tongue side), (c) mesial, (d) distal, and (e) incisal (or occlusal). Due to similarities between mesial and distal, these aspects will be discussed together in this text as the proximal surface.

In the study of any single type of human tooth, as for instance the maxillary central incisor, it is necessary to realize that this tooth varies in form in different people as much as different individuals vary from one another. One study of a collection of 100 maxillary central incisors showed considerable difference in such characteristics as size, relative proportions, and color (1). Information in this text on *crown length, crown width,* and *root length* is taken from measurements of extracted teeth by Dr. Woelfel and by his dental hygiene students at Ohio State University between 1974 and 1979. Teeth were collected from dentists in Ohio. The ranges indicate how greatly the same tooth can vary in size. See Tables 4.1**A** and **B**. For example, among the 398 maxillary central incisors measured, one central incisor was 16 mm longer than the shortest one. There was a lesser, but still considerable, range in crown length (6 mm) and in crown width (3 mm) from the smallest to the largest tooth found in this sample. Table 3.2 gives measurements for all teeth in the permanent dentition. **Specific data collected from Dr. Woelfel's studies are presented throughout the text in brackets [like this].**

### 1. MORPHOLOGY OF THE LABIAL SURFACE

Mamelons are usually seen on newly emerged incisor teeth. They are three scallops on the incisal edge centered beneath the three facial lobes (Fig. 4.1). Usually they are worn off after the tooth comes into functional position. (If you have the opportunity, observe a 7-year-old smile.) When mamelons remain on an adult, it is because

**Table 4.1A.** Size of Maxillary Incisors (Millimeters)

| Dimension Measured | 398 Centrals | | 295 Laterals | |
|---|---|---|---|---|
| | Average | Range | Average | Range |
| Crown length | 11.2 | 8.6–14.7 | 9.8 | 7.4–11.9 |
| Root length | 13.0 | 6.3–20.3 | 13.4 | 9.6–19.4 |
| Overall length | 23.6 | 16.5–32.6 | 22.5 | 17.7–28.9 |
| Crown width M-D | 8.6 | 7.1–10.5 | 6.6 | 5.0–9.0 |
| Root width (cervix) | 6.4 | 5.0–8.0 | 4.7 | 3.4–6.4 |
| Faciolingual crown size | 7.1 | 6.0–8.5 | 6.2 | 5.3–7.3 |
| Faciolingual root (cervix) | 6.4 | 5.1–7.8 | 5.8 | 4.5–7.0 |
| Mesial cervical curve | 2.8 | 1.4–4.8 | 2.5 | 1.3–4.0 |
| Distal cervical curve | 2.3 | 0.7–4.0 | 1.9 | 0.8–3.7 |

**Table 4.1B.** Size of Mandibular Incisors (Millimeters)

| Dimension Measured | 226 Centrals | | 234 Laterals | |
|---|---|---|---|---|
| | Average | Range | Average | Range |
| Crown length | 8.8 | 6.3–11.6 | 9.4 | 7.3–12.6 |
| Root length | 12.6 | 7.7–17.9 | 13.5 | 9.4–18.1 |
| Overall length | 20.8 | 16.9–26.7 | 22.1 | 18.5–26.6 |
| Crown width M-D | 5.3 | 4.4–6.7 | 5.7 | 4.6–8.2 |
| Root width (cervix) | 3.5 | 2.7–4.6 | 3.8 | 3.0–4.9 |
| Faciolingual crown size | 5.7 | 4.8–6.8 | 6.1 | 5.2–7.4 |
| Faciolingual root (cervix) | 5.4 | 4.3–6.5 | 5.8 | 4.3–6.8 |
| Mesial cervical curve | 2.0 | 1.0–3.3 | 2.1 | 1.0–3.6 |
| Distal cervical curve | 1.6 | 0.6–2.8 | 1.5 | 0.8–2.4 |

these teeth do not contact an opponent in function as may occur with an anterior open bite relationship where the incisors do not touch. The dentist could shave down the mamelons to make the incisal edge smooth and give it a more pleasing appearance.

*Developmental depressions*, seen most clearly on the tooth labeled #8 in Fig. 4.7, are the two shallow vertical depressions that help divide the labial surface into three portions. These three labial portions are sometimes called the mesial, middle, and distal *lobes*. Remember that there is a fourth lobe lingually that forms the cingulum (Figs. 3.12**B** and **C**).

Perikymata (pronounced per-i-kī´ mă-tă) are the fine horizontal lines on the crown surface (Figs. 4.2 and 4.3). Examine teeth and notice that these lines are closer together in the cervical part of the crown than they are nearer the incisal edge. Perikymata are found on the enamel of all newly erupted teeth. They are most easily seen on the labial surfaces of the anterior teeth because of their accessible location. Perikymata are more prominent on the teeth of young persons than on the teeth of older persons. They become lost with age due to abrasion in eating and from tooth brushing.

## C. Class Traits of All Incisors

Listed here are class traits that can be used to differentiate incisors from all other teeth (refer to appendix page 1).

1. **CROWNS, WHEN VIEWED FROM THE FACIAL:**

   a. are relatively rectangular, longer incisogingivally than wide mesiodistally (Appendix 1a).

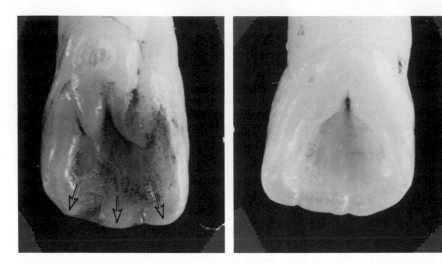

**Figure 4.1.** Lingual view of left and right maxillary central incisors. Both teeth have pronounced lingual marginal ridges and cingula and deeper lingual fossae than normal. They would be called "shovel-shaped" incisors. Both teeth have three rounded protuberances on their incisal edge called mamelons (*arrows*). The right tooth has a pit on the incisal border of the cingulum-the type of place that caries can penetrate without being easily noticed.

    b.  taper from the widest mesiodistal areas of proximal contact to the cervical line, i.e., are narrowest in the cervical third and broader toward incisal third (Appendix 1b).

    c.  are more convex on the distal than on the mesial sides (EXCEPT THE MANDIBULAR CENTRAL which is symmetrical) (Appendix 1c).

    d.  have contact areas (greatest crest of curvature proximally) that are mesially in the incisal third or near the junction of incisal and middle third; distally more cervical than the mesial (EXCEPT THE DISTAL OF THE MANDIBULAR CENTRAL which is at the same level as the mesial due to symmetry) (Appendix 1e, 2i, and 2r).

    e.  have a cervical line that is convex (dips) toward the apex on the facial and lingual sides (Appendix 1.L).

  2.  **ROOTS, WHEN VIEWED FROM THE FACIAL:**

    a.  taper (become more narrow) from the cervical line to the apex (Appendix 1f).

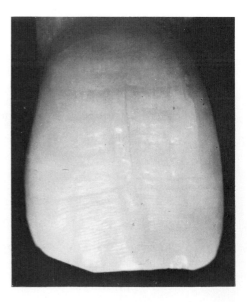

**Figure 4.2.** Perikymata on the labial surface of a maxillary right central incisor.

# Perikymata

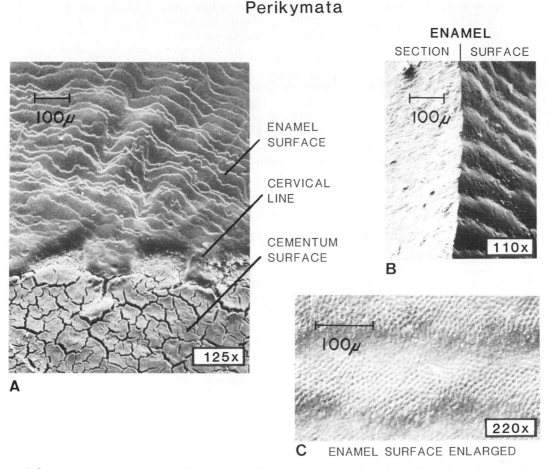

ENAMEL

SECTION | SURFACE

A

B

C ENAMEL SURFACE ENLARGED

**Figure 4.3. A.** View of perikymata (imbrication lines) near the cementoenamel junction where they are closest together. Notice their wave-like pattern. The cervical line is quite irregular at this magnification, and the cementum is thin, not necessarily extending to the enamel at every point. **B.** Cross-section of enamel showing perikymata waves on the right and the long enamel rods packed tightly and extending inward from the surface on the left. **C.** Higher magnification (x220) of enamel surface shows enamel rod ends on the perikymata waves. Enamel rods are about 4 μm in diameter. (These scanning electron micrographs were made and kindly provided by Dr. Ruth B. Paulson, Associate Professor Emeritus, Division of Oral Biology, Ohio State University, College of Dentistry.)

    b. are wider faciolingually than mesiodistally (EXCEPT MAXILLARY CENTRAL which has the mesiodistal width approximately the same as the faciolingual thickness) (Appendix 1g and Table 4.1A root width MD and FL both averaged 6.4mm).

    c. may bend in the apical one-third (EXCEPT MAXILLARY CENTRAL); when they bend, it is usually to the distal (Appendix 1h).

    d. are longer than crowns (CLOSEST IN LENGTH FOR MAXILLARY CENTRAL) (Appendix 1i).

3. **CROWNS, WHEN VIEWED FROM THE LINGUAL:**

    a. have a narrower lingual surface because the mesial and distal sides converge lingually (Appendix 1j seen on incisal view).

    b. have mesial and distal marginal ridges that converge toward the cingulum (Appendix 1k).

4. **CROWNS, WHEN VIEWED FROM THE PROXIMAL:**

    a. are wedge-shaped (Appendix 1m).

    b. usually have the incisal edge labial to the root axis line for the maxillary incisors and lingual to it on the mandibular incisors (Appendix 2o).

c. have a labial crest of curvature (greatest bulge) that is in the cervical third just incisal to the cervical line, and are therefore more convex cervically than incisally on their labial surfaces (Appendix 1n on facial view).

d. have a lingual crest of curvature in the cervical one-third on the cingulum, but the contour is concave from cingulum area to the incisal edge. Therefore, the lingual outline is S-shaped, being convex over the cingulum and concave from the cingulum nearly to the incisal edge (Appendix 1p). The lingual concavity on the maxillary anterior teeth is a most important guiding factor in the closing movements of the lower jaw, because the mandibular incisors fit into the fossae and against marginal ridges of the maxillary incisors as maximum closure or occlusion is approached. The "S" shape is more gradual in the mandibular incisors due to a smaller cingulum.

e. the cervical line proximally is convex, and curves incisally. The resultant curve is greater on the mesial surface than on the distal (Appendix 1o and Table 4.1).

5. **THE ROOTS, WHEN VIEWED FROM THE PROXIMAL:**

a. are widest at the cervical and taper to a rounded apex (Appendix 1f).

b. have a longitudinal depression in middle third of the *mesial* root surface. (The mandibular central and lateral incisors also have a prominent longitudinal depression on the distal surface.)

6. **THE CROWNS WHEN VIEWED FROM THE INCISAL:**

a. have a lingual fossa that is a shallow concavity just incisal to the cingulum.

b. have an incisal ridge that terminates mesiodistally at the widest portion of the crown (Appendix 1q).

c. have a labial outline (curve) that is broader and less curved, than the lingual outline (Appendix 1r).

## D. Arch Traits

Arch traits distinguish maxillary incisors from mandibular incisors: (Refer to Table 4.2 for a summary of incisor arch traits.)

The *mandibular* incisors differ from the maxillary incisors in many ways (arch traits). They (a) are smaller than maxillary incisors (Appendix 2p), (b) look more alike, (c) are nearly the same size, (d) have smaller roots, (e) are flatter on mesial and distal sides (Appendix 2q), (f) have crowns and roots that are relatively wider faciolingually than mesiodistally (Appendix 2n), (g) have contact areas located nearer the incisal ridge, (h) have smoother lingual surfaces (Appendix 2m), (i) have incisal ridges that are on or lingual to the root axis line (Appendix 2o), (j) have wear or attrition found only on the incisal edges, none on the lingual surface, and (k) have roots that are longer in proportion to the crowns.

Incisal edges of *maxillary* incisors are usually labial to the root axis line, whereas the incisal edges of *mandibular* incisors are usually lingual to the root axis line (Appendix 2o). Attrition on the incisal edges of incisors that occurs when shearing or incising food results in a wear pattern that is different on maxillary incisors compared to mandibular incisors (Fig. 4.4). This wear pattern occurs when the labial part of the incisal edge of mandibular incisors slides downward and forward while contacting the lingual part of the incisal edge of opposing maxillary incisors. The result is an incisal edge on worn *mandibular* incisors that slopes cervically toward the labial, whereas the incisal edge of *maxillary* incisors slopes cervically toward the lingual fossa.

**SECTIONS II-V AND TABLE 4.3 INCLUDE TYPE TRAITS THAT DISTINGUISH CENTRAL INCISORS FROM LATERAL INCISORS**

**Table 4.2.** How to Distinguish Between Maxillary and Mandibular Incisors (Arch Traits)

| Maxillary Incisors | Mandibular Incisors |
| --- | --- |
| **Labial View (Figs. 4.7 and 4.17)** | |
| Wider, less symmetrical crown | Long narrow, symmetrical crown |
| Mesial contacts are more incisally located than distal contacts | Mesial and distal contacts are at about the same level |
| More rounded distoincisal angles | Mesial and distal incisal angles are sharp |
| Common labial depressions | Less frequent labial depressions |
| More cervically located contacts | Contacts very near incisal edge (both mesial and distal) |
| Level of mesial and distal contacts vary | |
| **Lingual View (Figs. 4.8 and 4.18)** | |
| Pronounced marginal ridges | Lingual smooth, almost no marginal ridges |
| Deeper lingual fossa | Shallower lingual fossa |
| Sometimes lingual pits | No pits |
| Larger cingulum | Smaller cingulum |
| Central has cingulum to distal | Central almost perfectly symmetrical (Lateral has cingulum to distal) |
| **Proximal View (Figs. 4.9 and 4.19 A and B)** | |
| Incisal edge labial to root axis | Incisal edge on or lingual to root axis lines |
| Wear facets on lingual slopes of incisal edge and in lingual fossa | Wear facets slope labially on incisal edge, none on lingual surface |
| Elevated cingulum | Small cingulum |
| Roots narrower, especially in apical third | Roots noticeable wider faciolingually (with depressions on both sides of roots) |
| Mesial root surfaces are convex | |
| **Incisal View (Figs. 4.10 and 4.20)** | |
| Crowns wider mesiodistally than faciolingually | Crowns wider faciolingually than mesiodistally |
| Incisal edge labial to mid-root axis | Incisal edge is lingual to or centered on mid-root axis |
| Central cingulum is to distal | Central cingulum is centered |
| Lateral cingulum is centered | Lateral cingulum is to distal |
| Lateral has almost round crown outline | Lateral crown is oblong faciolingually |
| Central has more triangular crown outline | Central crown is oblong faciolingually |
| Lateral is convex labially near incisal | Lateral (and central) are nearly flat labially near incisal |

# SECTION II. MAXILLARY CENTRAL INCISOR (VIEWED IN FIGS. 4.5 AND 4.6)

## A. Labial Aspect of Maxillary Central Incisor

### LEARNING EXERCISE

*Examine several extracted maxillary incisors and/or tooth models as well as the examples in Fig. 4.7, top row, as you read. Hold these teeth root up and crown down, as they are positioned in the mouth. Also, tear out and refer to pages 1 and 2 found in the Appendix.*

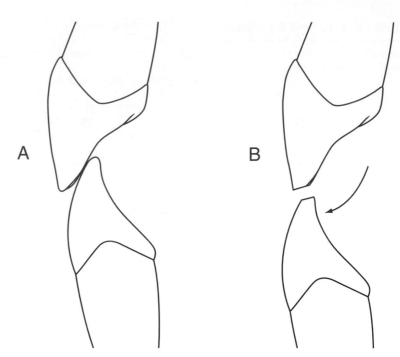

**Figure 4.4. A.** The relationship of incisors during centric occlusion. **B.** The wear pattern on the incisal edges of maxillary and mandibular incisors that occurs as these teeth move over one another during incision. Note that the facial of the incisal edge on the *maxillary* incisor is more incisal than the lingual; the facial of the incisal edge of the *mandibular* incisor is more cervical than the lingual due to functional attrition.

## 1. CROWN FROM THE LABIAL

### a. Crown Shape and Size

The crown is the longest [average: 11.2 mm] of all human tooth crowns, including that of the canines, and is also the widest of all incisors. The crown is usually longer (incisogingivally) than wide (mesiodistally) [averaging 2.6 mm longer] (Appendix 2a). The crown is narrowest in the cervical third and becomes broader toward the incisal third. Move your fingers over the sides of the crown from the cervical line to the incisal edge.

The distal outline of the crown is more convex than the mesial outline.

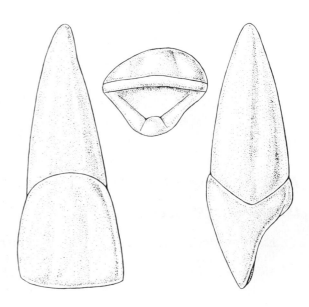

**Figure 4.5.** Maxillary right central incisor; labial incisal and mesial views.

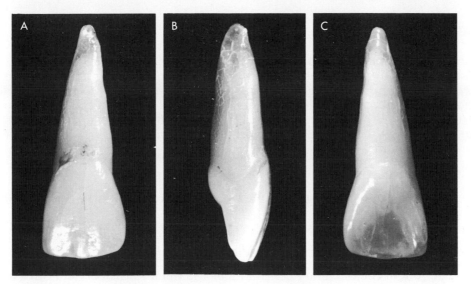

**Figure 4.6.** Maxillary left central incisor. **A.** Labial surface. **B.** Mesial surface. **C.** Lingual surface. In this tooth are clear, but not prominent, lingual marginal ridges which converge into the cingulum, and a distinct, but shallow, lingual fossa.

### b. Incisal Proximal Angles

The slightly rounded mesioincisal angle, where these two sides of the tooth join, nearly forms a right angle. The distoincisal corner is more rounded and the angle is somewhat obtuse (Appendix 1d and 2b). The incisal edge slopes cervically toward the distal (Appendix 2c).

### c. Contact Areas

Mesial—In the incisal third, very near the incisal edge.

Distal—Near the junction of the incisal and the middle thirds; i.e., distal contact is more cervical (right vs. left characteristic).

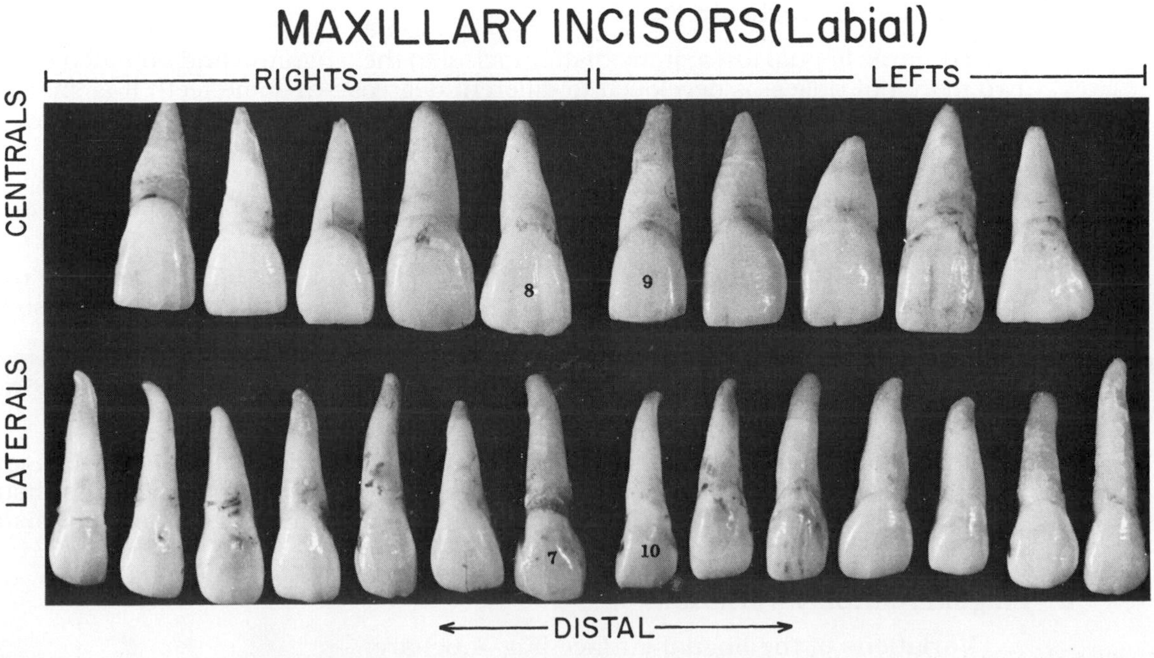

# MAXILLARY INCISORS(Labial)

RIGHTS LEFTS

CENTRALS

8    9

LATERALS

7    10

DISTAL

**Figure 4.7.** Maxillary incisors (labial view).

*Examine the teeth of several persons and notice the location of contact areas. Sometimes the distal contact area is in the middle third. It should be understood that the location of contact areas for any tooth may vary slightly among different individuals and according to the alignment and rotation of teeth in the arch. For all human teeth, contact areas are located in one of three places: in the incisal (occlusal) third, at the junction of the incisal and middle thirds, or in the middle of the crown. Contact areas are never located in the cervical third of permanent teeth.*

### d. Tooth Proportions

The root is just slightly longer than the crown [root to crown ratio is 1.16:1] (Appendix 2d).

## 2. ROOT SHAPE FROM THE LABIAL VIEW

The root of the maxillary central incisor is thick in the cervical third and narrows through the middle to a blunt apex. Its outline and shape is much like an ice cream cone. An apical bend is not common in the maxillary central incisor.

The central incisor root is the only maxillary tooth that is as thick at the cervix mesiodistally as faciolingually [6.4 mm]. The seven other maxillary tooth roots are thicker faciolingually than mesiodistally [ranging from 1.1 to 3.4 mm thicker for the lateral incisors and premolars, respectively]. Because of its shortness and conical shape, the maxillary central incisor root is generally considered to be a poor risk to help support a false tooth when making a dental bridge (i.e., a false tooth anchored to two adjacent surrounding teeth, one on either side of a lost tooth space).

## B. Lingual Aspect of Maxillary Central Incisor

### 1. CROWN FROM THE LINGUAL

#### a. Lingual Fossa: Varies in Depth

The large lingual fossa, immediately incisal to the cingulum and bounded by the two marginal ridges, is developed to different degrees—in some teeth it is shallow; in others, deep. Maxillary incisors with a deep lingual fossa and prominent mesial and distal marginal ridges are called "shovel-shaped incisors" (Fig. 4.1) (2–6).

#### b. Cingulum: Off-center Toward the Distal (Appendix 2e)

The *cingulum* on this tooth is usually well-developed and is located off-center toward the distal (right vs. left characteristic). The cingulum lies distal to the root axis line that bisects the root longitudinally in the cervical third. This can also be seen from the incisal view.

#### c. Marginal Ridges: Mesial Marginal Ridge Is Longer than the Distal Marginal Ridge (Appendix 2f)

The *mesial* and *distal marginal ridges* vary in prominence on central incisors from one person to another. They converge at the cingulum. Due to the distal placement of the cingulum, the mesial marginal ridge is longer than the distal marginal ridge (right vs. left characteristic).

#### d. Lingual Anatomy Variations

Variations of the lingual surface (Fig. 4.6c) are:

1. The fossa may be deep but smooth, i.e., no lingual ridges bordering the fossa.

# Maxillary Incisors (Lingual)

Lefts                                        Rights

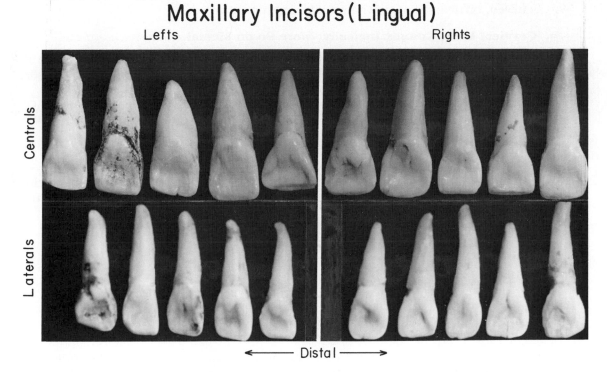

Centrals

Laterals

← Distal →

**Figure 4.8.** Maxillary incisors (lingual view).

2. *Accessory lingual ridges,* if present, are small or narrow and extend vertically from the cingulum toward the center of the fossa. These ridges may be 1, 2, 3, or 4 in number (see Fig. 2.9, tooth 9). Tiny grooves separate these ridges. [Inspection of 506 maxillary central incisors by Dr. Woelfel revealed 36% with none of these ridges, 27% with one small ridge, 28% with two accessory ridges, 9% with three ridges, and only three teeth with four small ridges.]

3. There may be a *lingual pit* at the incisal border of the cingulum where the mesial and distal marginal ridges come together in this location (Fig. 4.8).

## 2. ROOT FROM THE LINGUAL

The lingual surface of the root (Fig. 4.8), like for all anterior teeth, is convex, and is narrower mesiodistally than the labial surface. The root is flattened on the mesial side approaching the lingual side. Often there is a longitudinal depression on the mesial side of the root. The surface of the distal side of the root is convex, like the labial side.

## C. Proximal (Mesial and Distal) Aspects of Maxillary Central Incisor (Similarities and Differences)

### 1. CROWN (FROM THE PROXIMAL)

#### a. Incisal Edge

As is the tendency in the maxillary incisors, the incisal edge is slightly labial to the root axis line but may be mid-root axis. When viewed from the distal, the distoincisal edge may be on or just lingual to the axis line because of a slight distolingual twist of the incisal edge. (seen incisally in Appendix 2g).

The labial outline of the crown is convex in the cervical third and broadly curved, or nearly flat, in the middle and incisal thirds.

### b. Cervical Line: Convex Incisally; More So on Mesial

As on all anterior teeth, the cervical line (is convex) curves incisally on the mesial and distal surfaces of the tooth. As on most teeth, the curvature is greater on the mesial surface than on the distal surface (right vs. left characteristic), extending incisally one-fourth of the crown length. The mesial curvature of the cervical line of the maxillary central incisor is larger than for any other tooth [average: 2.8 mm]. The distal cervical line curves on the average 2.3 mm.

### c. Crest of Curvature

On the labial surface, the crest is in the cervical third just incisal to (below) the cervical line. On the lingual, it is also in the cervical third on the cingulum.

## 2. ROOT FROM THE PROXIMAL

### a. Root Outline

The root is thick or wide at the cervix and tapers evenly to a rounded apex. The lingual outline is nearly straight in the cervical third, then curves labially in the middle and apical thirds. The labial outline is slightly convex.

### b. Root Depression

The *mesial* surface of the root is somewhat flattened with a longitudinal depression in the middle third. This depression is located at the junction of the middle and lingual thirds of the root. Try to feel this mesial root depression.

The shape of the *distal* root surface is similar to the shape from the mesial aspect except that its surface is convex rather than flattened, and it does *not* have a depression (right vs. left characteristic) (Fig. 4.9, *top*)

## D. Incisal Aspect of Maxillary Central Incisor

*LEARNING EXERCISE*

*To follow this description, a maxillary incisor should be held in such a position that the incisal edge is toward you, the labial surface is at the top, and you are looking exactly along the root axis line. You should see slightly more lingual surface than labial surface because the incisal ridge is located somewhat labial to the root axis line. (refer to figs. 4.5, center and 4.10, upper two rows.*

## 1. CROWN WIDTH FACIOLINGUALLY VERSUS MESIODISTALLY

The crown outline is noticeably wider mesiodistally than faciolingually (average: 1.5 mm) (Appendix 2h).

## 2. CROWN OUTLINE

The crown is roughly triangular, with a somewhat curved labial outline forming the base that converges toward the cingulum.

## 3. INCISAL RIDGE CONTOUR

The incisal ridge or edge is 1.5–2 mm thick and is slightly curved from mesial to distal, the convexity being on the labial side. It terminates mesially and distally at the widest portion of the crown.

# Maxillary Incisors

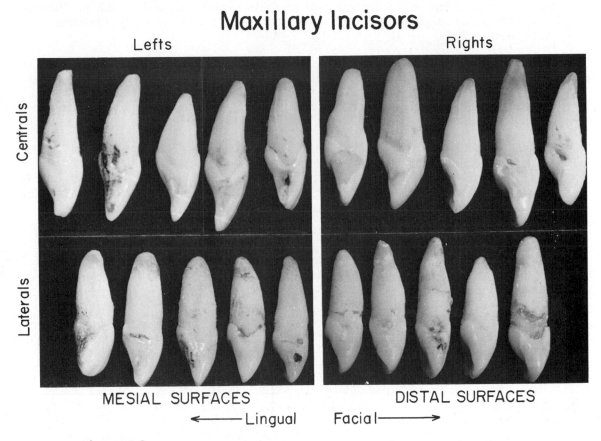

**Figure 4.9.** Maxillary incisors (proximal view). Facial surfaces are on the right.

# Maxillary Incisors (Incisal)

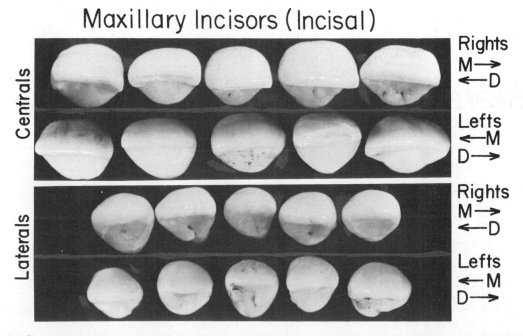

**Figure 4.10.** Maxillary incisors (incisal view). Facial surfaces of crowns are face up, lingual surfaces face down. *M* indicates mesial surfaces; *D* indicates distal surfaces. Three of the lateral incisors have pits in the cingulum region. Can you find them?

The position of the distoincisal angle is slightly lingual to the position of the mesioincisal angle, which then gives the incisal edge a slight distolingual twist (Appendix 2g).

## 4. CINGULUM

The cingulum is off-center to the distal, resulting in the mesial marginal ridge measuring longer than the distal marginal ridge (Appendix 2e and 2f) (right vs. left characteristic).

## 5. LABIAL CONTOUR

The labial outline of the crown usually appears broadly convex. On some teeth, a portion may be nearly flat. You can observe the two slight depressions (mesial and distal) on the labial surface located in the middle and incisal thirds.

### *LEARNING EXERCISE*

*Review the characteristics that distinguish a maxillary central from lateral incisor in Table 4.3.*

**Table 4.3.** How to Distinguish Between Maxillary Central and Lateral Incisors (Type Traits)

| Central Incisors | Lateral Incisors |
| --- | --- |
| **Labial View (Fig. 4.7)** | |
| Larger crown, wider cervically | Smaller crown, tipped distally at cervix |
| More symmetrical | Less symmetrical |
| Mesial incisal angle is 90° | Mesial incisal is rounded and acute angle |
| Mesial contact near incisal | Distal contact is near middle third |
| Root is wide cervically tapering to blunt apex | Longer and narrower root |
| Less root apex bend to distal | Root tip often bends to distal |
| **Lingual View (Fig. 4.8)** | |
| Large shallow lingual fossa | Deep but small fossa |
| Cingulum distally positioned | Cingulum is centered |
| Incisal edge outline curves less mesiodistally (is flatter) | Rounded incisal edge slopes up distally |
| Shorter distal than mesiolingual marginal ridge | Mesiolingual ridge is straight with distal curved |
| Less frequent lingual pits | Common lingual pits |
| **Proximal View (Fig. 4.9)** | |
| Greater cervical line curve | Slightly less cervical line curve |
| Evenly tapered root with mesial side only root depression | Root outlines more convex |
| Deeper lingual fossa outline | Slightly shallower lingual fossa |
| **Incisal (View (Fig. 4.10)** | |
| Crown noticeably wider mesiodistally | Crown size M-D and F-L almost the same |
| Crown outline roughly triangular | Crown outline round or oval |
| Incisal ridge curves mesiodistally | Shorter incisal ridge is straighter mesiodistally |
| Cingulum is off center to distal | Cingulum is centered |
| Labial developmental depressions | Sometimes labial depressions |

In determining a right from a left central incisor, look at the labial surface for the shape of the incisal angles (more rounded on distal) and position of contact points (more cervical on distal), the amount of cervical line curvature on the mesial and distal sides (more curved on mesial), as well as the flatter mesial or convex distal root surfaces. From the incisal view, look for the length of the marginal ridges (mesial is longer), distolingual twist of the incisal edge, and for the distal location of the cingulum. (Refer to Table 4.4.)

# SECTION III. MAXILLARY LATERAL INCISOR

There is great morphologic variation in this tooth—it may be missing altogether (Fig. 11.2**A**) it may resemble a small, more slender version of a maxillary central incisor, it may be quite asymmetrical and it may be peg-shaped. For the ideal shape, refer to Fig. 4.11.

## A. Labial Aspect of Maxillary Lateral Incisor

### 1. CROWN FROM THE LABIAL

#### a. Morphology of the Labial Surface

The labial surface is much like that of the central incisor (Figs. 4.7 and 4.12), but it is more convex or less flat mesiodistally and it appears more oblong cervicoincisally. Mamelons, and particularly labial depressions, are less prominent and less common than on the central incisor.

**Table 4.4.** How to Differentiate Maxillary Incisors Right from Left

| View | Central Incisors | Lateral Incisors |
|---|---|---|
| Labial (Fig. 4.7) | Flat mesial but rounded distal crown outline | Asymmetrical crown outline shorter on distal |
| | Mesioincisal angle is 90° | Acute mesioincisal angle |
| | Slightly rounded distoincisal angle | More rounded distoincisal angle |
| | Distal contact more cervical | Distal contact is much more cervical |
| Lingual (Fig. 4.8) | Same as labial | Same as labial |
| | Cingulum toward distal | Longer and straight mesiolingual ridge |
| | Longer mesiolingual marginal ridge | Short and curved distolingual ridge |
| Proximal (Fig. 4.9) | Larger cervical line curve on mesial than distal | Larger cervical line curve on mesial than distal |
| | Flat mesial side of root with depression | |
| Incisal (Fig. 4.10) | Cingulum toward distal | Shorter curved distolingual marginal ridge |
| | Longer mesiolingual marginal ridge | Mesial crown outline flatter than distal on lingual taper |

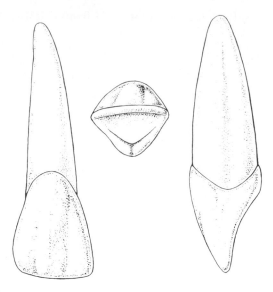

**Figure 4.11.** Maxillary right lateral incisor; labial, incisal, and mesial views.

### (1) Crown Shape and Size: More Oblong Cervicoincisally

The crown of the average lateral incisor is narrower [about 2 mm] than the crown of the central incisor, and the root is longer [about 0.5 mm], giving this entire tooth a long, slender look (Appendix 2a). The crown outline is less symmetrical than the central incisor.

### (2) Crown Incisal Proximal Angles

Both the mesioincisal and distoincisal angles are more rounded on the lateral incisor than on the central incisor (Appendix 2b).

The mesioincisal angle is more acute and the distoincisal angle is wider or more obtuse than on the central incisors. The incisal edge slopes cervically toward the distal (more so than on the maxillary central incisor) (Appendix 2c).

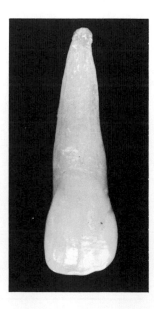

**Figure 4.12.** Maxillary left lateral incisor. Labial surface.

### (3) Crown Contact Areas from the Labial

Mesial—in the incisal third or near the junction of incisal and middle thirds.

Distal—more cervical than the mesial contact area; at the junction of incisal and middle thirds or in the middle third.

---

**LEARNING EXERCISE**

*Examine the teeth of several persons and notice the location of the contact areas. The mesial contact area will invariably be more incisally positioned than the distal contact area.*

### (4) Tooth Proportions

Like the crown, the root is 1.7 mm narrower mesiodistally, yet 0.4 mm longer than a central incisor, [comparing measurements of 398 maxillary central incisors and 295 lateral incisors]. This results in a root that is longer in proportion to the crown than on the maxillary central incisor (Appendix 2d, and nine of the 14 teeth in Fig. 4.7).

## 2. ROOT FROM THE LABIAL

The root tapers evenly toward the rounded apex, and the apical end is commonly bent distally (12 of the 14 teeth in Fig. 4.7, *lower row*).

# B. Lingual Aspect of Maxillary Lateral Incisor

## 1. CROWN FROM THE LINGUAL

### a. Lingual Fossa

The lingual fossa, although smaller in area, is more pronounced than on the central incisor (Fig. 4.8, lower row). However, it may be either shallow or deep, as on a shovel-shaped incisor.

### b. Cingulum

The cingulum is narrower than on the central incisor, and it is almost centered on the root axis line, not distally located as for the central incisors (Appendix 2e).

### c. Marginal Ridges

The mesial and distal marginal ridges are developed to different degrees on different teeth. Sometimes they are prominent and sometimes they are inconspicuous. They may also have been worn smooth from attrition (look for flattened wear areas which have a sheen called facets). The mesial marginal ridge outline is nearly straight; the shorter distal marginal ridge outline is curved cervicoincisally, as on the central incisor. It is shorter because the incisal edge slopes cervically from mesial to distal (Appendix 2f).

### d. Lingual Anatomy

As on the central incisor, there may be small vertical *accessory lingual ridges* on and incisal to the cingulum, only they are fewer in number and less common.

[Inspection of 488 maxillary lateral incisors by Dr. Woelfel revealed 64% with none of these small ridges, 32% with one small accessory ridge, and only 4% with two ridges.] Frequently, a lingual pit on a maxillary lateral incisor is present, and may need to be restored or filled by the dentist to arrest decay.

## 2. ROOT FROM THE LINGUAL

As with the maxillary central incisor, the root is narrower on the lingual side than on the labial side. There is a surface root depression on the mesial, but *not* on the distal (right vs. left characteristic).

## C. Proximal (Mesial and Distal) Aspect of Maxillary Lateral Incisor

### 1. CROWN: FROM THE PROXIMAL

#### a. Incisal Ridge

The incisal ridge or edge is 1.5–2 mm thick faciolingually, and is usually labial to the root axis line (as on maxillary central incisors). It is also sloped cervically toward the lingual from its most labial portion (like other maxillary anterior teeth).

#### b. Cervical Line

The curvature of the cervical line is deep, averaging 2.5 mm on the mesial (one-fourth of the crown length). It is more curved on the mesial surface than on the distal side, as is true for most teeth, but the difference is most pronounced on the anterior teeth.

### 2. ROOT FROM THE PROXIMAL

#### a. Root Outline

The root tapers gradually toward the apex, which appears blunt from these view. The root is slightly longer [0.4 mm] than that of the central incisor.

#### b. Root Depressions

Similar to the central incisor, a shallow longitudinal depression is often found on the middle of the *mesial* surface extending about half of the root length. The distal outline and surface are similar to the mesial outline and surface, except that usually there is no longitudinal depression on the distal. Thus, the distal root surface is slightly more convex than the mesial. The mesial surface of the root is least convex of the four sides (compare mesial and distal outlines in Fig. 4.9, *lower row*).

## D. Incisal Aspect of Maxillary Lateral Incisor

### 1. CROWN PROPORTION

Like the maxillary central incisor, the mesiodistal measurement of the lateral incisor crown is greater than the labiolingual measurement [average of 0.4 mm greater]. On some lateral incisors, the two dimensions are the same. In other words, the crown is almost the same size faciolingually as mesiodistally (Appendix 2h).

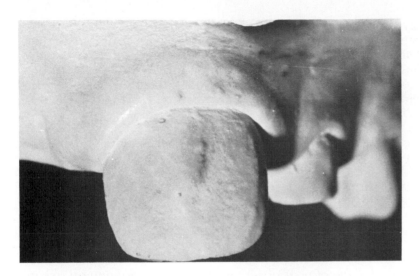

**Figure 4.13.** Maxillary left central incisor with a labial ridge.

## 2. CROWN OUTLINE FROM INCISAL

The lateral incisor is less symmetrical, but, in general, resembles the central incisor from this aspect. Its outline is more round or oval than triangular. The lateral incisor is more narrow mesiodistally. As was seen from the lingual view, its cingulum is nearly centered mesiodistally, unlike the central incisor (type trait).

## 3. INCISAL RIDGE CONTOUR

The incisal ridge is straighter mesiodistally than on the central incisors.

## 4. CINGULUM

The cingulum is centered mesiodistally (unlike maxillary central incisors; Appendix 2e), and the tooth tapers decidedly toward the cingulum from the contact points.

## 5. LABIAL CONTOUR

The labial outline of the crown is noticeably more convex than that of the central incisor (type trait). This characteristic difference is clearly seen in Figure 4.10.

## Variations in Maxillary Incisors

Racial differences in the maxillary incisor teeth have been reported in dental literature. For example, a high incidence of *shovel-shaped incisors* has been observed in Mongoloid peoples, including many groups of American Indians (2, 4, 5, 8). (Mongoloid pertains to a major racial division marked by a fold from the eyelid over the inner canthus, prominent cheekbones, straight black hair, small nose, broad face, yellowish complexion. Included are Mongols, Manchus, Chinese, Koreans, Eskimos, Japanese, Siamese, Burmese, Tibetans, and American Indians.) Caucasian and Negro peoples are reported to have less frequent occurrences of this characteristic. *Shovel-shape* is the term commonly used to designate incisor teeth that have prominent marginal ridges and a deep fossa on their lingual surfaces (Fig. 4.1). [Dr. Woelfel examined the maxillary incisors on casts of 715 dental hygiene students and found that 32% of the central incisors and 27% of the lateral incisors have some degree of shoveling. The rest had smooth concave lingual surfaces without prominent marginal ridges or deep fossae.]

A study of the skulls of American Indians who lived in Arizona about 1100 AD, has disclosed the occurrence of incisor teeth that have a mesial marginal ridge on the *labial* surface and a depression, or concavity, on the mesial part of the labial surface just distal to this ridge (9). In these teeth, the distal part of the labial surface is rounded in an unusual manner. Such teeth have been referred to as "three-quarter double shovel-shaped"—a descriptive, if ponderous, term. A central incisor with a labial ridge is seen in Figure 4.13. Labial "shoveling" has been reported also in some Eskimo peoples.

Palatal gingival grooves (cingulum and root) on maxillary lateral incisors are seen in Figures 8.15**A** and **B.**

A peg lateral incisor is seen in Figure 4.14. It developed with several lobes missing, possibly three of the normal four lobes. Peg or missing lateral incisors are not a rare occurrence.

## LEARNING EXERCISES

*It is interesting to keep a record of some of your observations as you examine an assortment of teeth. A sketch of any anomalies you find is of interest. Among items of significance might be the following:*

*Do you find any maxillary incisors with a pit at the incisal border of the cingulum?*

*If so, is there any evidence of dental decay (caries) in the lingual pit?*

*How many teeth have a deep lingual fossa and prominent marginal ridges? If you found some, would you call them "shovel-shaped"?*

*How many maxillary incisors have the incisal edge labial to the root axis line (as seen from the proximal aspect)?*

*How many have the incisal edge on the root axis line (as viewed from the proximal or incisal aspects)?*

*Can you find evidence of wear (shiny spots called facets) on the incisal edges and lingual surfaces of every tooth? Why are the wear facets sometimes on the incisal edge and at other times in the lingual fossa?*

*Can you find a maxillary lateral incisor that has the faciolingual crown dimension larger than the mesiodistal crown dimension? You should be able to find some, but you will not find any central incisors with this characteristic.*

*See if you can find an incisor that is larger or smaller than the dimensions given for range in size in Tables 4.1. and 4.1B.*

*Can you find an incisor with the crown longer than its root?*

*Do any of your specimens have perikymata or mamelons?*

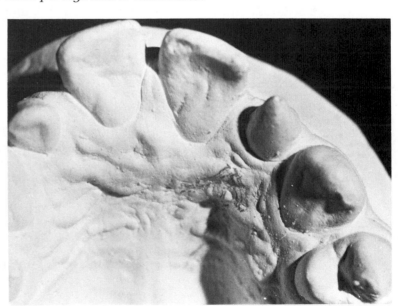

**Figure 4.14.** Incisal view of a peg-shaped maxillary left lateral incisor. Note the wide diastemata (spaces) between the teeth.

*Scrutinize each extracted tooth and attempt to determine why the patient had to have it taken out. Possible causes include dental decay (caries), loss of supporting bone, poor occlusion, looseness, drifting, dark color, pain, unable to be restored, a periapical abscess, a lateral abscess, or being the last tooth remaining in that part of the mouth. (All of these causes cannot be determined by the extracted tooth alone.) Are there are any clues as to how long or well the tooth served the patient (mamelon, hypercementosis, erosion, abrasion, attrition, wear on root surface, cracks in enamel, restoration, etc.)? Be a tooth detective and see what you can determine. You may even want to become a forensic dentist (Chapter 14).*

*Refer to the Table 4.3 comparison chart for distinguishing characteristics between maxillary central and lateral incisors. Then refer to the Table 4.2 comparison chart for distinguishing characteristics between maxillary and mandibular incisors, which should help you as you continue to learn the specific morphology of the mandibular incisors.*

# SECTION IV. MANDIBULAR CENTRAL INCISOR (FOR AVERAGE SIZES, REFER TO TABLE 4.1B)

## A. Labial Aspect of Mandibular Central Incisor

### LEARNING EXERCISES

*Examine several extracted teeth and/or models as you read. Also tear out and refer to the pages from the appendix on mandibular incisors. Hold mandibular teeth root down and crown up, the position of the teeth in the mouth. An ideal mandibular central incisor is seen in Figure 4.15.*

## 1. CROWN FROM THE LABIAL

### a. Morphology of the Labial Surface

The surface of the crown is nearly smooth. There may be two shallow developmental depressions in the incisal third if you scratch or examine the surface closely. [Dr. Woelfel found these depressions on 48% of 793 centrals and on 51% of 787 lateral incisors.]

*Mamelons* are usually present on newly emerged incisors (Fig. 4.16**A**). Ordinarily, they are soon worn off by functional contacts against the maxillary incisors (attrition).

### (1) Crown Shape and Size from the Labial (Fig. 4.17, Upper Row)

The crown is on average only five-eighths or 62% as wide as the crown of the maxillary central incisor. This crown is very narrow with respect to its length (Appendix 2p).

This tooth is so symmetrical that it is difficult to tell lefts from rights unless on casts or in the mouth. About the only difference to be found is the greater mesial than distal curvature of the cervical line (visible only on extracted teeth). The mesial and distal outlines of the crown are fairly straight near the almost flat incisal edge; then the crown tapers, becoming narrower from the incisally located contact areas toward the evenly convex cervical line.

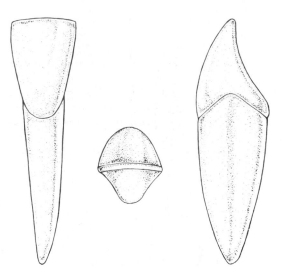

**Figure 4.15.** Mandibular right central incisor: labial, incisal, and mesial views.

The labial surface of the crown is convex mesiodistally in the cervical third (best viewed from the incisal) but nearly flat in the incisal third (feel it).

## LEARNING EXERCISE

*Examine someone's mouth and ask him to place his anterior teeth edge to edge and align the arch midlines over one another. Notice that the maxillary central incisor extends distal to the mandibular central incisor because it is the wider tooth by about 3.3 mm (Table 4.1).*

### (2) Incisal Proximal Angles from the Labial

The crown is nearly bilaterally symmetrical, and the mesioincisal and distoincisal angles are sharp, nearly right angles, or only a little rounded (Appendix 1d and 2j). The distoincisal angle is barely more rounded than the mesioincisal angle.

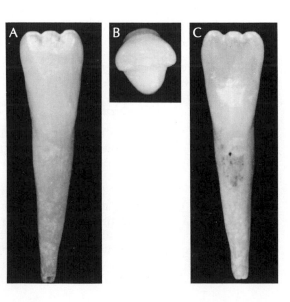

**Figure 4.16.** Mandibular right central incisor. **A.** Labial surface. The mamelons are unworn. The tip of the root may be resorbed or, more likely, its formation was not quite competed when it was lost. Notice the opening of the root canal at the root tip. **B.** Incisal aspect. The labial side is toward the top. The incisal ridge is perpendicular to the faciolingual dimension of the crown. **C.** Lingual surface. The crown surface is concave in the middle and incisal thirds, convex over the cingulum, and nearly smooth.

FACIAL

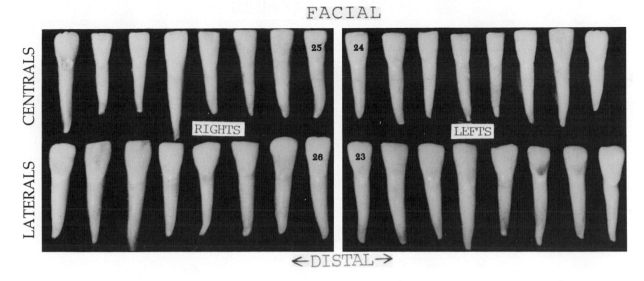

**Figure 4.17.** Facial view of mandibular central incisors (*upper row*) and mandibular lateral incisors (*lower row*).

### (3) Contact Areas from the Labial

*Mesial*—in the incisal third (Appendix 2i) near the mesioincisal angle almost level with the incisal edge.

*Distal*—in the incisal third, about the same level as the mesial contact area which is unique to mandibular central incisors (type trait).

### (4) Tooth Proportions from the Labial

The root-to-crown ratio is larger than for the maxillary central incisors [1.43 and 1.16] (arch trait). This means that mandibular incisor roots appear longer compared to their crown length.

## 2. ROOT SHAPE FROM THE LABIAL

The root is very narrow mesiodistally, but wide faciolingually (ribbon-like) (Appendix 2n), and tapers uniformly on both sides from the cervical line to the apex. The apical end *may* curve slightly to the distal (Fig. 4.17, upper row).

## B. Lingual Aspect of Mandibular Central Incisor

### 1. CROWN SHAPE (OUTLINE)

The outline of this tooth is much more symmetrical than either of the maxillary incisors or the mandibular lateral incisors (Fig. 4.18, upper row).

#### a. Lingual Fossa

The lingual surface is smooth and shallow, just slightly concave in the middle and incisal thirds.

#### b. Cingulum

The cingulum is convex, small, and centered.

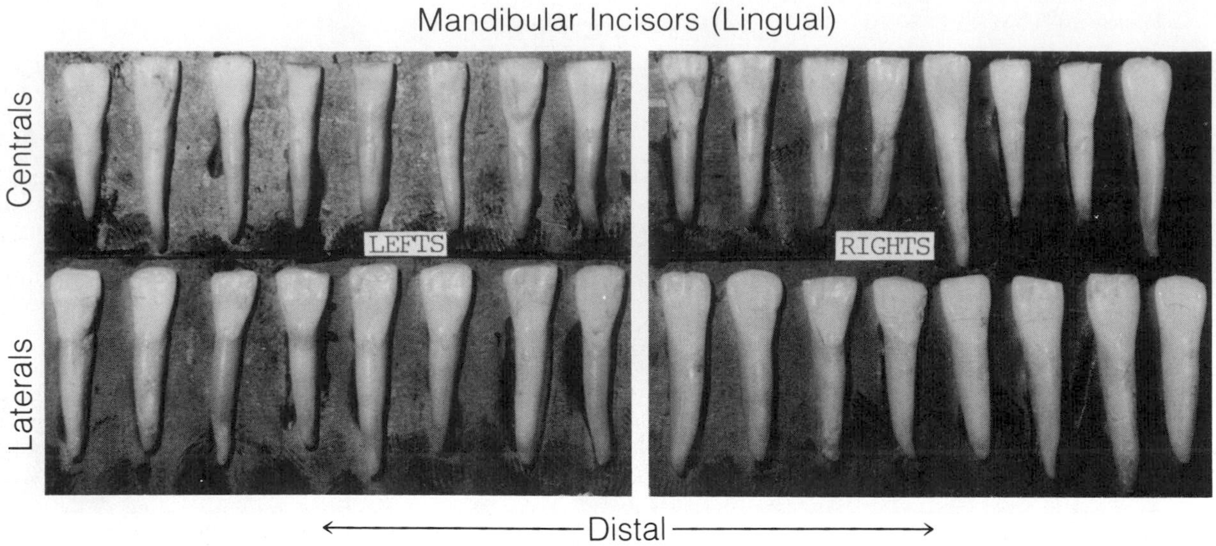

Mandibular Incisors (Lingual)

**Figure 4.18.** Lingual view of mandibular central incisors (*above*) and lateral incisors (*below*).

### c. Marginal Ridges

The marginal ridges and the lingual fossa usually are scarcely discernible, if at all, unlike the maxillary incisors (arch trait).

### d. Lingual Anatomy

The lingual surface does not have any grooves, accessory ridges, or pits.

## 2. ROOT FROM THE LINGUAL

As with other incisor roots, the root is slightly narrower on the lingual side than on the labial side. There are longitudinal depressions on *both* sides of the root (unlike the maxillary incisors which normally only have mesial root depressions).

## C. Proximal Aspect of the Mandibular Central Incisor

## 1. CROWN FROM THE PROXIMAL IS WEDGE-SHAPED LIKE ALL ANTERIOR TEETH

### a. Incisal Edge from the Proximal

As on other mandibular anterior teeth, the incisal edge is on or lingual to the mid-root axis.

### b. Cervical Line

The cervical line on the mesial has a deep curvature of 2 mm extending incisally over one-fourth of the short crown length. The curvature on the distal is 0.4 mm less (compare Figs. 4.19A and B, upper rows).

### c. Crest of Curvature from the Proximal

As on the other anterior teeth, the crest of curvature or greatest bulge on the *labial* surface of the crown is just incisal to the cervical line. The crest of curvature of the *lingual* surface is also in the cervical third, on the cingulum.

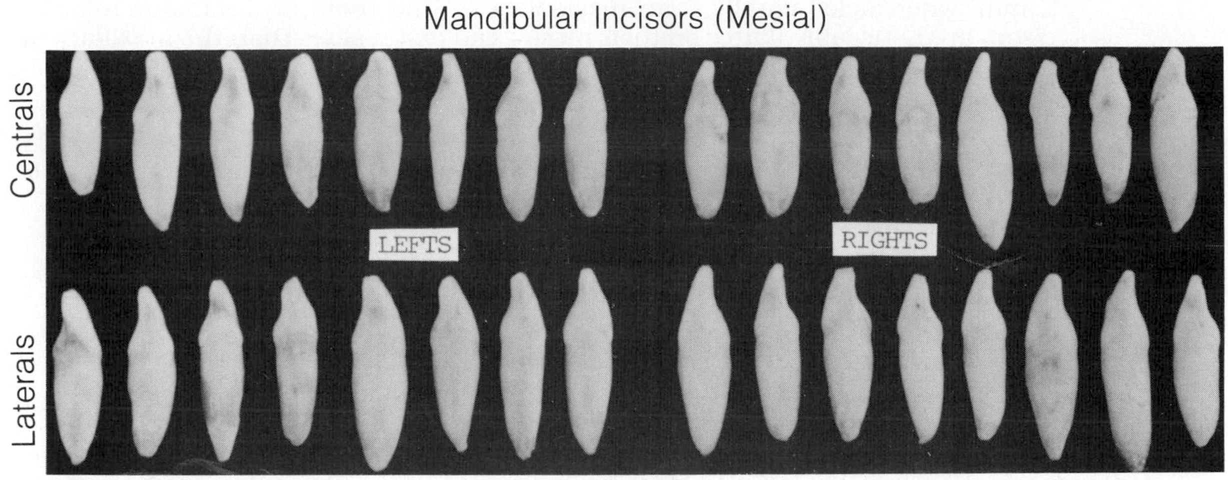

## Mandibular Incisors (Mesial)

**Figure 4.19. A**. *Mesial* view of mandibular central incisors (*above*) and lateral incisors (*below*).

The *labial* contour of the crown from the crest of curvature to the incisal edge is so slightly curved that often it seems to be nearly flat, especially in the incisal half (feel it). The *lingual* contour or outline is convex over the cingulum, concave in the middle third, and straighter in the incisal third (a shallow "s" outline), similar to all anterior teeth.

## 2. ROOT FROM THE PROXIMAL

### a. Root Outline from the Proximal

The facial and lingual sides of the root are nearly straight from the cervical line to the middle third; then the root tapers with its apex on the axis line (Figs. 4.19A and B, upper rows).

The relatively large faciolingual dimension of the root at the cervix is apparent in this view. The cervical portion of the roots on the mandibular incisors are

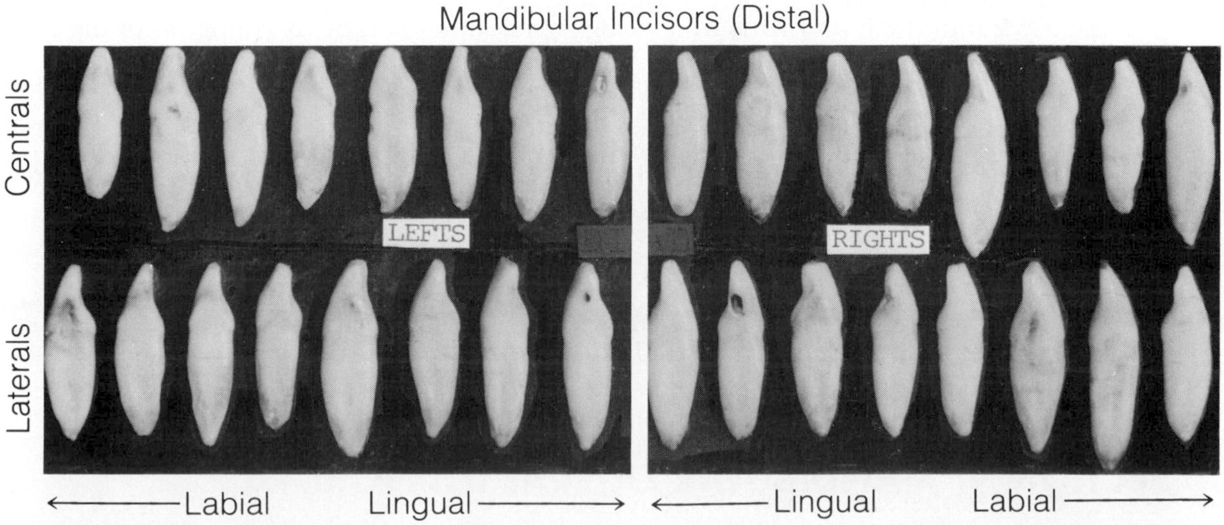

## Mandibular Incisors (Distal)

←——Labial    Lingual——→    ←——Lingual    Labial——→

**Figure 4.19. B**. Mandibular central incisors (*upper row*) and lateral incisors (*lower row*), *distal* aspect. Observe the position of the incisal ridge, often lingual to the root axis line, and the wide roots in the cervical and middle thirds.

2 mm wider faciolingually than mesiodistally. The roots of the mandibular incisors are noticeably flatter on their mesial and distal sides than the maxillary incisors (arch trait).

### b. Root Depressions from the Proximal

There is a longitudinal depression on the middle third of the *mesial and distal* root surfaces with the distal depression more distinct.

## D. Incisal Aspect of Mandibular Central Incisor

### LEARNING EXERCISE

*To follow this description the tooth should be held in such a position that the incisal edge is toward the observer, the labial surface is at the top, and the observer is looking exactly along the root axis line (Fig. 4.20A and B, top row). You should see slightly more of the labial than the lingual surface because the incisal ridge is just lingual to the root axis line.*

### 1. CROWN PROPORTIONS FROM THE INCISAL

The *labiolingual measurement of the crown is greater* than the mesiodistal measurement by about 0.4 mm. (This is quite different from the measurements of the maxillary incisors, especially the maxillary central incisors which are a lot wider mesiodistally than faciolingually).

### 2. CROWN OUTLINE FROM THE INCISAL

The mandibular central incisor is practically bilaterally symmetrical with little to differentiate the mesial half from the distal half. The greatest crest of curvature labially and lingually is centrally located.

### 3. INCISAL RIDGE CONTOUR FROM THE INCISAL

The incisal ridge or edge is at right angles to the *labiolingual root axis plane*. It is nearly 2 mm thick and runs in a straight line mesiodistally. It is lingual to the mid root axis.

### 4. CINGULUM FROM THE INCISAL

The cingulum is centered, smooth, and makes a narrow convex outline (Appendix 2k).

### 5. LABIAL CONTOUR FROM THE INCISAL

The labial surface is slightly convex in the incisal third labial to the incisal edge and makes a noticeably convex outline in the cervical third (Fig. 4.20A).

## SECTION V. MANDIBULAR LATERAL INCISOR

The mandibular lateral incisor is a little larger in all dimensions than the mandibular central incisor in the same mouth (for size, refer to Table 4.1B.). The crown is less symmetrical than the mandibular central incisor, especially from the incisal view but also from the

A **MANDIBULAR CENTRAL INCISORS (Incisal)**

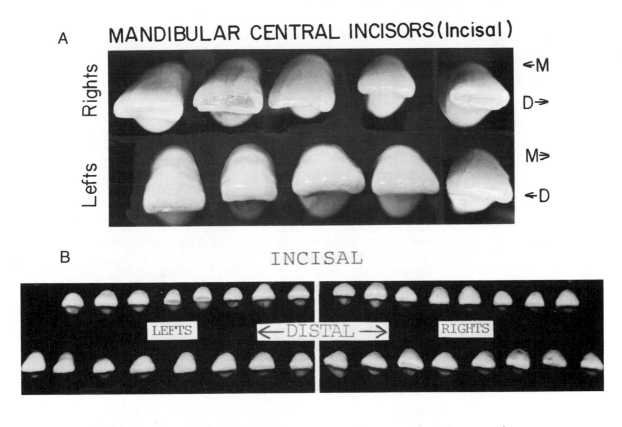

B INCISAL

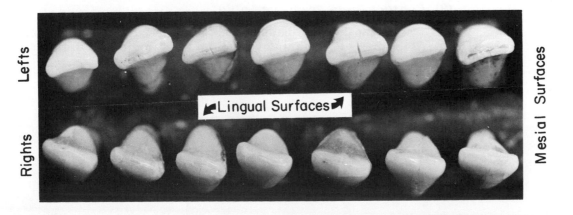

C Mandibular Lateral Incisors (Incisal)

**Figure 4.20. A.** Close-up incisal aspect of 10 mandibular (central) incisors. Observe the position of the thick incisal ridge relative to the labial and lingual crown outlines and the almost complete symmetry in form. The labial surfaces are toward the top. *M* and *D* denote the direction of the mesial and distal surfaces. **B.** Incisal view of 16 mandibular *central* incisors (*upper row*) and 16 mandibular lateral incisors (*lower row*). **C.** Close-up incisal aspect of mandibular *lateral* incisors. Observe the asymmetric outlines and the counter-clockwise twist to the incisal ridges on the left lateral incisors (*upper row*). Then turn this page upside down to easily see the clockwise twist on the right lateral incisors. This distolingual twist is helpful in determining rights from lefts on lower lateral incisors.

labial and lingual views (type trait). The crown is also tipped slightly distally on its root base when viewed from the labial (Appendix 2.l).

## A. Labial Aspect of Mandibular Lateral Incisor

### 1. CROWN FROM THE LABIAL

#### a. Morphology of the Labial Surface

The labial surface of the mandibular lateral incisor is similar to that of the mandibular central incisor—smooth with minimal depressions (Fig. 4.21, Left). About half of them will have two shallow depressions near the incisal third. The labial surface of the crown is convex mesiodistally, more in the cervical third and less toward the incisal edge. Feel these contours with your finger and fingernail.

##### (1) Shape and Size from the Labial

The crown of the mandibular lateral incisor resembles that of the mandibular central incisor, but it is *not* as bilaterally *symmetrical*. The distal side of the crown can be seen to bulge slightly compared to a somewhat flatter mesial crown outline (Fig. 4.17, *lower row*)

The crown of the lateral incisor is tilted distally on the root, giving the impression that the tooth has been bent at the cervix (Appendix 2l). This makes the distal outline of the crown shorter than the mesial outline.

##### (2) Incisal Proximal Angles from the Labial

The distoincisal angle is noticeably more rounded than the mesioincisal angle (before attrition) (Appendix 2j). This helps to distinguish rights from lefts prior to attrition.

##### (3) Contact Areas from the Labial

The mesial and distal contact areas of the lateral incisor are not at the same level, a condition different from that found in the central incisor (type trait) (Appendix 2i).

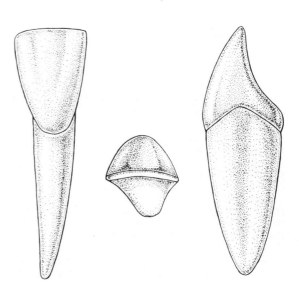

**Figure 4.21.** Mandibular right lateral incisor: labial, incisal, and mesial views.

*Mesial*—in the incisal third, fairly near the incisal edge.

*Distal*—in the incisal third, but cervical to the level of the mesial contact area.

### (4) *Proportions of the Crown from the Labial*

Like on the mandibular central incisor, the crown is narrow with respect to its length (Appendix 2p).

## 2. ROOT SHAPE FROM THE LABIAL

The root appears very narrow mesiodistally, and tapers gradually from the cervical line toward the apex which may curve slightly to the distal.

# B. Lingual Aspect of Mandibular Lateral Incisor

## 1. CROWN FROM THE LINGUAL

The shape resembles that of the mandibular central incisor, but lacks bilateral symmetry. (Fig. 4.18, Lower Row) The crown is tilted distally on the root and tapers lingually in the middle and cervical thirds.

As seen from the lingual and incisal views, the small smooth cingulum lies slightly distal to the axis line of the root similar to the maxillary central incisor, making the mesial marginal ridge slightly longer than the distal marginal ridge.

As with the mandibular central incisor, the marginal ridges and the lingual fossa usually are not conspicuous with the generally smooth lingual surface (arch trait) (Appendix 2m).

## 2. ROOT FROM THE LINGUAL

The lingual surface of the root is convex, smooth, and narrower on the lingual than labial sides. Sometimes the longitudinal depressions on the proximal surfaces can often be seen from this view.

# C. Proximal Aspect of Mandibular Lateral Incisor

## 1. CROWN FROM THE PROXIMAL

### a. Incisal Edge

The incisal edge is on or lingual to the mid-root axis (Appendix 2o). From the mesial side, the distolingual twist of the incisal ridge places the distal portion at the ridge somewhat more lingual than on the mesial.

### b. Cervical Line (Appendix 1o)

Mesially, the cervical line has a deep curvature (2 mm), extending incisally over one-fourth of the crown length. The curvature averaged 0.6 mm greater on the mesial surface than on the distal surface [234 teeth measured]. (Compare Fig. 4.19**A** with Fig. 4.19**B**, Lower Rows).

### c. Crest of Curvature

As with other incisors, the labial crest is near the cervical line in the cervical third; the lingual crest is on the cingulum.

The labial outline and surface become nearly flat through the middle and incisal thirds of the crown.

The *mesial* surface is nearly flat from the middle third to the cervical line and convex faciolingually in the incisal third (feel it).

## 2. ROOT OUTLINE AND DEPRESSIONS

The root outline is nearly straight from the cervical line to the middle third; then it tapers. (Fig. 4.19, *lower rows*) There is a slight longitudinal depression on the *mesial* surface of the root, and on the *distal* surface of the root where it is a little more distinct than the depression on the mesial surface.

## D. Incisal Aspect of Mandibular Lateral Incisor

### 1. CROWN PROPORTIONS

As with the mandibular central incisor, but unlike the maxillary incisors, the crown is broader labiolingually than mesiodistally [by 0.4 mm].

### 2. CROWN OUTLINE

The mandibular lateral incisor is not bilaterally symmetrical, and this fact makes it easy to select rights from lefts and to determine centrals from laterals especially from this view (Figs. 4.20**B**, lower row, and **C**).

If you hold a tooth correctly, slightly more of the labial than lingual surface is visible because of the lingually positioned incisal ridge (Appendix 2k, *proximal view*).

### 3. INCISAL RIDGE CONTOUR: A DISTOLINGUAL TWIST (FIG. 4.20**C**)

Usually the incisal edge does not follow a straight line mesiodistally, but rather it has a *distolingual twist:* that is, the distal half of the incisal edge is bent lingually, so that the distoincisal angle is more lingual in position than the mesioincisal angle (Appendix 2k). The twist of the incisal edge corresponds to the curvature of the mandibular dental arch—a tooth on the right side of the arch is twisted clockwise; one on the left is twisted counterclockwise.

### 4. CINGULUM: OFF-CENTER DISTALLY

The cingulum is slightly off-center to the distal, like that of the maxillary central incisor, but unlike that of the mandibular central incisor (Appendix 2k). The lingual fossa is barely discernible.

### 5. LABIAL CONTOUR

The labial outline is slightly convex in the incisal third labial to the incisal ridge and is decidedly so in the cervical third.

## VARIATIONS IN MANDIBULAR INCISORS

There is more uniformity of shape in the mandibular incisor teeth than in other teeth. Occasionally, but rarely, a mandibular lateral incisor is found to have a labial and a lingual root division in the cervical third. More commonly, they may have two canals in the single root.

In some Mongoloid peoples, the cingulum of mandibular incisors is characteristically marked by a short, deep groove running cervicoincisally. This groove is often a site of dental caries.

In Chapter 11, you will see fused mandibular incisors, a missing central incisor, and lateral incisors emerged distally to the canines (see Fig. 11.33).

## LEARNING EXERCISES

Compare the location and slopes of facets (wear spots from attrition) on the mandibular incisors with those you found on the maxillary incisors. Why can't you find any facets on the lingual surfaces of the mandibular incisors?

Should you find a mandibular incisor with attrition on the lingual surface, how can this be accounted for? The only possible explanation is an anterior crossbite (Fig. 10.11). **A far more likely explanation would be that you are looking at a maxillary, not a mandibular, incisor.**

Have you found any mandibular incisors with a vertical groove on the cingulum, either in your examination of mouths or in extracted teeth? If so, did the groove show evidence of caries?

Have you found, among your extracted teeth, a mandibular incisor with conspicuous mamelons? If you have one, and if you carefully grind off the facial surface in the incisal third of the crown (see Chapter 8 for method of grinding) you may find a deep pit between the center mamelon and the mesial and distal mamelon. There may be some evidence of early caries in such a pit.

Can you find any two-rooted mandibular lateral incisors? They are rare and would be considered anomalies. Try to find some mandibular incisors that are larger or smaller than the dimensions in Tables 4.1**A** and **B** under the range column.

Review the characteristics that distinguish mandibular central and lateral incisors in Table 4.5.

TEST YOUR NEWLY ACQUIRED KNOWLEDGE BY ANSWERING THE FOLLOWING QUESTIONS:

The incisal edge of mandibular incisors usually lies lingual to the mid-root axis. T___ F___

Is this true on your tooth models? Yes___ No___ Is this true on the natural extracted teeth in your tooth collection? Yes___ No___

What are the best features to use in a tooth identification test to distinguish between the following teeth (list two or three for each set of teeth):

1. Maxillary from mandibular incisors

2. Maxillary central incisor from maxillary lateral incisor

3. Mandibular right lateral incisor from mandibular left lateral incisor

4. Maxillary right central incisor from left central incisor

Which incisor is most likely to have a bifurcated root?

Which incisor is most likely to be missing in Caucasian dentitions?

Shovel-shaped incisors are associated with dentitions in what ethnic group?

What geometric outlines do the labial and proximal views of incisors resemble?

Labial _____

Proximal _____

**Table 4.5.** How to Distinguish Between Mandibular Central and Lateral Incisors (Type Traits) (Refer to Figs. 4.15 through 4.21 plus Appendix page 2.)

| Central Incisors | Lateral Incisors |
|---|---|
| More symmetrical | Less symmetrical (labial, lingual, incisal views) |
| Smaller overall and shorter root: Crown is 0.6 mm shorter, root is 0.9 mm shorter in same mouth | Crown larger overall (especially mesiodistally by 0.4 mm) with longer root (0.9 mm longer) |
| **Labial and Lingual Views** | |
| Same level contacts | Lower distal contact |
| Crown *not* bent distally on root | Crown tipped distally on root |
| No distal side bulge on crown | Distal side bulge on crown |
| **Incisal and Lingual Views** | |
| Cingulum centered | Cingulum distal to center |
| Same length marginal ridges | Longer mesial marginal ridge |
| No distolingual twist of incisal edge | Distolingual twist of incisal edge |

## References

1. Hanihara K. Racial characteristics in the dentition. J Dent Res 1967;46:923–926.
2. Carbonelli VM. Variations in the frequency of shovel-shaped incisors in different populations. In: Brothwell DR, ed. Dental anthropology. London: Pergamon Press, 1963:211–234.
3. Brabant H. Comparison of the characteristics and anomalies of the deciduous and the permanent dentitions. J Dent Res 1967;48:897–902.
4. De Voto FCH. Shovel-shaped incisors in pre-Columbian Tastilian Indians. J Dent Res 1971;50:168.
5. De Voto FCH, Arias NH, Ringuelet S, Palma NH. Shovel-shaped incisors in a northwestern Argentine population. J Dent Res 1968;47:820.
6. Taylor RMS. Variations in form of human teeth: I. An anthropologic and forensic study of maxillary incisors. J Dent Res 1969;48:5–16.
7. Ash MM. Wheeler's dental anatomy, physiology and occlusion. 7th ed. Philadelphia: W.B. Saunders, 1993.
8. Dahlberg AA. The dentition of the American Indian. In: Laughlin WS, ed. The physical anthropology of the American Indian. New York: The Viking Fund, 1949.
9. Snyder RG. Mesial marginal ridging of incisor labial surfaces. J Dent Res 1960;39:361.

## General Reference

Goose DH. Variability of form of maxillary permanent incisors. J Dent Res 1956;35:902.

# Morphology of Permanent Canines

Using the maxillary right canine as a representative example for all canines, refer to the Appendix, page 3, while reading Section I of this chapter. Throughout this chapter, "Appendix" followed by a number and letter (e.g., Appendix 3a) is used to denote reference to the page (number 3) and item (letter a) being referred to on that appendix page. The appendix pages are designed to be torn out to facilitate study and minimize page turns. Other appendix pages will be referred to throughout this chapter.

## SECTION I. GENERAL DESCRIPTION OF CANINES

There are four canines: one on either side in the maxillary (#6 and #11) and mandibular (#22 and #27) arches. They are longest of the permanent teeth [26.3 mm and 25.9 mm, respectively].

The canines are distal to the lateral incisors and are the third teeth from the midline. The mesial surface of the canine is in contact with the distal surface of the lateral incisor. The distal surface of each canine contacts the mesial surface of the first premolar.

The four canines are justifiably termed cornerstones of the arches as they are located at the corners of the mouth or dental arches. They are often referred to as cuspids, eyeteeth, and fangs (nicknames and slang terminology). The use of such slang terminology should be greatly discouraged.

Frequently, the canines are the last teeth to be lost from dental disease (decay or periodontal problems). Have you known or seen an elderly person who is edentulous (toothless) except for one or more of the canines?

The name canine is of Greek origin and is found in the writings of Hippocrates and Aristotle of 2350 years ago. Aristotle first described canine anatomy, stressing the intermediate nature of it between incisors and molars: it is sharp like an incisor and wide at the base like a molar. Celsus was the first writer to mention the roots of teeth, saying the canine was monoradicular (1, 2). The word cuspid in Spanish means "to spit." Therefore the term cuspid would mean "spit tooth," a most unfair name for such an important tooth.

## A. Functions

In dogs, cats, and other animals with long, prominent canine teeth, the functions of these teeth are catching and tearing food and defense. Canines are essential to their survival.

In human beings, these teeth usually function with the incisors (a) to support the lip and the facial muscles, (b) to cut, pierce, or shear food morsels. The canines (c) act as important guideposts in occlusion, their deep vertical overlap serving as a protective mechanism relieving the posterior teeth from excessive and potentially damaging horizontal forces during lateral excursions of the mandible (canine protected occlusions). A steep vertical overlap of the maxillary and mandibular canines, when present, causes all of the posterior teeth to separate (disclude) when the mandible moves to either side as the longer opposing canines touch edge-to-edge. Canine guidance or protection thus relieves the premolars and molars from lateral forces while chewing.

Canines, because of their large, long roots, are good anchor teeth (abutments) for a fixed dental bridge or removable partial denture when other teeth have been lost. As such, they often continue to function as a prime support for the artificial teeth for many years.

## B. General Characteristics or Class Traits (Similarities) of Canines (Both Maxillary and Mandibular)

### 1. SIZE

The canines are the longest teeth in the mouth. They have particularly long [average: 16.2 mm] thick roots (faciolingually) that help to anchor them securely in the alveolar process. See Table 5.1 and Figures 5.1 and 5.2.

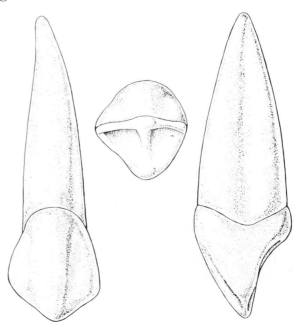

**Figure 5.1.** A maxillary right canine: labial, incisal, and mesial views.

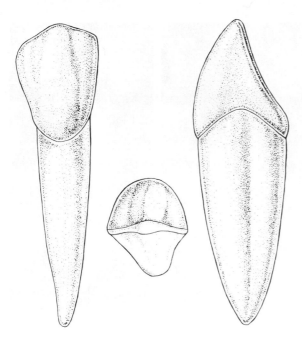

**Figure 5.2.** A mandibular right canine: labial, incisal, and mesial views.

## 2. INCISAL RIDGE

The incisal ridge of a canine is divided into two inclines or slopes by a cusp rather than being nearly straight across as in the incisor, therefore resembling a pentagon shape (Appendix 3a). The *mesial slope* or cusp ridge of the cusp is shorter than the *distal slope* or cusp ridge (Appendix 3b; Fig. 3.5**A**). (In older individuals, the lengths of the cusp slopes are often altered by attrition.)

Canine teeth do not ordinarily have mamelons, but may have a notch on either cusp slope, as seen in Figure 5.3**A.** Figure 5.12 shows an accentuated mesial notch.

## 3. LABIAL CONTOUR

The labial surface of a canine is prominently convex with a vertical *labial ridge* (Appendix 3c). Canines are the only teeth with a labial ridge although premolars have a similar ridge called the buccal ridge.

**Table 5.1.** Size of Canines (Millimeters) (Measured by Dr. Woelfel and his dental hygiene students 1974–1979)

| Dimension Measured | 321 Maxillary Canines Average | Range | 316 Mandibular Canines Average | Range |
|---|---|---|---|---|
| Crown length | 10.6 | 8.2–13.6 | 11.0 | 6.8–16.4 |
| Root length | 16.5 | 10.8–28.5 | 15.9 | 9.5–22.2 |
| Overall length | 26.4 | 20.0–38.4* | 25.9 | 16.1–34.5 |
| Crown width M-D | 7.6 | 6.3–9.5 | 6.8 | 5.7–8.6 |
| Root width (cervix) | 5.6 | 3.6–7.3 | 5.2 | 4.1–6.4 |
| Faciolingual crown size | 8.1 | 6.7–10.7 | 7.7 | 6.4–9.5 |
| Faciolingual root (cervix) | 7.6 | 6.1–10.4 | 7.5 | 5.8–9.4 |
| Mesial cervical curve | 2.1 | 0.3–4.0 | 2.4 | 0.2–4.8 |
| Distal cervical curve | 1.4 | 0.2–3.5 | 1.6 | 0.2–3.5 |

*In the 1962 issue of the Journal of the North Carolina Dental Society (46:10), there is a report of an extraction, without incident, of a maxillary left canine 47 mm long.

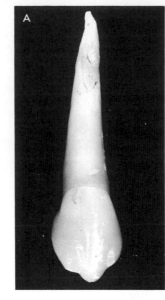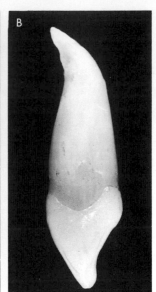

**Figure 5.3.** Maxillary right canine. **A.** Labial surface. Both this tooth and the tooth in Figure 5.4**A** are of shapes frequently found. Notice the difference. **B.** Mesial surface. Compare the facial and lingual outlines with the same curvatures of the tooth in Figure 5.4**C**. Observe the unusual labial root curvature near the apex. The cervical line is clear in this picture. Notice that the enamel fits onto the crown somewhat like a cap, and at the cervical border it appears as a beveled edge. Examine your extracted teeth carefully and notice the form of this cementoenamel junction.

## 4. PROPORTIONS

The measurement of the crown is greater labiolingually than it is mesiodistally, [on the uppers by 0.5 mm and on the lowers by 0.9 mm; averages from 637 teeth] (Appendix 3d). The root cervix measurements are even more oblong faciolingually [by 2.0 mm on uppers and 2.3 mm on lowers]. They taper lingually to be narrower on the lingual than on the labial side. See the average measurements in Table 5.1.

## 5. SIMILARITIES WITH INCISORS

a. Similar to most incisors (EXCEPT the mandibular central, where contacts are at the same level), the distal contact area is more cervical in position than the mesial (Appendix 3g).

b. Canines are wedge-shaped proximally (Appendix 3o).

c. From the proximal view, the crest of curvature on the lingual surface is on the rather bulky cingulum, which makes up the cervical third of the crown length. The remaining outline of the lingual surface (lingual ridge) is slightly concave in the middle third and is straight or slightly convex in the incisal third. Combined, the lingual outline is "s"-shaped, as in all other anterior teeth (Appendix 3q).

## C. How to Distinguish Maxillary from Mandibular Canines (Arch Traits)

Compare Figs. 5.1 and 5.2 and check the specific differences in Table 5.2

When compared to the crown of the incisor teeth, the canine crown appears thick from the mesial aspect. The cusp tip of the *maxillary* canine is located *labially* to the root axis line as on maxillary incisors, a not unexpected position, since this tooth overlaps the mandibular teeth when the jaws are closed. (Examine someone's mouth or a set of casts that fit together.) This labial to center cusp tip position from this view is an excellent criterion to use in telling maxillary from mandibular canines (arch trait; Appendix 4h). Do not forget to look for this (Figs. 3.5**B,** 5.4, and 5.7, *top row*). There are exceptions to this (see Fig. 5.3**B** where the cusp tip is on the root axis line).

**Table 5.2.** How to Distinguish Maxillary from Mandibular Canines (Arch Traits)*

| | |
|---|---|
| Labial view (Fig. 5.5) | • More acute cusp angle on uppers (maxillary about 105°, mandibular 120°)<br>• Crown of uppers is more squatty (short and wide)<br>• Length of cusp slopes (mesial is shorter, much shorter on lowers)<br>• Extra mesial bulge of crown beyond root on uppers<br>• Both contact points nearer level of cusp tip on lowers<br>• Continuous mesial crown to root outline on lowers<br>• Labial ridge more pronounced on uppers<br>• Straighter shorter root and more blunt root tip on lowers<br>• More pointed root tip and distal bend in apical one-third on uppers |
| Lingual view (Fig. 5.6) | • More pronounced lingual marginal ridges with two fossae on uppers<br>• Smooth lingual surface on lowers<br>• Attrition on uppers; none lingually on lowers<br>• Cingulum centered on uppers; off toward distal or centered on lowers<br>• Lingual ridge most prominent on uppers (46%); distal marginal ridge most elevated on lowers (63%)<br>• Wider mesial crown bulge on uppers |
| Proximal view (Fig. 5.7) | • Less prominent cingulum on lowers<br>• Location of cusp tip to root axis line—labial on uppers, lingual on lowers<br>• Labial crest of curvature closer to cervical line on lowers<br>• Slope of wear on incisal ridges—located toward labial and downward on lowers, toward lingual and upward on uppers (due to attrition) |
| Incisal view (Fig. 5.8) | • Asymmetrical crown outline on uppers—more symmetrical and oblong faciolingually on lowers<br>• Location of cusp and cusp ridges—labial to center uppers; lingual to or on center for lowers<br>• Greater faciolingual bulk compared to mesiodistal width on lowers<br>• Cingulum centered on uppers, off to distal (or centered) on lowers<br>• Distolingual crown twist on lowers<br>• Attrition on cusp ridges of lowers but on lingual surfaces of uppers<br>• Mesiodistal direction of cusp ridges—straight on uppers; distal cusp ridge is bent slightly toward lingual on lowers<br>• More bulky cusp tip on uppers due to heavy lingual ridge |

*Carefully scrutinize Figures 5.4 through 5.8 to determine how many of these suggested differences you can recognize. Some differences will be subtle, others will be readily apparent. YOU SHOULD NEVER RELY ON ONLY ONE CHARACTERISTIC DIFFERENCE between teeth to name them; rather, make a list of possibly six clues that suggest the tooth is a maxillary one to perhaps only one that makes you think it belongs in the mandible. This way you can play detective and become an expert at recognition at the same time.

Notice from the proximal view that the highest part of the *mandibular* canine cusp tip and cusp ridge after the teeth have been worn is on the lingual border, not the labial border of the cusp ridge, as it is on the maxillary canines. Wear facets on mandibular canines are found to have a labiocervical angulation or slope (facets) because they wear against the lingual surfaces of the upper teeth. You will rarely find any wear facets on the lingual surfaces of mandibular canines. (Refer to Fig. 4.4.)

# SECTION II. MAXILLARY CANINE, TYPE TRAITS

## A. Labial Aspect of the Maxillary Canine

While reading this section, refer to Figs. 5.1, *left*, 5.4, *left*, and 5.5, *top row*, for viewing similarities and the range of differences.

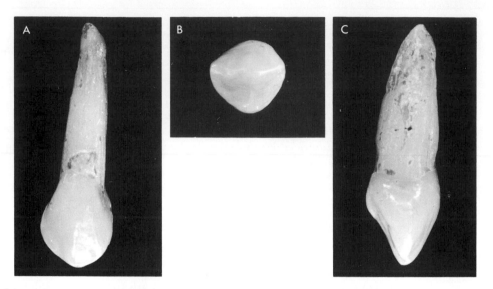

**Figure 5.4.** Maxillary right canine. **A.** Labial surface. The scar on the cervical part of the root is damage, possibly due to tooth removal. It is not part of the tooth anatomy. **B.** Incisal aspect. The labial side is toward the *top;* mesial at *right.* Note the concavity on the distal half of the labial surface, which is characteristic of this tooth. **C.** Distal surface. Notice the curvatures of the facial and lingual surface and the breadth of the root faciolingually.

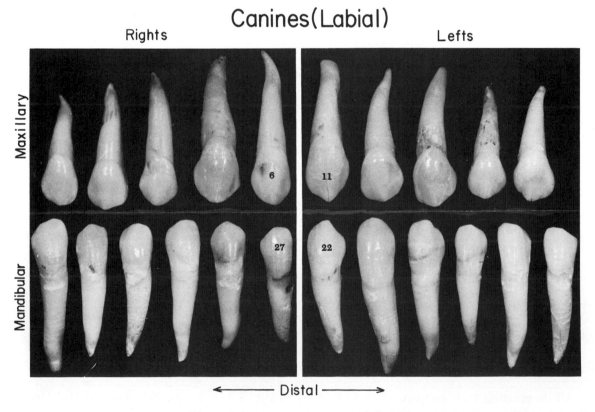

**Figure 5.5.** Canines (labial or facial view).

## *LEARNING EXERCISE*

*Examine several extracted canines and/or models as you read. Hold maxillary canines with crowns down as you examine them. Also, tear out and refer to the study pages on canines from the appendix.*

## 1. CROWN

### a. **Morphology of the Labial Surface**

The facial side of the crown is made up of three labial lobes like the incisors (Figs. 3.12**A** through **C**). (The cingulum on the lingual side of the crown is the fourth lobe.) The middle lobe on the facial forms the prominent labial ridge. Canines are the only teeth that have labial ridges. The *labial* ridge runs cervicoincisally near the center of the crown in the middle and incisal thirds. *Shallow depressions* lie mesial and distal to the labial ridge.

#### *(1) Shape and Size*

The outline of the <u>mesial</u> side of the crown is broadly convex in the middle third becoming nearly flat in the cervical third (Appendix 4b; Fig. 5.1, *left*). The *distal* side of the crown outline makes a shallow "s," being convex in the middle third and slightly concave in the cervical third (Fig. 5.1, *left*).

#### *(2) Cusp: Incisal Ridges*

The cusp has a *mesial slope* and a *distal slope* (called the mesial and distal cusp ridges or cusp arms). The mesial slope is *shorter* than the distal slope.

The *cusp tip* is usually facial to or centered on the root axis line (unless the tooth is worn). The cusp slopes and the cusp make up nearly one-third of the cervicoincisal length of the crown because the angle of the cusp approaches that of a right angle (105°) (Appendix 4c).

#### *(3) Contact Areas*

Mesial—at the junction of the incisal and middle thirds, closer to the cusp tip than is the distal contact point.

Distal—in the middle third, just cervical to the junction of the incisal and middle thirds, thereby following the characteristic of most anterior teeth where the distal contact is more cervically located than the mesial contact point. (Appendix 3g).

#### *(4) Tooth Proportions*

The crown is nearly as long as the maxillary central incisor, but the root is much longer [3.5 mm longer on the average on 719 teeth] (Appendix 3k).

## 2. ROOT

The root is long, slender, and conical. The apical third is narrow mesiodistally and the apex may be pointed or sharp. The apical third of the root often bends distally. [On 100 maxillary canines examined by Dr. Woelfel, 58 bent distally, 24 were straight, and 18 had the apical end of their roots bending slightly toward the mesial.] Three roots can be seen bending mesially in Figure 5.5 and two more can be seen in Figure 5.11. The labial surface of the root is convex (feel it).

## B. Lingual Aspect of Maxillary Canine

Refer to Figure 5.6, *upper row*, for similarities and differences.

### 1. CROWN

#### a. Lingual Ridges and Fossae

There is a lingual ridge running cervicoincisally from the cusp to the cingulum (Appendix 4d). The mesial and distal lingual fossae lie on either side of the lingual ridge and are usually shallow.

#### b. Cingulum: Centered

The *cingulum* is large. Its incisal border is sometimes pointed in the center (Fig. 11.16), resembling a small cusp or tubercle. The cingulum and the tip of the cusp are usually centered mesiodistally (Appendix 4e).

#### c. Marginal Ridges

The elevated *mesial* and *distal marginal ridges* usually are of moderate size, and the *lingual ridge* is often more prominent. The distal marginal ridge is slightly more elevated than the mesial marginal ridge (prior to attrition). [Dr. Woelfel's dental hygiene students inspected 455 maxillary canines on dental stone casts. The lingual ridge was found to be the most elevated of the three lingual ridges

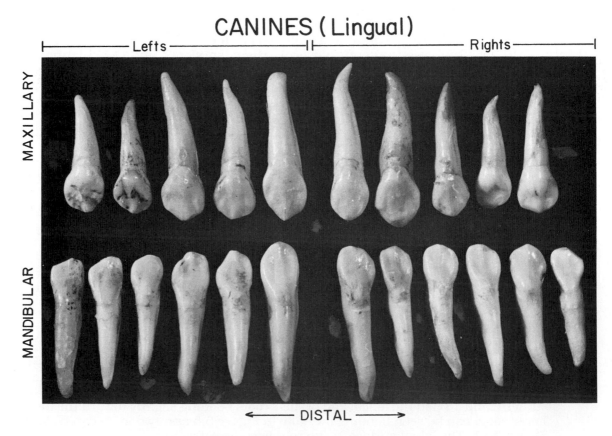

**Figure 5.6.** Canines (lingual view).

46% of the time, the distal ridge was most elevated 36% of the time, and the mesial marginal ridge was most elevated only 18% of the time.]

The mesial marginal ridge is longer than the distal marginal ridge because of the shorter mesial cusp slope and the location of the mesial contact area near the incisal third.

### d. Lingual Anatomy

Sometimes the lingual surface is naturally smooth or worn smooth from attrition so that the lingual ridge and the two fossae on either side of it are not easily discernible. By examining a number of specimens you will find some with considerable wear or attrition on the lingual surface, sometimes entirely obliterating the lingual ridge.

## 2. ROOT

The root is narrower on the lingual side than on the labial side. Therefore, it is possible to see both sides of the root and one or both of the longitudinal root depressions from this view.

## C. Proximal Aspect of Maxillary Canine

Refer to Figures 5.1, *right*, 5.3**B,** Fig. 5.7, *upper row,* for similarities and differences.

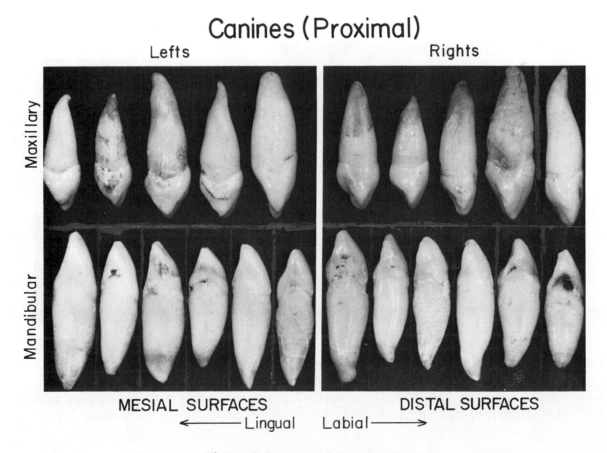

**Figure 5.7.** Canines (proximal view).

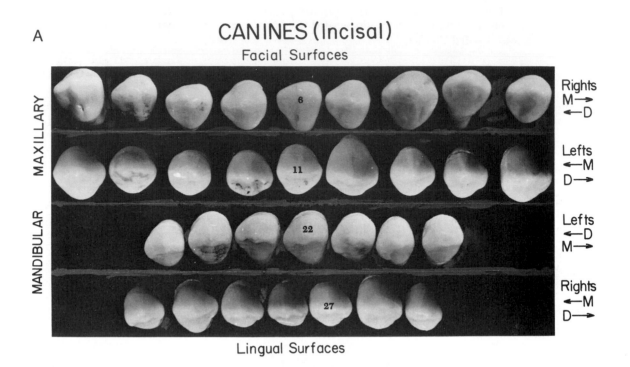

## CANINES (Incisal)
### Facial Surfaces

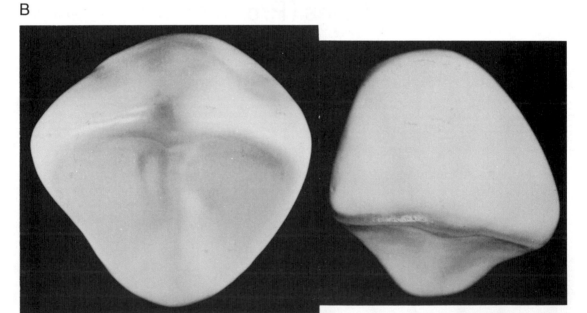

**Figure 5.8. A.** Canines (incisal view). *M* indicates the direction of the mesial sides and *D* denotes the direction of the distal sides of the 32 teeth. **B.** Incisal view of the two large, ideally shaped canine plastic tooth models. Both are right-side teeth; the smaller, more symmetric tooth is a mandibular canine. Notice that its cusp ridges are positioned lingual to the root axis line, that it has a distally located cingulum, and that it has a less prominent lingual morphology than the larger maxillary canine (*left side*).

## 1. CROWN

The wedge-shaped crown has a bulky cusp because of the labial and lingual ridges.

### a. Crest of Curvature

As with all teeth, the *labial* crest of curvature is in the cervical third of the crown (Fig. 3.5**B**) but it may not be as close to the cervical line as the corresponding curvature on the incisor teeth or on the mandibular canine. The labial surface is much more convex than on the incisors (feel it and compare the curvatures of the incisors and the canines). As with all *anterior* teeth, the *lingual* crest of curvature is in the cervical third on the cingulum.

### b. Cervical Line

The cervical line mesially curves (dips) incisally quite a bit (over 2 mm) (Fig. 5.1, *right*). The curvature is greater on the mesial surface than on the distal surface, and it is less on the canines than on the incisors. [Of the 321 maxillary canines measured by Dr. Woelfel's dental hygiene students, the mesial cervical curvature averaged 2.1 mm, with a range from 0.3–4.0 mm; the distal curvature averaged 1.6 mm with a range of 0.2–3.5 mm.] Such variability is not unusual.

## 2. ROOT

### a. Root Outline

The root is noticeably broad faciolingually in its cervical third and frequently in the middle as well (Figs. 5.1, *right*, and 5.7). The labial outline of the root is slightly convex and the lingual outline is more convex although this varies.

### b. Root Depressions; Mesial and Distal

The *mesial* root surface is broad and has a vertical depression running cervicoapically. [On 100 maxillary canines examined by Dr. Woelfel, 70 had a longitudinal depression on the mesial root surface (six fairly deep), 23 were flat, and only eight had convex mesial root surfaces.] A depression also often runs longitudinally on the *distal* aspect of the root that is more distinct than the depression on the mesial side. [Of 100 teeth examined by Dr. Woelfel, 90 had a longitudinal depression on the distal surface, 20 were rather deep, and only 10 had no distal root depression.]

## D. Incisal Aspect of Maxillary Canine

Refer to Figs. 5.1, *center*, 5.8**A,** *upper two rows*, and 5.8**B,** *left*, for similarities, differences, and comparison to a mandibular canine viewed this way.

### LEARNING EXERCISE

*To follow this description, the tooth should be held in such a position that the incisal edge (cusp tip) is toward the observer, the labial surface is at the top, and the observer is looking exactly along the root axis line. You should see more of the lingual surface because the cusp tip and the cusp slopes are labial to the root axis line.*

## 1. CROWN PROPORTIONS

The *crown outline* is not *symmetrical*. The labiolingual dimension of the crown is slightly greater than mesiodistally (0.5 mm) (Appendix 3d). This is like all mandibular anteriors but *not* like the maxillary incisors.

## 2. INCISAL EDGE (CUSP TIP) CONTOUR

The cusp tip and thick cusp slopes lie slightly labial to the mesiodistal axis line of the root, and they traverse in almost a straight line mesiodistally (Appendix 4f).

## 3. CINGULUM

The cingulum is large and is located in the center mesiodistally (Appendix 4e).

## 4. LABIAL CONTOUR

The labial surface is convex, more than either maxillary incisor, since the labial ridge is often prominent. The mesial half of the labial outline is quite convex, whereas the distal half of the labial outline is frequently somewhat concave, giving this portion of the crown the appearance that it has been pinched faciolingually (Appendix 4g). This observation is most helpful and is a reliable guide in determining right from left maxillary canines (Fig. 5.1, *center*).

## 5. LINGUAL CONTOUR

The lingual ridge divides the lingual surface in half with a shallow fossa on each side.

## SECTION III. MANDIBULAR CANINE

### A. Labial Aspect of Mandibular Canine

Refer to Figures 5.2, *left*, 5.5, *lower row*, and 5.9**A** for similarities and differences.

#### LEARNING EXERCISE

*Always hold mandibular canines with their crowns up and roots down as you examine them. This is the way they are oriented as in the mouth.*

The mandibular canine is considerably larger than either of the mandibular incisors, particularly in length and in mesiodistal width (class trait).

### 1. CROWN OUTLINE

#### a. Morphology of the Labial Surface

The labial surface is smooth and convex. A labial ridge is often present, but not as pronounced as on the maxillary canines (arch trait). In the incisal third, the crown surface is convex but slightly flattened mesial to the labial ridge, and a little more flattened distal to the ridge. (Feel it.) There may even be shallow vertical depressions on either side of the labial ridge in this region (Fig. 5.2, *left*).

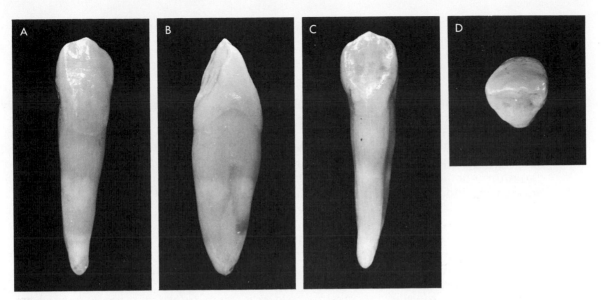

**Figure 5.9.** Mandibular left canine. **A.** Labial surface. The cusp tip is a wide angle (less steep cusp slopes); the mesial slope, to the left is shorter than the distal. **B.** Mesial surface. The crest of curvature of the facial side of the crown is close to the cervical line. **C.** Lingual side. The slight, but continuous, curvature of the full length of the tooth that results in a convex line along the mesial (*right*) side is a frequent characteristic of this tooth. (Of course, there are exceptions.) **D.** Incisal aspect. Labial side at *top;* mesial at *right.*

### (1) Crown Shape and Size

The crown appears long and narrow compared with the crown of the maxillary canine (Appendix 4a; compare Fig. 5.1, *left*, with Fig. 5.2 *left*). [It is actually 0.4 mm longer and 0.8 mm narrower; averages from 637 teeth.] The *mesial* side of the crown is slightly convex to almost flat, nearly in line with the mesial side of the root, and not projecting beyond it (Appendix 4b). This is a *conspicuous feature of this tooth* and is not seen on maxillary canines (arch trait). In other words, the mesial side of the crown does *not* bulge or project beyond the root outline.

The *distal* side of the crown may be slightly concave in the cervical third; it is convex in the incisal two-thirds. There is noticeably more of the crown distal to the root axis line than mesal to it. This often makes the crown appear to be tilted or bent distally when the root is held in a vertical position.

### (2) Cusp Tip

The *cusp tip* is usually on the root axis line and forms a more obtuse angle (120°) than the maxillary canine (Appendix 4c; compare Fig. 5.1, *left*, to Fig. 5.2, *left*). As with the maxillary canine, the *mesial slope of the cusp* is noticeably shorter than the *distal slope*, more so than on maxillary canines. (Wear on the incisal edge may alter the length of the cusp slopes, sometimes even completely obliterating the cusp.) The mesial cusp slope is also in a more nearly horizontal plane compared to the longer distal cusp ridge, which slopes more severely in an apical direction (Figs. 5.2, *left*, and 5.9**A**).

### (3) Contact Areas (Slightly More Incisal than on Maxillary Canines)

*Mesial*—in the incisal third just below the mesioincisal angle.

*Distal*—at the junction of the middle and incisal thirds, more cervically located than the mesial contact area.

## 2. ROOT

The root (Fig. 5.5, *lower row*) is convex on the labial surface and tapers apically to a somewhat blunt apex. The apical end of the root is more often straight than curving toward the mesial or distal sides. [On 100 mandibular canines inspected by Dr. Woelfel, 45 had absolutely straight roots, 29 had the apical third bending mesially, and 26 bent slightly toward the distal.] Therefore, *on mandibular canines, the root curvature should not be used to differentiate rights and lefts* (Fig. 5.5, *lower row*). Roots were shorter than the roots of upper canines [0.6 mm shorter on 637 teeth].

## B. Lingual Aspect of Mandibular Canine

Refer to Figures 5.6, *lower row*, and 5.9**C** for similarities and differences.

## 1. CROWN

The crown and the root both taper toward the lingual surface, making it narrower than the labial surface. Both sides of the roots are usually visible.

### a. Lingual Ridge and Fossae

The lingual ridge and the two lingual fossae are not prominent (Appendix 4d).

### b. Cingulum

The cingulum is low, less bulky, and less prominent than on maxillary canines. The cingulum lies just distal to the root axis line.

### c. Marginal Ridges

The marginal ridges are not prominent, and much of the lingual surface appears smooth when compared to that of the maxillary canines (arch trait).

The somewhat inconspicuous mesial marginal ridge may be longer and straighter than the shorter, more elevated and curved distal marginal ridge because the cingulum rests distal to the center. The distal marginal ridge is usually slightly more prominent or elevated than either the lingual ridge or the mesial marginal ridge. [Of 244 mandibular canines on dental stone casts inspected by dental hygiene students, the distal marginal ridge was the most prominent of the three lingual ridges on 63% of the teeth and the mesial marginal ridge was the most prominent on only 18%. The lingual ridge was most prominent only on 19% of these teeth.] On *maxillary* canines we often expect to find a more conspicuous lingual ridge [46%].

## 2. ROOT

The lingual surface of the root is convex. As with all anterior teeth, the root is narrower on the lingual side throughout its length and we can usually see an indication of the longitudinal depressions on the mesial and distal surfaces from this aspect.

## C. Proximal (Mesial and Distal) Aspects of Mandibular Canine

Refer to Figures 5.2, *right*, 5.7, *lower row*, and 5.9**B** for similarities and differences.

## 1. CROWN

The crown is wedge-shaped but thinner in the incisal portion than the crown of the maxillary canine because of a less bulky lingual ridge.

### a. Incisal Ridge

*Incisal ridge* is lingual to root axis line (Appendix 4h).

The cusp tip is most often located slightly lingual to the root axis line, but it may be centered over it. This is a good distinguishing point between mandibular and maxillary canines (arch trait). Remember that the maxillary canine cusp tip is labial to the root axis line as shown on the majority of teeth in Figure 5.7 (upper row).

The distoincisal angle is slightly more lingual in position than the cusp tip because of the distolingual twist of the crown so that much of the lingual surface is visible from the mesial aspect (similar to the mandibular lateral incisors). (Appendix 4f).

### b. Cervical Line

The cervical line appears to curve more incisally on mandibular compared to maxillary canines. The fact that the mandibular canine crown is narrower faciolingually than the maxillary canine [by 0.4 mm] and has a greater cervical line curve [by 0.3 mm] accentuates the apparent depth of the curve [averages from 637 canines]. One of the mandibular canines had a mesial cervical curvature of 4.8 mm. Another one's curve was almost flat [0.2 mm]. So, once again, the tremendous variation between the same kind of teeth is evident.

As with most other teeth, the cervical line curves [0.8 mm] less on the distal surface than on the mesial surface [curvature average 1.6 mm on 316 teeth].

### c. Crest of Curvature

The crest of curvature of the labial surface of the crown is closer to the cervical line than on a maxillary canine (compare Fig. 5.1, *right*, to Fig. 5.2, *right*). Lingually, the cingulum is low and somewhat flattened. There is an almost continuous crown-root outline on mandibular canines with minimal facial or lingual crown bulge when viewed from the proximal aspects (see Figs. 5.7, *lower row*, and 5.9**B**).

## 2. ROOT

The root has a clear depression longitudinally on the mesial and distal surfaces. The vertical longitudinal depression on the distal side of the root is often deeper than the depression on the mesial side. [Of 100 mandibular canines examined by Dr. Woelfel, 88 had a middle third mesial root depression (28 were fairly deep), eight were flat, and four were considered to be convex; of 100 mandibular canines examined by Dr. Woelfel, 97 had a longitudinal depression on the distal surface (40 were fairly deep), and only three had flat distal root surfaces. None of the distal root surfaces were judged to be convex on the middle third of the root.] See Figure 5.7, *lower row.*

## D. Incisal Aspect of Mandibular Canine

Refer to Figures 5.2, *middle*, 5.8**A**, *lower two rows*, 5.8**B**, *right tooth*, and 5.9**D** for similarities and differences.

## 1. CROWN PROPORTIONS

The labiolingual dimension of the crown is noticeably larger than the mesiodistal measurement (by an average of 0.9 mm on 316 teeth). This oblong faciolingual outline is characteristic for mandibular canines.

## 2. CROWN OUTLINE

The outline of the crown is more symmetrical than a maxillary canine (Fig. 5.8**B**). However, the labial crown outline mesial to the center line is noticeably more convex whereas the distolabial outline is more flat or concave (Figs. 5.8**B** and 5.9**D**). The crown tapers lingually, making the lingual portion considerably narrower than the labial.

## 3. CUSP TIP OR INCISAL EDGE—DISTOLINGUAL TWIST

The cusp tip is near the center labiolingually, or it may be lingual to the center. The distal cusp slope is directed slightly lingually from the cusp tip, placing the distoincisal angle in a position lingual to the position of the cusp tip (Appendix 4f). This lingual placement of the distoincisal angle gives the incisal part of the crown a slight *distolingual twist* like the mandibular lateral incisor. From this view, the distolingual twist of the crown would match closely the curvature of the dental arch (right vs. left characteristic).

## 4. CINGULUM—CENTERED OR DISTAL

On the lingual outline, the crest of curvature of the cingulum is centered or slightly distal to the center line (Appendix 4e). Thus, the mesial marginal ridge is longer than the distal marginal ridge because of the distolingual twist (which places the distal cusp ridge to the lingual) and the slight distal placement of the cingulum.

### LEARNING EXERCISE

*At this time, refer to Table 5.3 for an overview of characteristics that distinguish right from left canines.*

# SECTION IV. VARIATIONS IN CANINE TEETH

Probably the most conspicuous variation in canine teeth is found in the mandibular canine. It is not surprising to find a mandibular canine tooth with the root divided into labial and lingual parts. The division may be only in the apical third or it may extend into the cervical third of the root (Fig. 5.10). It is rare to find a maxillary canine tooth with the root similarly divided, but this division is known to occur.

Observe the enormous variation in size and shape among several maxillary and mandibular canines in Figure 5.11. Referring to the measurements of 637 canines in Table 5.1 of under the range column: maxillary canine crowns from shortest to longest varied by 5.4 mm, root length by 17.7 mm, and overall length by 18.4 mm; on mandibular canines, these respective ranges varied by 9.6, 12.7, and 18.4 mm. Can you imagine one mandibular canine with a crown 9.6 mm longer than another one? The shortest mandibular canine (cusp tip to root apex) was only 16.1 mm long. Two of the mandibular canine crowns in Figure 5.11 are 16.1 mm. See if you can spot these teeth.

**Table 5.3.** How to Differentiate Rights from Lefts

| View | Maxillary Canine | Mandibular Canine |
|---|---|---|
| Labial (Fig. 5.5) | • Mesial cusp ridge is shortest<br>• Mesial side of crown is flatter than distal<br><br>• Root tip MAY bend distally<br>• Distal contact is in a more cervical position | • Mesial cusp is shortest<br>• Mesial side of crown is in line with mesial side of root<br>• More distal bulge of crown<br>• Crown tipped distally on root<br>• Apical bend of root is POOR GUIDE<br>• Distal contact is in a more cervical position |
| Lingual (Fig. 5.6) | • Cingulum centered<br>• Strong lingual ridge (46%), then distal (36%) | • Cingulum is distal to center<br>• Prominent distal marginal ridge (63%) |
| Proximal (Fig. 5.7) | • More distinct distal than mesial root depression<br>• Greater mesial than distal cervical line curvature | • Only slight distal root depression<br><br>• Greater mesial than distal cervical curvature |
| Incisal (Fig. 5.8) | • BEST JUDGMENT OF ALL is from this view: Asymmetrical crown outline with more F-L bulk in mesial half; distal half extends out farther and seems pinched in labiolingually | • Difficult to determine except for shorter mesial cusp ridge and distal placement of cingulum |

A maxillary canine with an unusual notch on its mesial cusp slope is seen in Figure 5.12. A palatal gingival groove on the lingual side of a maxillary canine crown and root is seen in Figure 8.15**C.** A very unusual maxillary canine with a shovel-shaped lingual surface is seen in Figure 7.32.

## LEARNING EXERCISES

*Have you seen a maxillary canine with a cusp-like projection on the incisal border of the cingulum?*

*Have you seen a maxillary canine with a sharp cusp tip, a prominent labial ridge, and deep depressions mesial and distal to the ridge?*

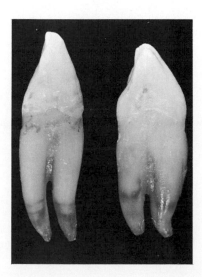

**Figure 5.10.** Two mandibular canines. The furcated root (facial and lingual) is found rarely enough to be interesting, but frequently enough not to be amazing. It would be interesting to learn the frequency of occurrence of this characteristic in different populations.

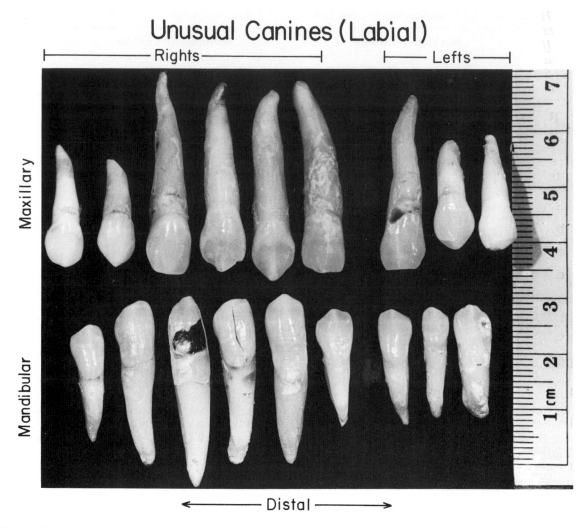

**Figure 5.11.** Unusual canines (labial view). Although sizes can vary, the shorter ones probably belonged to women and the very long ones to men.

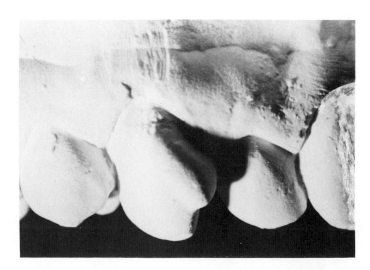

**Figure 5.12.** Maxillary right canine with an overdeveloped mesiolabial lobe and a deep notch mesial to the cusp tip.

*Have you found a mandibular canine with a facial and a lingual root? If so, how far cervically is the root divided?*

*If you have found a maxillary canine with a root divided into facial and lingual parts, you have a "real find."*

*See if you can find any canines that are longer, shorter, thicker, or thinner than the extremes given under ranges in Table 5.1.*

## QUIZ:

In the space to the left of each statement, indicate the letter of the best response from the four selections provided. Selections may be used more than once to address all the statements: *no more than one selection per statement.*

a. Maxillary central incisor

b. Maxillary canine

c. Mandibular canine

d. All of the above

( ) This tooth exhibits less cervical line curvature on the distal aspect than on the mesial aspect.

( ) The cingulum is centered mesiodistally.

( ) There is an almost continuous crown-root outline on the mesial surface of this tooth.

( ) The mesial contact area is located more incisally than the distal contact area on the same tooth.

( ) The cusp tip is positioned lingual to the root axis line from the proximal view.

( ) Mamelons could be observed on this tooth.

( ) On which tooth is the cusp angle more acute?

( ) The mesiodistal width of this tooth is greater than its labiolingual width.

( ) The mesial and distal marginal ridges are positioned more vertically than horizontally on the lingual surface.

( ) This tooth develops from four lobes.

( ) One of these teeth occludes with teeth #21 and #22.

## References

1. Cootjans G. The cuspid in Greaco-Latin literature. Rev Belge Med Dent 1971;26(3):387–392.
2. Year Book of Dentistry. Chicago: Year Book Medical Publishers, 1973:354.

## General References

Taylor RMS. Variations in form of human teeth: II. An anthropologic and forensic study of maxillary canines. J Dent Res 1969;48:173–182.

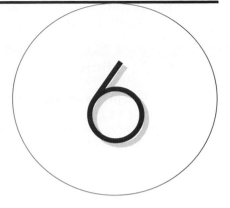

# Morphology of Permanent Premolars

The term premolar is used to designate any tooth in the permanent dentition of mammals that succeeds a primary molar.

## SECTION I. OVERVIEW OF PREMOLARS

Using the maxillary right second premolar as a representative example for all premolars, refer to the Appendix, page 5, while reading Section I of this chapter. Throughout this chapter, "Appendix" followed by a number and letter (Appendix 5a) is used to denote reference to the page (number 5) and item (letter a) being referred to on that appendix page. The appendix pages are designed to be torn out to facilitate study and minimize page turns. Other appendix pages will be referred to throughout this chapter.

### A. General Description of Premolars

There are eight premolars: four in the maxillary arch and four in the mandibular arch. They are the fourth and fifth teeth from the midline in each quadrant. The maxillary premolars can be identified by the universal numbering system as teeth #5 and #12 (maxillary right and left first premolars, respectively) and #4 and #13 (maxillary right and left second premolars, respectively). The mandibular right and left first premolars are #28 and #21, respectively, with the right and left second premolars numbered #29 and #20, respectively.

The mesial surfaces of the *first* premolars contact the distal surfaces of adjacent canines, whereas distal surfaces contact the mesial surfaces of adjacent second premolars. The distal sides of the *second* premolars are in contact with the mesial sides of the adjacent first molars.

## B. Functions

The premolars (upper and lower) function with the molars (a) in the mastication of food and (b) in maintaining the vertical dimension of the face. The first premolars (c) assist the canines in shearing or cutting food morsels and all premolars (d) support the corners of the mouth and cheeks to keep them from sagging. This is more discernible in older people.

Patients who unfortunately have lost all of their molars can still masticate or chew quite well if they still have four to eight occluding premolars.

## C. Comparison of Morphology of Premolars to Anterior Teeth

### LEARNING EXERCISE

*Compare the similarities of premolars, and differences with anterior teeth by examining ideal models of the entire arch as you read the following.*

### 1. PREMOLARS ARE SIMILAR TO ANTERIOR TEETH IN THE FOLLOWING CHARACTERISTICS

#### a. Number of Developmental Lobes

The facial or buccal surface of all premolars develop from three facial lobes, usually evidenced by two depressions separating a center ridge on the facial surface of the crown from mesial and distal portions. This buccal ridge is most pronounced in the maxillary arch (similar to the maxillary canine) and may be less conspicuous in mandibular premolars (Appendix 5a). Also, like anteriors, most premolars have one developmental *lingual* lobe. In premolars, this lobe forms one lingual cusp; in anterior teeth, it forms the cingulum. An EXCEPTION to this rule occurs in one variation of the mandibular second premolar, the three-cusp type, which develops from three facial and *two* (not one) lingual lobes (Fig. 3.12), forming two lingual cusps (not one lingual cusp, as with the other premolars). Due to the variation of this mandibular second premolar sometimes having three cusps, the term bicuspid is hardly appropriate for this group of teeth.

#### b. Taper Cervically from Proximal Crest of Curvature

From the facial, crowns are narrower in the cervical third than occlusally (Appendix 5m). This a reflection of the location of the proximal crest of curvature (or contact areas) in the incisal or occlusal to middle third.

#### c. Cervical Lines

Cervical lines (when viewed from the proximal) are convex coronally (curving toward the occlusal or incisal) (Appendix 5o) and, when viewed from the facial or lingual, the cervical line is convex toward the apex (Appendix 5n). Also, the amount of curvature is slightly greater on the mesial than on the distal.

### d. Root Shape

Lingual and facial surfaces are convex. The lingual side of the root and crown are narrower than the facial side.

## 2. PREMOLARS ARE DIFFERENT THAN ANTERIOR TEETH IN THE FOLLOWING CHARACTERISTICS

### a. Terminology Related to Tooth Surface

Compared to the anterior teeth, the *facial* surfaces of the posterior teeth are called *buccal* (resting against the cheeks) instead of *labial,* and they have *occlusal* surfaces instead of *incisal* edges. Occlusal surfaces have cusps, ridges, and grooves and are oriented in a horizontal plane.

### b. Occlusal Cusps Versus Incisal Edges

Unlike anterior teeth with incisal edges or ridges and a cingulum, premolars have one buccal or facial cusp, and most have one lingual cusp (Appendix 5b). The EXCEPTION is the mandibular second premolar which has *two* lingual cusps 54% of the time.

### c. Marginal Ridges

The marginal ridges of premolars are oriented in a horizontal plane (versus a more vertical plane in the anterior teeth) (Appendix 5c).

### d. Crown Length

The maxillary premolar crowns are *shorter* than the maxillary anterior teeth [by 0.8–3.5 mm]. The premolar roots are about the same length as the maxillary incisor roots but are shorter than the roots of the maxillary canine [by 2.5–3.1 mm for 1472 teeth]. (See Table 6.1**A**.)

### e. Crest of Curvature: Generally More Occlusally Positioned on Buccal and Lingual than on the Anterior Teeth

From both mesial and distal aspects, the crests of curvature of the buccal and lingual surfaces of the crown are more occlusal in position than the corresponding crests of curvature in the anterior teeth (Appendix 5d). In other words, the greatest bulge is farther from the cervix. An *exception* is the buccal crest of contour of the mandibular *first* premolar which may be located as far cervically as in the anterior teeth.

### f. Contact Areas

The proximal contact areas are more cervically located and broader than on anterior teeth.

## D. Other Class Traits Characteristic of all Premolars

### *LEARNING EXERCISE*

*Evaluate these similarities of all premolars while comparing models or extracted specimens of all four types of premolars from the views indicated. Also, use the study pages from the Appendix to identify the class traits. It is important to note that although general characteristics are described in this book, there is considerable variation from these de-*

*scriptions in nature (1–3) (see Table 3.2). Please remember when studying the maxillary premolars to hold them with their facial side toward you, crown down and roots upward. With lowers, have the crowns upward and the roots below. In this manner, the tooth will be oriented as it was in the mouth.*

## 1. BUCCAL ASPECT OF PREMOLARS

### a. Crown Shapes (Outline)

#### (1) *Outline shape: Pentagon (Appendix 5g)*

The crown from the buccal is broader at the level of the contact areas and more narrow at the cervix: shaped roughly like a pentagon. The mesial and distal sides of the crown from contact areas to the cervical line are nearly straight to convex.

#### (2) *Cusp Slope Size*

As with canines, when viewed from the facial, the tip of the buccal cusp is often slightly mesial to the vertical axis line of the tooth (Appendix 5h) with the mesial slope of the buccal cusp shorter than the distal slope (Appendix 5i). The EXCEPTION to this general rule is the maxillary first premolar where the buccal cusp tip is located slightly to the distal of the vertical axis line.

#### (3) *Convex Contact Areas*

Both mesial and distal sides of the crown are convex around the contact areas. Mesial proximal contacts are near the junction of the occlusal and middle thirds and the distal contacts are normally slightly more cervical, in the middle third, EXCEPT on mandibular first premolars where mesial contacts are more cervical than the distal contacts (Appendix 5e).

### b. Crown Morphology (Contours)

#### (1) *Convex*

The buccal surface is convex.

#### (2) *Buccal Ridge*

There is usually an elevation running cervico-occlusally in the middle of the crown called the buccal ridge (Appendix 5a). (This ridge is least prominent in mandibular second premolars.)

### c. Root

#### (1) *Outline*

The buccal surface of the root is convex and tapers apically (Appendix 5q).

#### (2) *Distal Bend*

The apical third is usually bent distally (Appendix 5p).

## 2. LINGUAL ASPECT OF PREMOLARS

### a. Crown Shape (Outline)

#### (1) *Taper to Lingual*

The crown is narrower on the lingual side than on the buccal side. (EXCEPTION: some three-cusp mandibular second premolars may be wider on the lingual.)

### (2) Convex

The lingual surface is convex.

## b. Root

### (1) Convex and Tapered Lingually

The lingual surface of the root is convex, and narrower mesial-distally than on the buccal.

## 3. PROXIMAL ASPECT OF PREMOLARS

### a. Triangular Ridges Form Transverse Ridges

Buccal and lingual *triangular ridges* slope from each cusp to the occlusal sulcus meeting at the central groove (Fig. 6.9). The buccal and lingual triangular ridges meet and together make up the transverse ridge, which can be best observed from the occlusal aspect. An EXCEPTION: the three triangular ridges on the three-cusped mandibular second premolar do not meet to form a transverse ridge (Fig. 6.21).

### b. Crest of Curvature

The crest of curvature of the *buccal* surface of the crown is usually at or near the junction of the middle and cervical thirds. EXCEPTION: mandibular first premolars where the buccal crest is near cervical line. The crest of curvature of the *lingual* surface of the crown is usually in the center occlusogingivally (considerably different than on the anterior teeth).

### c. Marginal Ridges

The mesial marginal ridge (Appendix 5j) is more occlusally positioned than the distal marginal ridge, so if you first look at the mesial side and then the distal side of this tooth, you should be able to see less of the triangular ridges from this mesial view. An EXCEPTION is the mandibular first premolar where the distal marginal ridge is more occlusal than the mesial marginal ridge.

## 4. OCCLUSAL ASPECT OF PREMOLARS

Refer to Figures 6.9, 6.18, and 6.21.

### a. Tooth Proportions: Wider Faciolingually than Mesiodistally

Premolars are considerably wider faciolingually than mesiodistally (Appendix 5k). (Measuring 923 premolars, their crowns were wider faciolingually by 1.2 mm and roots by 2.8 mm.)

### b. Cusp Slopes and Marginal Ridges Bound the Occlusal Table (Appendix 5l)

Both the buccal and lingual cusps have mesial and distal cusp slopes that join or meet at the tip of the cusp and merge laterally with the marginal ridges.

### c. Triangular Ridges

As seen from the proximal view (Figs. 6.7 and 6.15), the *buccal and lingual triangular ridges* extend from the tip of their respective cusps across the occlusal surface to the *central groove*. Combined, these two triangular ridges make up the transverse ridge EXCEPT on the three-cusp mandibular second premolar (Fig. 6.21).

### d. Grooves and Fossae

*The central developmental groove* runs mesiodistally across the occlusal surface. (TWO EXCEPTIONS: the mandibular first premolar and the three-cusp mandibular second premolar, which both have a distal and mesial groove instead of a central groove as seen in Figures 6.18 and 6.21.) A central groove ends mesially and distally in pits in the mesial and distal fossae. These fossae are bounded by the buccal and lingual triangular ridges, which form the sloping sides of the triangle, and the marginal ridge, which forms the base of the triangular fossa. In the distal triangular fossa, the distal end of the central groove meets the *distobuccal and distolingual supplemental or developmental grooves* and, at the point of union, there may be a distal pit.

In the mesial triangular fossa, the mesial end of the central groove meets the mesiobuccal and mesiolingual supplemental or developmental grooves and, at the point of union, there may be a mesial pit (Fig. 6.19).

### f. Proximal Contacts from the Occlusal View

Proximal contacts from the occlusal view are either on or slightly buccal to the mid-root axis (Appendix 5f).

## E. Characteristics That Differentiate Maxillary from Mandibular Premolars (Arch Traits)

Refer to Figure 6.1 while reading about differences between maxillary and mandibular premolars.

The maxillary first and second premolars are more alike than the mandibular premolars, and unlike the mandibular premolars, the maxillary first premolar is larger than the second.

### 1. LINGUAL TILT IN MANDIBULAR PREMOLARS ONLY (MAXILLARY CROWNS AND ROOT ARE ALIGNED ALONG SAME AXIS)

From either proximal aspect, the *mandibular* premolar crowns appear to be tilted lingually from the roots (the first noticeably more so than the second). This lingual tilting of the crown is characteristic for all mandibular posterior teeth and enables their buccal cusps to fit and function both beneath and lingual to the maxillary buccal cusps. (Appendix 6a; Figs. 6.7 and 6.15.)

### 2. CUSP SIZE AND LOCATION

The buccal cusp is larger than the lingual cusp (or cusps) on premolars more so on mandibular premolars (Appendix 6c and 6p). Lingual cusp tips are positioned off center to the mesial most often on maxillary premolars, and may be centered to the mesial in mandibular first and second (two-cusp) premolars.

### 3. DISTAL TILT ON MANDIBULAR PREMOLARS

From the buccal and lingual aspects, many mandibular premolar crowns, especially the first mandibular premolar, appear to be tilted distally at the cervix. This distal tilting is characteristic of all mandibular posterior teeth (including the three molars) and the mandibular canines.

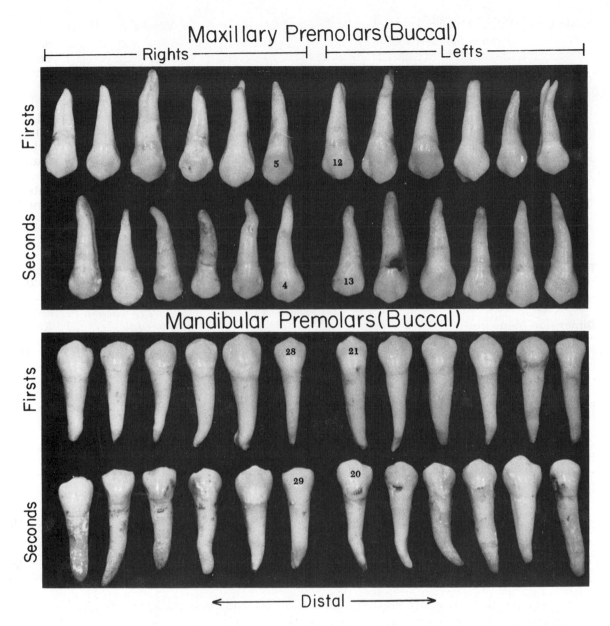

**Figure 6.1.** Maxillary and mandibular premolars (buccal view). Compare similarities and differences.

## 4. BUCCAL RIDGE PROMINENCE

The buccal ridge is not as prominent on the mandibular first premolar as on the maxillary first premolar.

## 5. PROPORTIONS

From the occlusal view, maxillary premolars are more oblong faciolingually, whereas mandibular premolars are more square (Appendix 6d).

The buccolingual and mesiodistal dimension of the mandibular premolars are more nearly equal than these dimensions on maxillary premolars where the buccolingual dimension is noticeably greater (see Table 6.1**B**).

**Table 6.1A.** Size of Maxillary Premolars (Millimeters) (Measured by Dr. Woelfel and His Dental Hygiene Students 1974–1979)

| Dimension Measured | 234 First Premolars | | 224 Second Premolars | |
|---|---|---|---|---|
| | Average | Range | Average | Range |
| Crown length | 8.6 | 7.1–11.1 | 7.7 | 5.2–10.5 |
| Root length | 13.4 | 8.3–19.0 | 14.0 | 8.0–20.6 |
| Overall length | 21.5 | 15.5–28.9 | 21.2 | 15.2–28.4 |
| Crown width M-D | 7.1 | 5.5–9.4 | 6.6 | 5.5–8.9 |
| Root width (cervix) | 4.8 | 3.6–8.5 | 4.7 | 4.0–5.8 |
| Faciolingual crown size | 9.2 | 6.6–11.2 | 9.0 | 6.9–11.6 |
| Faciolingual root (cervix) | 8.2 | 5.0–9.4 | 8.1 | 5.8–10.5 |
| Mesial cervical curve | 1.1 | 0.0–1.7 | 0.9 | 0.4–1.9 |
| Distal cervical curve | 0.7 | 0.0–1.7 | 0.6 | 0.0–1.4 |

**Table 6.1B.** Size of Mandibular Premolars (Millimeters) (Measured by Dr. Woelfel and His Dental Hygiene Students 1974–1979)

| Dimension Measured | 238 First Premolars | | 227 Second Premolars | |
|---|---|---|---|---|
| | Average | Range | Average | Range |
| Crown length | 8.8 | 5.9–10.9 | 8.2 | 6.7–10.2 |
| Root length | 14.4 | 9.7–20.2 | 14.7 | 9.2–21.2 |
| Overall length | 22.4 | 17.0–28.5 | 22.1 | 16.8–28.1 |
| Crown width M-D | 7.0 | 5.9–8.8 | 7.1 | 5.2–9.5 |
| Root width (cervix) | 4.8 | 3.9–7.3 | 5.0 | 4.0–6.8 |
| Faciolingual crown size | 7.7 | 6.2–10.5 | 8.2 | 7.0–10.5 |
| Faciolingual root (cervix) | 7.0 | 5.5–8.5 | 7.3 | 6.1–8.4 |
| Mesial cervical curve | 0.9 | 0.0–2.0 | 0.8 | 0.0–2.0 |
| Distal cervical curve | 0.6 | 0.0–1.6 | 0.5 | 0.0–1.3 |

# SECTION II. CHARACTERISTICS THAT DIFFERENTIATE MAXILLARY FIRST FROM MAXILLARY SECOND PREMOLARS

For this section, compare Figure 6.2**A** with 6.2**B,** and compare Figure 6.3**A** with 6.3**B.**

## A. Buccal Aspect of Maxillary Premolars

From the buccal view, compare the maxillary first and second premolars in Figure 6.4.

### LEARNING EXERCISE

*Compare tooth models and/or extracted maxillary premolars as you read the following characteristics, holding the crown down, root up, just as they are oriented in the mouth. The premolars, along with the molars, are known collectively as the* posterior *teeth.*

### 1. RELATIVE SIZE AND SHAPE OF CROWN: (PENTAGON SHAPE)

The crown of the maxillary first premolar is wider [by 0.5 mm] and longer [by 0.9 mm] than the second maxillary premolar crown, and its overall length is longer [by 1.3 mm; measurements on 458 teeth].

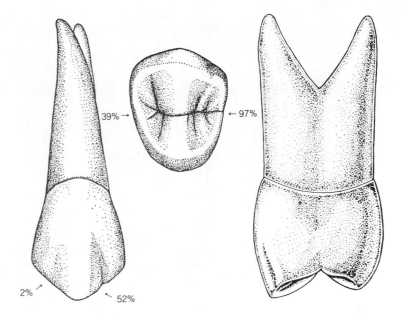

**Figure 6.2. A**. Maxillary right first premolar: buccal, occlusal, and mesial aspects. The percentages by the *arrows* give the frequency of a deeper depression in the occlusal third of the crown (buccal view) and the frequency of marginal ridge grooves (occlusal view).

The mesial and distal sides of the crown, from the contact areas to the cervical line, converge more noticeably on the maxillary first premolar than second premolar. This makes the cervical portion of the crown of the second premolar appear relatively wider.

The shoulders (junction of cusp slopes and proximal surfaces) seem more broad, bulging, and angular (especially on the mesial) on the first premolar than on the second.

### a. Contacts: Same for Both Maxillary Premolars (Appendix 5e)

Mesial contacts are usually in the middle third, near the junction of the occlusal and middle thirds. Distal contacts are slightly more cervical, still in the middle third.

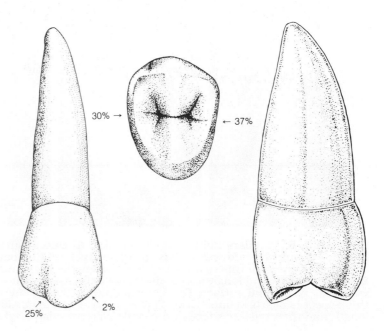

**Figure 6.2. B**. Maxillary right second premolar: buccal, occlusal, and mesial aspects. Percentages give frequency of a deeper depression in the occlusal third of the crown (buccal view) and of marginal ridge grooves (occlusal view).

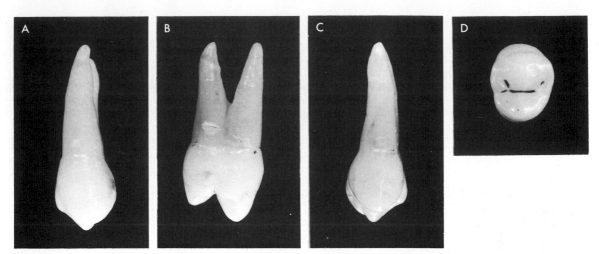

**Figure 6.3. A**. Maxillary left first premolar. **A.** Buccal surface. Notice the sharp angle formed by the two cusp slopes, and the flatter mesial than distal side of the crown. **B.** Mesial surface. Notice how short the lingual cusp is compared to the buccal cusp. Study the curvatures of the crown outline. **C.** Lingual surface. The lingual sides of the crown are convex. **D.** Occlusal surface that is not symmetric, the buccal side is at the *top,* the mesial side is at the *left.* The mesial marginal groove is clear. The lingual cusp tip is mesial to the center line. The central groove is noticeably longer than that of the maxillary second premolar (Fig. 6.8, *lower rows*).

### b. Location of Buccal Cusp Tip

The maxillary *first* premolar has its buccal cusp tip placed slightly to the distal of the vertical axis line with a longer mesial cusp slope compared to distal cusp slope (Appendix 6e) (an EXCEPTION to all other premolars and canines which have their buccal cusp tip placed more to the mesial or centered with their mesial slope shorter than their distal.) See Figures 6.3, *left,* and 6.4.

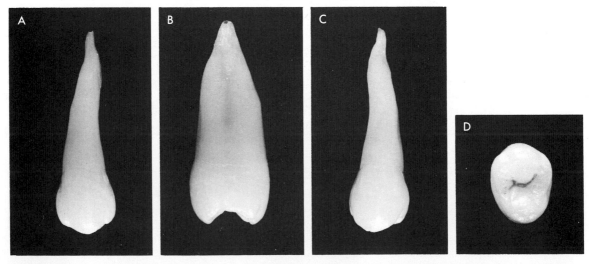

**Figure 6.3. B**. Maxillary right second premolar. **A.** Buccal surface. Note the wide cusp angle (130°), rounded shoulders, and wide cervix. **B.** Distal surface. Compare the relative lengths of the buccal and lingual cusps in this tooth with the cusp lengths in the maxillary first premolar (Fig. 6.3**A,** view **B**). Notice the typical longitudinal distal root depression without any crown depression near the cervical line. **C.** Lingual surface. **D.** Occlusal surface (mesial side toward the right). The contour from this aspect is nearly symmetrical. This is not true of the maxillary first premolar. Notice the short length and the irregular shape of the central groove compared to that of a first premolar.

# Maxillary Premolars (Buccal)

Rights        Lefts

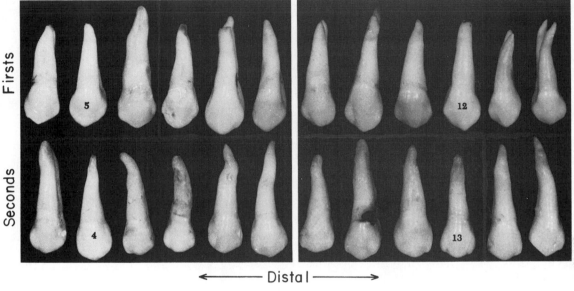

Firsts

Seconds

⟵ Distal ⟶

**Figure 6.4.** Maxillary premolars (buccal view).

### c. Shape of the Buccal Cusp

The buccal cusp of the *first* premolar is relatively long and pointed or *sharp* (Appendix 6f), resembling a maxillary canine, with the mesial and distal slopes meeting at almost a right angle (100–110°) compared to the *second* premolar, which is less pointed and *more obtuse* (125–130°).

## 2. MORPHOLOGY (CONTOURS) OF CROWN

### a. Buccal Ridge and Depressions

The buccal ridge is prominent on the maxillary first premolar (Appendix 6g). A shallow vertical depression mesial to the buccal ridge in the occlusal third of the crown was found about half of the time in the first premolars [52% of 452], but rarely on the distal [2%]. The buccal ridge is less prominent on the second premolar, and depressions were found only 27% of the time on second premolars [506 teeth].

## 3. ROOT FROM THE BUCCAL VIEW

### a. Number of Roots

Most of the time, the *first* maxillary premolar has a divided root with buccal and lingual portions or roots coming off a common trunk in the apical third (Appendix 6h; Fig. 6.3**A**). [On 200 teeth, 61% had two roots, 38% had one root, and 1% had three roots (see Fig. 6.5)]. On the maxillary first premolar (with two roots), sometimes you can see the tip of the lingual root when it is straighter or bends in a different direction than the buccal root.

### b. Length

The root of the *second* premolars is *longer* on the average than first premolars by 0.6 mm and is nearly twice as long as the crown. The root to crown ratio is 1.8:1, which is the highest for any maxillary tooth.

## MAXILLARY RIGHT FIRST PREMOLAR

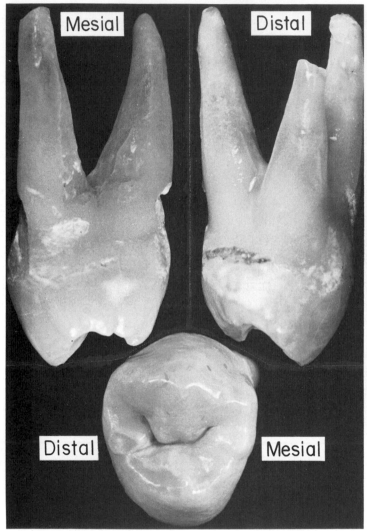

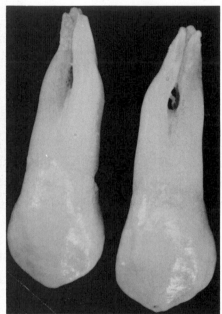

**Figure 6.5.** *Left side:* Three views of a maxillary right first premolar with two buccal roots and one lingual root (mesiobuccal, distobuccal, and lingual). There is nothing unusual about the crown of this tooth, but the roots are unusual. Except for the fact that they are less spread apart, the roots resemble those of a maxillary molar. This would be called an anomaly, but it still occurs in about 1% of maxillary first premolars. In anthropoid apes, this condition is the usual one (6). Notice the mesial crown concavity, marginal ridge groove, and typical occlusal shape. In the occlusal view, part of the mesiobuccal root is seen, an indication of its spread laterally from the distobuccal root. *Right side:* Buccal view of two other three-rooted maxillary first premolars. The roots are not as widely spread, but still show the less common division into two buccal roots.

**c. Distal Bend**

The apical end of the root of both premolars frequently bends distally [58% of 343 second premolars and 66% of 426 first premolars], but these roots may also be straight or bend mesially.

## B. Lingual Aspect of Maxillary Premolars

Compare the lingual view of maxillary first and second premolars in Figure 6.6, as well as in Figure 6.3.

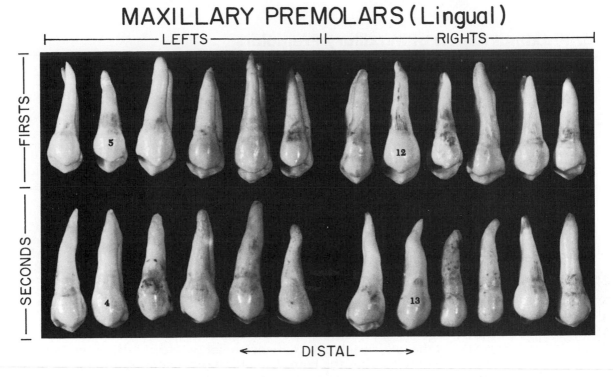

**Figure 6.6.** Maxillary premolars (lingual view). Notice the difference in lingual cusp lengths between first and second premolars.

## 1. CROWN SHAPE

### a. Taper to Lingual

The crown is a little narrower on the lingual side than on the buccal side, more on the first premolar than second premolar.

### b. Relative Cusp Size

The lingual cusp is shorter than the buccal cusp, noticeably so on the first premolar. [Maxillary first premolar lingual cusps were 1.3 mm shorter on the average, ranging from 0.3 to 3.3 mm shorter on 317 teeth; second premolar lingual cusps averaged only 0.4 mm shorter on 300 teeth.]

### c. Cusp Slopes

The mesial and distal slopes of the *lingual* cusp of the maxillary first premolars meet at the cusp tip at a somewhat rounded angle, but the angle is still sharp or steep compared to the molar cusps. The tip of the lingual cusp of the second premolar is relatively sharp.

### d. Lingual Cusp Positioned Mesially

*The tip of the unworn lingual cusp of both maxillary premolars always bends toward the mesial* (Appendix 6i). This makes it easy to tell rights from lefts.

## 2. ROOT

The lingual roots of two-rooted maxillary first premolars are shorter than the buccal roots [0.8 mm for 93 teeth]. The apical end of the *lingual* root of the teeth may bend toward either the mesial or the distal. Both first and second premolar roots taper to the lingual.

## C. Proximal Aspect of Maxillary Premolars

Compare the proximal views of maxillary first and second premolars in Figures 6.2, 6.3, and 6.7.

### 1. CROWN SHAPE (TRAPEZOID-LIKE)

#### a. Crown Morphology

Maxillary *first* premolars have a prominent *mesial concavity* cervical to the contact area; second premolars do not (Appendix 6j).

#### b. Relative Cusp Height

From this view, the buccal cusp is *noticeably longer* than the lingual cusp on maxillary first premolars. This is one of the characteristics that distinguish the maxillary first premolar from the second premolar, which has two cusps of nearly equal length [only 0.4 mm different for 300 teeth] (Appendix 6c).

#### c. Distance Between Cusps

The average distance between the cusp tips of maxillary first premolars of 5.9 mm is 65% of the total faciolingual dimension [for 243 teeth]. However, both cusp tips are located well within the boundary of the root contour, an important relationship for good functional support for a large chewing area. The second premolar distance between cusps is slightly less at 5.7 mm [on 243 teeth] or 63% of the total faciolingual dimension.

#### d. Marginal Ridge Location

The distal marginal ridge of both maxillary premolars is more cervical in position than the mesial marginal ridge, so that more of the occlusal surface is seen from the distal aspect. This phenomenon is true of all posterior teeth, with the EXCEPTION of the mandibular first premolar where the distal marginal ridge is the more occlusal one.

#### e. Marginal Ridge Grooves: Mesial Is More Common than Distal

The mesial marginal ridge of maxillary *first* premolars is almost always crossed by a developmental groove [97% of 600 maxillary first premolars] (Fig. 6.2**A**). This marginal ridge groove serves as a spillway for food during mastication (Appendix 6k). There is a distal marginal ridge groove less frequently [39% of 600 teeth].

A short mesial marginal ridge groove was found crossing the ridge of *second* premolars [37% of 641 teeth]. This is much less frequent than on maxillary first premolars. Also, a short distal marginal ridge groove is sometimes found crossing the distal marginal ridge [30% of 641 maxillary second premolars] which is slightly less common than on the mesial side (Fig. 6.2**B**).

#### f. Cervical Line

The cervical line on the mesial of the *first* premolar curves occlusally in a broad, but shallow, curvature [averaging only 1.1 mm on 234 teeth]. The curvature was slightly greater on the mesial than on the distal side of these teeth [by 0.4 mm]. The cervical line at the lingual border is in a more occlusal position than on the buccal border. This accentuates the appearance that the lingual cusp is definitely shorter than the buccal cusp.

# Maxillary Left Premolars
## Mesial Surfaces

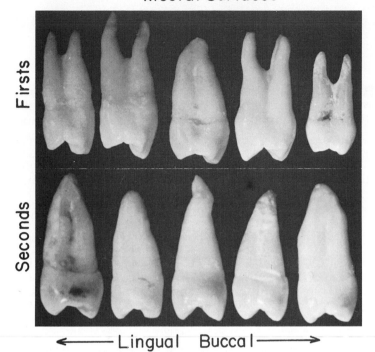

Firsts

Seconds

⟵ Lingual    Buccal ⟶

**Figure 6.7. A**. Maxillary left premolars (mesial surfaces). The first premolar roots have a deep depression compared to second premolars, which have a deeper depression on their distal root surfaces (shown below in Fig. 6.7**C**).

# Maxillary Right First Premolars
## (Distal Surfaces)

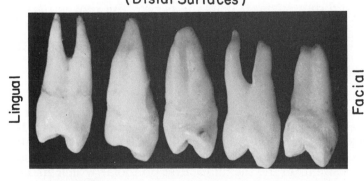

Lingual

Facial

**Figure 6.7. B**. Maxillary right first premolars (distal surfaces). Observe the shallower depressions on these root surfaces compared to the mesial sides as seen in the upper row shown in Figure 6.7**A**.

# Maxillary Left Second Premolars
## (Distal Surfaces)

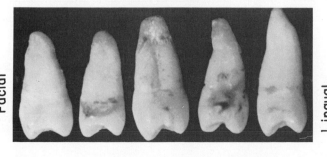

Facial

Lingual

**Figure 6.7. C**. Maxillary left second premolars (distal surfaces). Notice the deeper distal than mesial root depression (compare with the lower row in Fig. 6.7**A**).

### g. Crest of Curvature

Like most posterior teeth, buccally it is in the cervical third near the junction of the middle and cervical third; lingually it is more occlusal—in the center of the crown.

## 2. ROOT

### a. Root Outline

Frequently maxillary first premolars have *two* roots [61% of 200 teeth], one buccal and one lingual, which are distinguishing characteristics of these teeth. [On 93 two-rooted teeth, the lingual root averaged 0.8 mm shorter than the buccal root.] The bifurcation occurs in the apical third to half of the root.

In the two-root type of maxillary first premolar, the buccal and lingual roots are usually relatively straight, except for a frequent distal curvature of the buccal root near the apex (facial view). Second premolars usually have one root.

### b. Root Depressions

The roots of the premolars, when viewed from the mesial or distal aspect, often have root depressions of varying depths (Fig. 6.7**A–C**). Knowledge of the frequency with which these depressions occur, as well as the relative location and depth of these depressions, can be helpful clinically when evaluating root surfaces for the presence of calcified depositions which contribute to periodontal disease, and when identifying areas of decay on the roots.

The maxillary *first* premolar, as stated previously, is the only premolar with an obvious concavity or depression on the mesial surface of the *crown,* and this depression continues onto the root [100% of teeth studied]. Recall that this tooth usually has two roots [61% of 100 teeth] with a bifurcation in the apical third of the root. Even when there is only one root, there is a *mesial root depression.* On the *distal* root surface, near the cervix, the root is usually convex or flat with little or no depression. However, apical to the convex area, on the middle third of the undivided portion of the root, there is a depression that is found on both double- and single-rooted teeth [100% of 100 teeth]. This distal longitudinal root depression is less deep than the one on the mesial side.

The maxillary *second* premolar is likely to have a longitudinal depression on the mesial root surface [78% of 100 teeth], **but it does not extend onto the crown**. On the distal surface, there is usually a longitudinal depression in the middle third of the root, where it tends to be deeper than on the mesial root surface. This feature is the opposite from the maxillary first premolar which usually has the deepest mid-root depression on the mesial.

## D. Occlusal Aspect of Maxillary Premolars

Compare occlusal views of maxillary first and second premolars in Figures 6.2, 6.3, and 6.8.

### *LEARNING EXERCISE*

*To follow this description, the tooth should be held as those displayed in Figure 6.8, so that the buccal surface is at the top and you are sighting down the center of the vertical axis.*

# Maxillary Premolars (Occlusal)

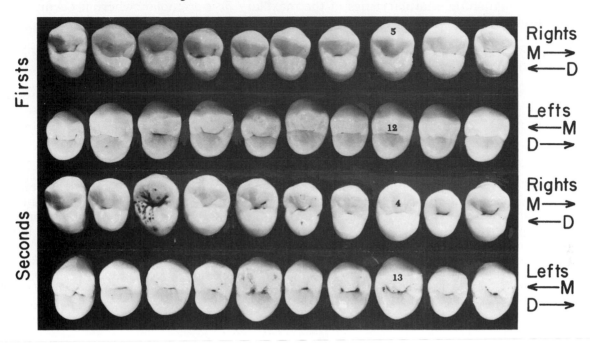

**Figure 6.8.** Maxillary premolars (occlusal view). Buccal surfaces face up, lingual surfaces face down. *M* indicates mesial surfaces; *D* indicates distal surfaces. Look for symmetry and asymmetry, central developmental groove length, the mesial marginal ridge groove, and all characteristics that help distinguish first from seconds and rights from lefts.

## 1. RELATIVE SIZE

In the same mouth, the second premolar was judged to be smaller than the first premolar in 55% of the specimens examined and larger than the first premolar in only 18% [1392 comparisons were made on dental stone casts].

## 2. GROOVES AND FOSSAE

Characteristically, a central developmental groove runs mesiodistally across the center of the tooth with a pit at both ends. The length of the central groove of the maxillary *first* premolar is *more than one-third* the mesiodistal width of the occlusal surface [average length was 2.7 mm of 408 teeth]. This length is one of the distinguishing characteristics of the maxillary first premolar (longer than the central groove on the maxillary second premolar). The groove of the second premolar averaged 2.1 mm, shorter than on first premolars by 0.6 mm [818 teeth averaged] (Appendix 6l). Compare relative groove lengths on the teeth in Figure 6.8.

Because the central groove is longer on the maxillary first premolar, the mesial and distal pits are relatively closer to the marginal ridges than on maxillary second premolars. In other words, the pits are farther apart on maxillary first premolars.

There are *fewer* supplemental grooves on maxillary *first* premolars than on maxillary *second* premolars (type trait). On seconds, there are usually supplementary grooves radiating buccally and lingually from the pit at the depth of each triangular fossa. These are named mesiobuccal supplementary groove, mesiolingual supplemental groove, distobuccal supplementary groove, and distolingual supplementary groove.

On the first premolar, a *mesial marginal groove* crosses the mesial marginal ridge on [97% of 600 first premolars]. The mesial marginal groove connects with the central groove in the mesial triangular fossa. The mesial marginal groove is one of the distinguishing characteristics of the maxillary *first* premolar, where it occurs with much greater frequency [97%] than on second premolars [39%].

Distal marginal grooves also may be found [on 39% of first premolars and 30% of second premolars], which is less frequent than *mesial* marginal grooves.

The distal triangular fossa was largest on 55% of the 184 maxillary first premolars and 53% of 209 maxillary second premolars. The mesial triangular fossa was largest on 27% of first premolars and 17% of second premolars.

## 3. RELATIVE PROPORTIONS

The asymmetrical oblong crown of the maxillary *first* premolar outline is greater buccolingually than mesiodistally [by 2.1 mm on 234 teeth]. From the occlusal aspect, the shape of the *buccal* surface is a wide and inverted V because of the prominent buccal ridge (Fig. 6.9). This is the only part of the occlusal outline that looks symmetrical. The lingual three-fourths portion of the tooth seems to be bent mesially. This asymmetrical occlusal design is a distinguishing feature of maxillary *first* premolars and is not found on most second premolars (type trait) (Appendix 6m). The mesiobuccal cusp ridge joins the mesial marginal ridge at an almost right angle (not so on second premolars). The *second* premolars are less angular, more oval shaped.

## 4. TAPER TO LINGUAL

On *first* premolars, the lingual side of the tooth is narrower than the buccal side. This lingual side taper is slight in second premolars.

## 5. LINGUAL CREST OF CURVATURE

The lingual crest of curvature is usually mesial to the center line of the tooth for both first and second premolars, with the *tip of the lingual cusp always mesial to the center of the tooth.*

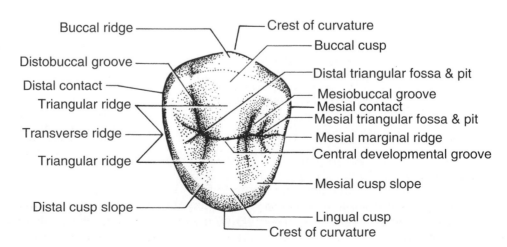

**Figure 6.9.** Maxillary right first premolar; occlusal surface. Notice proximal contact locations.

**Table 6.2.** How to Differentiate First from Second Maxillary Premolars (Type Traits)

| View | First Premolar | Second Premolar |
|---|---|---|
| Buccal (Fig. 6.4) | Shallow depression mesial to buccal ridge (occlusal one third) in 52% | Shallow depression distal to buccal ridge in 25% |
| | Larger (55%), longer, sharper buccal cusp (105°) | Smaller (55%), shorter crown, more blunt buccal cusp angle (125°) |
| | Bulging shoulders and angular outline | Narrow, more rounded shoulders |
| | Mesial cusp arm longest | Mesial cusp arm shortest |
| | Prominent buccal ridge | Smoother buccal surface (less ridge) |
| | Tapers more from contacts to cervix | Less taper from contacts to broad cervix |
| Lingual (Fig. 6.6) | Can see both cusps; lingual shorter | Both cusps nearly same length and width |
| | Crown narrower on lingual | Less taper toward lingual |
| Mesial (Fig. 6.7**A**) | Buccal cusp 1.3 mm longer than lingual | Buccal and lingual cusps same length |
| | Cusp tips seem close together | Cusp tips look spread apart |
| | Mesial crown and root depression | No crown depression near cervix |
| | Two roots or divided root often* | Single root |
| | Deep root depression | Mesial root surface relatively flat near cervix |
| | | Less deep root depression |
| | Mesial marginal ridge groove often (97%) | |
| | Cervical enamel wider than cusp tips | |
| Distal (Figs. 6.7 **B** and **C**) | Shallower distal than mesial root depression | Deeper distal than mesial root depression |
| Occlusal (Fig. 6.8) | Crown profile hexagonal and asymmetrical | Crown outline oval and symmetrical |
| | Strong lingual convergence of proximals | Little tapering toward lingual |
| | Buccal cusp inclines longer than lingual | Lingual cusp inclines almost as long as buccal |
| | Longer central groove | Short central groove |
| | Mesial marginal ridge groove often (97%) | Less common mesial marginal ridge groove (37%) |
| | Prominent buccal ridge | Less bulge for buccal ridge |
| | Mesiobuccal cusp ridge and marginal ridge meet at right angle | Obtuse angle at mesiobuccal corner |
| | Distal contact is most buccal | Mesial contact is most buccal |
| | Few supplemental grooves | More supplemental grooves |
| | Mesial side concave or flat and short; distal side curved or convex and longer | Two sides of crown are more symmetrical |
| | Triangular fossae close to marginal ridges | Triangular fossae smaller and farther in from marginal ridges |

*Not always; don't be fooled. Look for other features as well. As many as 38% have only one root.

## 6. OUTLINE (COMPARE TO HEXAGON)

The mesial outline of the *first* premolar and the mesial marginal ridge form a nearly straight or concave (bent inward) outline buccolingually, which is shorter buccolingually than the more convex distal marginal ridge (compare this characteristic in Fig. 6.9).

**Table 6.3.** How to Differentiate Right from Left Maxillary Premolars

| View | First Premolar | Second Premolar |
|------|----------------|-----------------|
| Buccal (Fig. 6.4) | Longer mesial cusp ridge<br>Depression mesial to buccal ridge 52% (occlusal third) (46% had none)<br>Root curves to distal (66%) | Shorter mesial cusp ridge<br>Depression distal to buccal ridge 25% (occlusal third) (73% had none)<br>Root curves to distal (58%) |
| Lingual (Fig. 6.6) | Lingual cusp is bent toward the mesial* | Lingual cusp is bent toward the mesial* |
| Proximal (Fig. 6.7) | Greater mesial than distal cervical line curvature<br>Height of marginal ridges (distal is more cervical)*<br>Deeper mesial than distal root depression<br>Mesial crown depression (100%) and mesial marginal ridge groove (97%)* | Greater mesial than distal cervical line curvature<br>Height of marginal ridges (distal is more cervical)*<br>Deeper distal than mesial root depression<br>No mesial crown depression, mesial marginal ridge groove only 37% of the time |
| Occlusal (Fig. 6.8) | Larger, deeper distal triangular fossa (55%)<br>Lingual cusp tip toward mesial<br>Mesial crown outline is flat, distal is curved (same for marginal ridges)*<br>Mesial marginal ridge groove (97%)<br><br>Longer more convex distal marginal ridge<br>Mesiobuccal corner is a right angle | Larger, deeper distal triangular fossa (53%)<br>Lingual cusp tip toward mesial<br>Slightly longer and more convex distal marginal ridge and crown outline<br>Infrequent marginal ridge grooves (mesial 37%, distal 30%)<br><br><br>Mesiobuccal corner is an obtuse angle |

*Most reliable guides for differentiating rights from lefts only (NOT for differentiating first from second premolars)

Seen from the occlusal aspect, the *second* premolar is typically much more symmetrical than the first premolar. The occlusal outline of the second premolar is less angular than that of the first premolar and has an oblong or oval shape. (Compare several first and second premolars from the occlusal view as in Figure 6.8.) The buccal ridge on the second premolar is less prominent than on the first premolar.

## 7. CONTACT AREAS FROM THE OCCLUSAL ASPECT

*Mesial* contacts are near or at the junction of the buccal and middle thirds (slightly more buccal on first premolars). Recall that one-third of the tooth from this aspect means one-third of the total buccolingual measurements of the crown, rather than one-third of the occlusal surface measurement (Fig. 6.9).

*Distal* contacts are in the middle third on *second* maxillary premolars, located more *lingually* than mesial contacts. Just the opposite is true on first premolars with their asymmetry, where the *distal* contact is more *buccal* than the mesial contact.

### LEARNING EXERCISE

*Review the summary of characteristics that differentiates the maxillary first from second premolars (Table 6.2) and the maxillary right from left premolars (Table 6.3).*

# SECTION III. CHARACTERISTICS THAT DIFFERENTIATE MANDIBULAR FIRST FROM MANDIBULAR SECOND PREMOLARS

For this section, compare mandibular first and second premolars in Figure 6.10**A** with 6.10**B**.

## A. Two Types of Mandibular Second Premolars

There are two common types of mandibular second premolars (3): a two-cusp type with one lingual cusp, and a three-cusp type with two lingular cusps. (Fig. 6.10**B**). The frequency of these two types on 808 dental hygiene students from Ohio is given in Table 6.4.

*LEARNING EXERCISE*

*Look in your own mouth and determine which of these categories matches your mandibular second premolars. Both types are seen in Figure 6.16 (lower three rows). The three-cusp type occurs with only slightly greater frequency than the two-cusp type [54.2% of 532 teeth for three cusps type versus 43.0% for the two-cusp type.]*

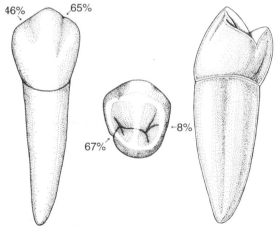

**Figure 6.10. A**. Mandibular right first premolar, buccal, occlusal, and mesial aspects. Percentages (buccal view) give frequency of notches on cusp ridges, and in the occlusal view (*center*) the occurrence of marginal ridge grooves.

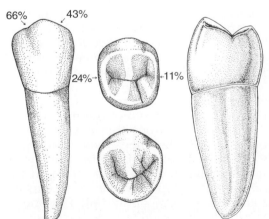

**Figure 6.10. B**. Mandibular right second premolar, buccal and mesial aspects (either type); occlusal aspect, three-cusp type (*above*) occur 54.2% of the time, compared to the two-cusp type (*below*) which are found in 43% of mandibular second premolars. Percentages shown list the frequency of cusp ridge grooves (*left*) and of marginal ridge grooves (*above center*). When comparing the two-cusp type (*below center*) and the three-cusp type (*above center*), the occlusal surface of the three-cusp type is more square or rectangular.

**Table 6.4.** Occurrence of Lingual Cusps on Mandibular Second Premolars (808 Females, 1532 Teeth)

| Number and Frequency | | Percentage | Comment |
|---|---|---|---|
| 2 lingual cusps on both sides | | 44.2% | Almost half |
| 1 lingual cusp on both sides | | 34.2% | One-third |
| 2 lingual cusps on one side | | 18.2% | One-fifth |
| 3 lingual cusps on both sides | | 1.7% | } 1 in 29 |
| 3 lingual cusps on one side | | 1.7% | |
| Overall frequency | 3-cusp type | 54.2% | } 1532 teeth |
| | 2-cusp type | 43.0% | |
| | 4-cusp type | 2.8% | |
| Same type on both sides | | 80.1% | } 702 comparisons |
| Different type on each side | | 19.9% | |

## B. Distinguishing Characteristics of Mandibular Premolars

The morphologic details of mandibular premolars are difficult to describe because of the great amount of variation. To list all of the frequent variations would lead to confusion rather than to clarification. Bear in mind while studying these teeth that one description will not exactly fit every tooth (1–3). Most descriptions in this book are for unworn teeth. Most extracted tooth specimens will have signs of attrition and caries.

In general, the *first* mandibular premolar has a longer crown [by 0.6 mm] and a shorter root [by 0.3 mm] than does the second premolar [average measurements of 465 teeth], and it is slightly longer overall than the second.

### LEARNING EXERCISE

*Examine several extracted mandibular premolars or models as you read. Hold them with the crowns up and the roots down.*

### 1. BUCCAL ASPECT OF MANDIBULAR PREMOLARS

Refer to views from the buccal of mandibular first and second premolars in Figures 6.10, 6.11, and 6.12.

#### a. Crown Shape

##### (1) Shape (Outline): Short Symmetrical Pentagon Shape with Slight Distal Tip

The mandibular *first* premolar appears nearly symmetrical except for the shorter mesial cusp ridge and the distal bulge of the crown. Some teeth have a slight *distal tilt* of the crown on the root. As with all premolars, the shape is roughly a pentagon. The crown of the second premolar has a more square (still a pentagon) appearance because it is shorter overall and is wider in the cervical third than the first premolar (Fig. 6.12).

The shape of the buccal surface of the *second* premolar is similar on both two-cusp and three-cusp type. The crown of the mandibular second premolar bears some resemblance from this aspect to the mandibular first premolar, but there are differences (type traits) that make second premolars easily distinguishable (Table 6.5). The buccal cusp of the mandibular *second* premolar is *less pointed* than on the mandibular first premolar, and the cusp slopes are less steep (meeting at a more obtuse angle of about 130°) (Appendix 6n). The buccal cusp of the mandibular *first* premolar appears long and sharp, is cen-

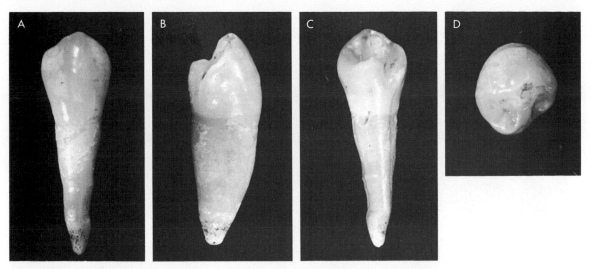

**Figure 6.11. A**. Mandibular left first premolar. **A.** Buccal surface. **B.** Mesial surface. The lingual cusp is very short. The mesiolingual groove lies between the lingual cusp and the mesial marginal ridge. Notice the curvature of the facial and lingual surfaces. The buccal cusp tip is about on the root axis line. **C.** Lingual surface. Much of the occlusal surface is visible because of the shortness of the lingual cusp. In this figure, you can see that the mesial marginal ridge (on the *right*) is more cervical in position than the distal marginal ridge. The distal half is more like a molar and the mesial half is more like a canine. This is a unique feature of this tooth. **D.** Occlusal surface. The mesial and distal fossae are circular, not triangular, and there is a large transverse ridge separating them. A barely visible central groove crosses the transverse ridge. Notice the greater bulk of tooth buccolingually in the distal half (on the *left*).

tered over the root, and looks much like a maxillary canine from this aspect. The cusp slopes meet at a nearly right angle (110°). The buccal cusp is longer, sharper, and more pointed than the buccal cusp on second premolars (type trait).

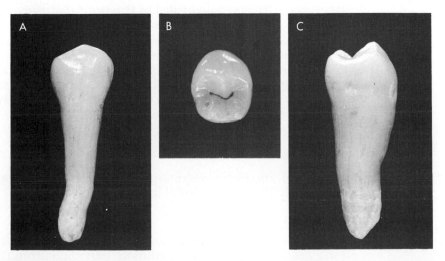

**Figure 6.11. B**. Mandibular right second premolar, three-cusp type. **A.** Buccal surface. **B.** Occlusal surface. Buccal side at *top*; mesial at *left*. The two lingual cusps of this tooth are nearly equal in size. Here, it is difficult to tell which is larger; but the mesiolingual cusp (on the left) is larger than the distolingual. Notice the configuration of the long mesial and shorter distal groove. There is no central groove. **C.** Distal surface. Notice the difference in buccal and lingual cusp height, and also the curvature of the buccal and lingual surfaces.

# Mandibular Premolars (Buccal)

Rights           Lefts

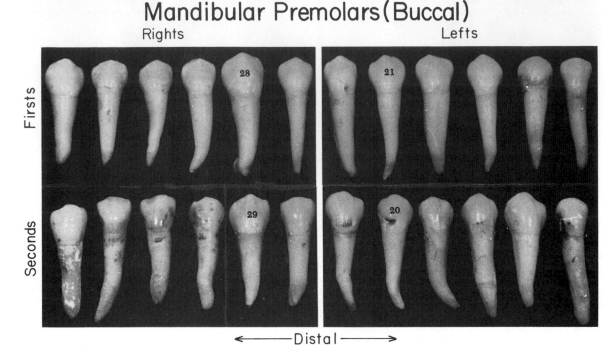

Firsts

Seconds

←——— Distal ———→

**Figure 6.12.** Mandibular premolars (buccal view).

### (2) Notches on Cusp Ridges: Common on Cusp Arms

Shallow notches are commonplace on both cusp ridges on unworn premolars. These notches serve as spillways for food during mastication (sometimes called Thomas notches named after a dentist, Peter K. Thomas, who strongly recommends carving them in all occlusal restorations and crowns because spillways for food are so important).

The most common occurrence and frequency of such notches and of depressions in the occlusal third of the buccal surface on the cusp ridges seen on mandibular premolars is evident in Figures 6.10 and 6.13. On the mandibular *first* premolar, the shorter mesiobuccal cusp slope is more likely to have a notch [65% of 1348 teeth] than the longer distobuccal cusp ridge [46% of 1348 teeth]. The notches on the mesial cusp ridges were most pronounced. On the mandibular *second* premolar, the frequency of notches is reversed. It is more likely to have a notch on the distal cusp slope [66% of 1522 teeth] than on the mesial cusp slope [43% of 1522 teeth].

### (3) Cervical Lines

The cervical line of the second premolar curves less (is more flat) mesiodistally than on first premolars.

### (4) Contact Areas

Because of the greater length of the buccal cusp, the contact areas on the *first* premolar are located more cervically from the cusp tip than they are on mandibular second premolars. On mandibular *second* premolars, both contact areas are positioned closer to the cusp tip, or are in a more occlusal position, than on the mandibular first premolars because the seconds' cusp slopes join at a less steep angle [Figs. 6.10 and 6.12].

**Table 6.5.** How to Differentiate First from Second Mandibular Premolars (Type Traits)*

| View | First Premolar | Second Premolar |
|---|---|---|
| Buccal (Fig. 6.12) | Longer crown<br>More pointed cusp (110°)<br>Notch on mesial cusp slope (65%)<br>Lower mesial than distal contact<br>More taper from contacts to cervix<br>Shorter root with pointed apex<br>Sometimes occlusal third depression mesial to buccal ridge (17%)<br>More prominent buccal ridge | Shorter wider crown<br>Less pointed cusp (130°)<br>Notch on distal cusp slope (66%)<br>Lower distal than mesial contact<br>Relatively wider at cervix<br>Longer root with blunt apex<br>Sometimes occlusal third depression distal to buccal ridge (25%)<br>Less prominent buccal ridge |
| Lingual (Fig. 6.14) | Crown much narrower on lingual<br>Lingual cusp very short and narrow<br>Can see most of occlusal surface<br>Nonfunctional lingual cusp<br><br>Can see lower mesial marginal ridge with mesiolingual groove | Crown quite wide on lingual<br>One or two functional lingual cusps, less short than first premolar<br>Cannot see much of occlusal surface<br>Mesiolingual cusp widest (three-cusp type)<br>Lingual groove if two lingual cusps<br>Lingual cusp or cusps are functional |
| Mesial (Fig. 6.15, *left*) | Crown tipped severely to lingual<br>Lingual cusp much shorter than buccal cusp (nonfunctional)<br>Low mesial marginal ridge is parallel to triangular ridge of buccal cusp<br>Can see much of occlusal surface<br>Root depression on 45%<br><br>Mesiolingual groove on 67%<br>Root may be divided in apical third | Less crown tilt toward lingual<br>Lingual cusp slightly shorter than buccal cusp<br>Mesial marginal ridge high and in horizontal plane<br><br>Cannot see much of occlusal surface<br>Mesial root surface is flat or convex on 81%<br>No mesiolingual groove<br>Root not divided |
| Occlusal (Figs. 6.16, 6.17, and 6.18 compared to 6.21) | Nonsymmetrical crown outline<br>Small occlusal, a nonfunctional surface<br>Convergence toward lingual, especially on mesial side<br>Mesial cusp arm and marginal ridge join at right angle<br>Mesiolingual groove (67%)<br>Two circular fossae-two grooves (mesial and distal)<br><br>Developmental grooves run buccolingually<br>Definite transverse ridge | Square crown outline<br>Larger occlusal surface (is functional)<br><br>Crown may be wider on lingual than buccal (three-cusp type)<br>May have lingual groove (three-cusp type)<br>No mesiolingual groove<br>Two-cusp type-two circular fossae<br>Three-cusp type-three fossae (three grooves: mesial, distal, lingual)<br><br>No transverse ridge |

*Because of the morphologic variations in mandibular premolars, you may not find all of these characteristics every time.

Mesial contacts of both mandibular premolars are near the junction of the occlusal and middle thirds (slightly more occlusal on second premolars).

The *distal* contact of the mandibular *second* premolar follows the general rule: slightly cervical to the mesial contact area (Appendix 6o). EXCEPTION TO ALL THE OTHER TEETH: *The distal contact area of the mandibular first premolar is usually slightly more occlusal in position than the mesial contact area (one of only two teeth that have a more*

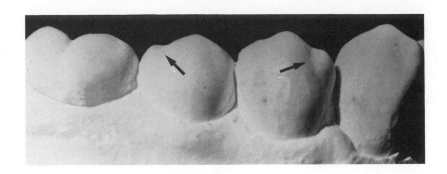

**Figure 6.13.** Mandibular first and second premolars depicting the most common type of notch on the buccal cusp ridges with a shallow depression beneath it on the buccal surface (see *arrows*). These depressions in these locations were found in 17% of first premolars and 25% of second premolars.

*occlusally [incisally] located distal than mesial contact;* the other tooth is the deciduous maxillary canine).

### (5) Morphology

The buccal ridge of both mandibular premolars is less discernible than on the maxillary premolars. On the *first* premolar there is a minimal tendency for a vertical depression in the occlusal third of the buccal surface on either side of the indistinct buccal ridge (Fig. 6.13) [80% of 285 teeth had a smooth buccal surface in the occlusal third without depressions, 17% had a deeper depression on the mesial side of the buccal ridge, and only 3% had a deeper distal depression].

On the *second* premolar, there may be either a flattened area or a slight depression on the occlusal third of the buccal surface mesial and distal to the buccal ridge. [Only 26% of 328 teeth had any discernible depressions; of these, 25% had a deeper distal than mesial depression, and only 1% had a deeper mesial depression.] This differs from the first premolar.

### (6) Root (Buccal Aspect)

The root of mandibular premolars tapers gradually to the apex. The root is noticeably more blunt on mandibular second premolars than on first premolars. As with most roots, there is a tendency for the apical third of the root to bend distally [on 58% of 424 teeth mandibular first premolars and 62% of 343 teeth mandibular second premolars. The tendency for a mesial bend was 23% and 17% on first and second premolars, respectively.]

### b. Root Shape (Two-Cusp Type and Three-Cusp Type)

The root of the mandibular second premolar appears thicker (0.2 mm wider mesiodistally) and is longer than the root of the first premolar. The root of the mandibular second premolar is nearly twice as long as the crown, with a root-to-crown ratio of 1.80:1, the highest of any permanent tooth except for the mandibular first and second molars and maxillary second premolars.

## 2. LINGUAL ASPECT OF MANDIBULAR PREMOLARS

For the lingual aspect, refer to lingual views of mandibular first and second premolars in Figures 6.11**A,** *view C,* and 6.14.

### a. Crown Shape

#### (1) Taper to Lingual

On mandibular *first* premolars, the crown is much narrower on the lingual side than on the buccal side. This can also be seen on

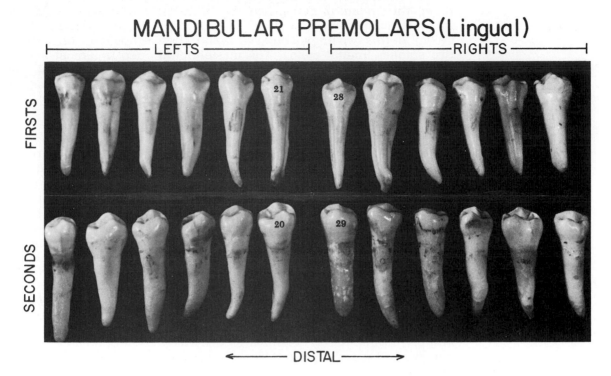

**Figure 6.14.** Mandibular premolars (lingual view). Note the different heights of the mesial and distal marginal ridges, the reduced height of the lingual cusps, and the marked taper of the crown toward the lingual side on first premolars. Observe the more blunt root apexes, higher lingual cusps, and wide lingual side of the crown on the second premolars. Not all of the roots bend toward the distal.

mandibular second premolars with one lingual cusp. The width of the lingual side of the second premolar with two lingual cusps is usually as wide or wider mesiodistally than the buccal side. Only this tooth and some maxillary first molars have their crowns wider on the lingual side than on the buccal side.

### (2) Lingual Cusp Size and Shape

The lingual cusp of the *mandibular first premolar* is small and is often pointed at the tip. It is nonfunctional, and could be considered a transition between the canine cingulum and prominent lingual cusp of the second premolar. Sometimes there are two or more lingual cusps or cusplets (Fig. 2.8**A**, *left side*). This tooth may have almost no lingual cusp or as many as four lingual cusplets. Much of the occlusal surface of this tooth can be seen from the lingual aspect because of the most obvious *shortness* of the lingual cusp. [Of 321 first premolars measured, the lingual cusp averaged 3.6 mm shorter than the buccal cusp (range from 1.7 to 5.5 mm shorter).]

On *second premolars with one lingual cusp,* the single lingual cusp is smaller than the buccal cusp, but it is larger (longer and wider) than the lingual cusp of the first premolar. This single lingual cusp is either just *mesial* to (often) or on the center line of the root (Appendix 6q). The mesial and distal slopes of the lingual cusp merge into the mesial and distal marginal ridges. There is sometimes a slight depression where the distal cusp slope joins the distal marginal ridge, perhaps a remnant of where the other lingual cusp would have been.

*On the second premolar with two lingual cusps* [present 54% of the time], the *lingual groove* passes between the mesiolingual and distolingual cusps and extends slightly onto the lingual surface of the crown. In this two lingual cusp variation, there is one large buccal and two smaller lingual cusps. The mesiolingual cusp is almost always larger and longer than the distolingual cusp [90% of 818 teeth]. The two lingual cusps were rarely equal in size [only on 3%] nor was the distolingual cusp larger [only 7%] (Fig. 6.20).

### (3) Marginal Ridges

As with most other posterior teeth, the distal marginal ridge of the *second* mandibular premolars is the slightly more cervically located of the two ridges (Fig. 6.14, *lower row*). An EXCEPTION to all other adult teeth is the mandibular *first* premolar, the only adult tooth where the mesial marginal ridge is more cervically located than the distal marginal ridge. See Figure 6.11**A.** This may be more apparent when comparing the mesial and distal aspects, than viewing the tooth from the lingual.

### (4) Mesiolingual Groove on Mandibular First Premolars

On mandibular first premolars there is frequently a *mesiolingual groove* separating the mesial marginal ridge from the mesial slope of the small lingual cusp (Fig. 6.11**A** and Appendix 6r) [present in 67% of 609 first premolars]. Rarely, a similar groove was present between the distal marginal ridge and the distal slope of the lingual cusp [8% of these 609 first premolars].

## b. Root

The root of second mandibular premolars is tapered and is slightly longer than the root of first premolars [0.3 mm longer on average for 465 teeth].

## 3. PROXIMAL ASPECT OF MANDIBULAR PREMOLARS

For the proximal views of mandibular first and second premolars, refer to Figures 6.10, 6.11, and 6.15.

### a. Crown Shape (Rhomboid Shape)

### (1) Lingual Tilt, Cusp Size and Proportion

As on all mandibular posterior teeth, the crown of the mandibular *first* premolar tilts noticeably toward the lingual surface at the cervix (much more than any other premolar). This tilt places the tip of the buccal cusp almost over the root axis line (*upper row* in Fig. 6.15). As seen from the lingual aspect, the lingual cusp of the mandibular first premolar is shorter than the buccal cusp by more than one-third of the total crown length [3.6 mm average for 321 teeth]. By virtue of being so short and narrow mesiodistally, it is a nonfunctioning cusp (Appendix 6p). The tip of the short lingual cusp results in the cusp tip location usually in line vertically with the lingual outline of the cervical portion of the root.

The mandibular *second* premolar crown (both types) also tips lingually, but not as much as the mandibular first premolar (*lower row* in Fig. 6.15). As with the first premolar, the tip of the lingual cusp (or of the mesiolingual cusp) of this second premolar is usually about on a line with the lingual surface of the root (Fig. 6.10**B,** *right*).

## Mandibular Right Premolars (Proximal)

MESIAL SURFACES                    DISTAL SURFACES

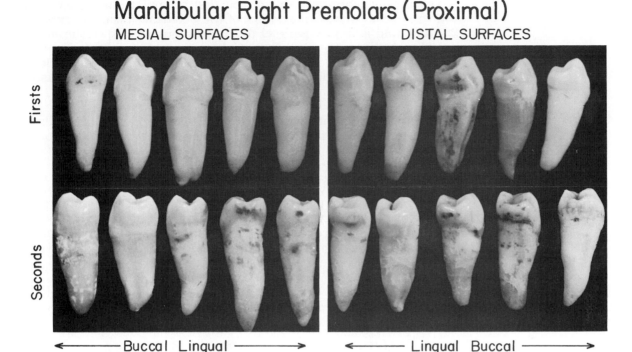

**Figure 6.15.** Mandibular right premolars (proximal view). Compare mesial and distal marginal ridge heights.

In the *two-cusp type of second premolar,* the lingual cusp is also shorter than the buccal cusp, but not as much so as in the first premolar. In the *three-cusp type of second premolar,* the mesiolingual cusp is shorter than the buccal cusp. From the mesial, the mesiolingual cusp conceals the still shorter distolingual cusp when the tooth is examined from the mesial aspect, while from the distal aspect, both lingual cusp tips are usually visible.

The lingual cusp (or mesiolingual cusp for three-cusp types) of *second* premolars is closer in length to the buccal cusp than on first premolars: [average of 1.8 mm shorter than the buccal cusp; range 0.1–3.8 mm for 317 teeth]. Remember that on the first premolars, the lingual cusps averaged 3.6 mm shorter than the buccal cusps. Compare this difference in Figure 6.15. The tip of the buccal cusp of the mandibular second premolar is usually located on a line that would divide the crown vertically into buccal and middle thirds.

### (2) *Marginal Ridge*

On the mandibular *first* premolar, the mesial marginal ridge is usually located more cervically than is the distal marginal ridge. *This is the ONLY posterior tooth in which this is true.* The relative positions and height of the mesial and distal marginal ridges on this tooth frequently put the mesial contact area cervical to the distal contact area. This is an EXCEPTION to the usual finding that mesial contacts are more occlusal (incisal) than distal contacts. The distal marginal ridge of this first premolar is longer from buccal to lingual than the mesial marginal ridge, and it is in a more horizontal position compared to the mesial marginal ridge which slopes cervically at nearly a 45° angle from the buccal cusp.

The mesial marginal ridge of the *first* premolar slopes cervically from the buccal toward the center of the occlusal surface at nearly a 45° angle and is nearly parallel to the triangular ridge of the buccal cusp (Appendix 6s, Fig. 6.11**A,** *mesial view,* and Fig. 6.23**B**). This feature alone is most helpful in differentiating rights from lefts (by identifying the mesial surface). *The triangular ridge of the lingual cusp* is short and is in a nearly *horizontal* plane (Fig. 6.15, *upper row*).

The mesial marginal ridge of the *second* premolar is occlusally located hiding much of the occlusal surface from view (*lower left row* in Fig. 6.15).

### (3) Marginal Ridge Grooves on Second Premolars

The *mesial marginal* ridge is *in*frequently crossed by a marginal ridge groove [21 of 100 teeth]. The *distal* marginal ridge is concave, somewhat longer buccolingually, and definitely in a more cervical position than the mesial marginal ridge (compare mesial and distal views in Fig. 6.15). Only rarely is it crossed by a marginal ridge groove [4 of 100 teeth].

### (4) Mesiolingual Grooves on First Premolars

When present [67% of the teeth studied] the *mesiolingual groove* on mandibular *first* premolars lies between the mesial marginal ridge and the mesial slope of the lingual cusp in the lingual third of the tooth (Figs. 6.10**A** and 6.11**A**). There is seldom a groove between the distal marginal ridge and the distal slope of the lingual cusp [8% of 609 mandibular first premolars]. This mesiolingual groove is not present on mandibular second premolars.

### (5) Crest of Curvature

In general, the crest of curvature of the mandibular premolar crown on the *buccal* is near the junction of the cervical and middle thirds. The mandibular first premolar is an EXCEPTION: the buccal crest of contour of the first premolar crown is just occlusal to the cervical line. The buccal outline of the mandibular second premolar crown is flatter or less convex than the first premolar from the crest of curvature to the cusp (Fig. 6.15, *lower left five teeth*).

For all premolars, the crest of curvature of the *lingual* surface of the crown is about in the *center* of the total crown length. In the mandibular first premolar, this is not far from the tip of the lingual cusp (Figs. 6.10**A,** *right,* and 6.15). Because of the extreme lingual tilting of the crown, the lingual surface of both mandibular premolar crown extends lingually beyond the lingual surface of the root.

### (6) Cervical Lines

Similar to other teeth, the occlusal convexity or the curve of the cervical line on premolars is greater on the mesial than on the distal. [The mesial cervical line of the mandibular first premolar curves an average of 0.9 mm for 238 teeth versus 0.6 mm on the distal; mesial of second mandibular premolar curves occlusally an average of 0.8 mm for 227 teeth versus 0.5 mm (almost flat) on the distal.] It is more occlusally located on the lingual than on the buccal, more so on *first* premolars, by as much as 2 mm. This makes the crowns appear to be quite short on the lingual side.

### (7) Root (From the Proximal)

On the mandibular *first* premolar, often the outline of the root is nearly straight on the buccal and lingual sides in the cervical third, or even in the cervical half, and then it tapers apically to a blunt end (Figs. 6.10**A** and 6.15). Occasionally, the mandibular first premolar will have a furcated root, i.e., the apical part of the root is divided into a buccal and lingual portion (Fig. 6.23).

On the *second* premolar (both types), the root also tapers apically with the least taper in the cervical third). Only rarely is the root of the second mandibular premolar furcated (Fig. 6.24).

### (8) Root Depressions

The mandibular *first* premolar has a shallow longitudinal depression in the apical and middle thirds of the *mesial* root surface about half of the time [45 of 100 teeth], but is even more likely to have a longitudinal depression on the *distal* surface [86 of 100 teeth]. Comparison depths of the depressions on mesial and distal root surfaces of this tooth are not a positive basis to determine rights from lefts.

The mandibular second premolar is *not* likely to have a longitudinal root depression on the *mesial* [only 19 of 100 teeth had a depression], but is likely to have a longitudinal depression in the middle third of the *distal* root surface [73 of 100 teeth], where it is usually detectable. This difference may be helpful in determining right from left mandibular *second* premolars (the distal surface more likely to be concave).

## 4. OCCLUSAL ASPECT AT MANDIBULAR PREMOLARS

For the occlusal view of mandibular first and second premolars, refer to Figures 6.10, 6.11, and 6.16 through 6.21.

### LEARNING EXERCISE

*To follow this description the tooth should be held with the occlusal surface toward the observer, the buccal surface up, and the observer looking exactly along the vertical axis of the root.*

#### a. Outline (Shape) (Crest of Curvature and Contacts)

There is much variation in the occlusal morphology of the mandibular *first* premolar (2). The outline of the crown is not symmetrical (more bulk in the distal half as seen in the *upper two rows* teeth in Fig. 6.16). It often looks as though the mesial side of the crown has been pushed inward on the mesiolingual corner (toward the distal) (Appendix 6u).

On mandibular *first* premolars, the *buccal* ridge is not prominent, and the buccal crest of curvature is slightly mesial to center (Fig. 6.18). The crest of curvature of the *lingual* surface is often distal to the center line of the tooth. The tip of the buccal cusp is near the center of the crown outline from the occlusal view (slightly buccal to tooth center from this view, Fig. 6.18). The cusp slopes of the buccal cusp are in a nearly straight line mesiodistally and both are frequently notched (Fig. 6.10**A**). The occlusal surface is broadest mesiodistally at a point just lingual to the line of the buccal cusp slopes and the cusp tip (Fig. 6.18). The *contact areas as seen from the occlusal aspect* are at the point of broadest mesiodistal dimension just lingual to the line of the buccal cusp slopes (Figs. 6.19**A** and **B** and 6.20).

## Mandibular Premolars (Occlusal)

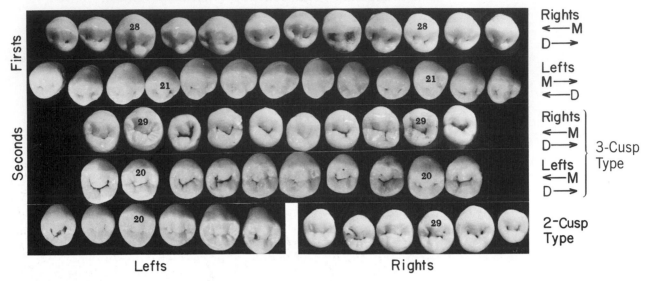

**Figure 6.16.** Mandibular premolars (occlusal view). Facial surfaces are above, lingual surfaces are below. The upper two rows of mandibular second premolars are the three-cusp type. *M* denotes mesial surfaces; *D* indicates distal surfaces. The *bottom row* (two-cusp type second premolars) have their distal surfaces away from the white area that divides rights from lefts.

The crown of the mandibular *first* premolar is somewhat diamond shape, converging lingually from the contact areas, somewhat more so on the mesial side. The mesial outline of the crown is flat or slightly curved. The distal crown outline is considerably more convex (Fig. 6.18). The shape is asymmetrical. The *distal* marginal ridge is often nearly at right angles to the distobuccal cusp slope or ridge, whereas the *mesial* marginal ridge meets the mesiobuccal cusp ridge at a more nearly acute angle. Sometimes the mesial and distal marginal ridges may converge lingually in such a way that the occlusal surface is nearly an equilateral triangle with the base made up of the buccal cusp slopes and the apex of the lingual cusp tip (Fig. 6.19**B**). On this type of tooth, it is more difficult to determine right from left by looking at the occlusal design. Compare several teeth.

On the *two-cusp second premolars,* the crown is *round or oval* shaped, but with a square occlusal table. The crown outline is rounded (less oval) on the lingual side than on the buccal side and also tapers to the lingual. There is slightly more buccolingual bulk of tooth in the mesial half than in the distal half of the crown (tooth tapers from mesial to distal) (Fig. 6.17).

On the *three-cusp second premolars,* the occlusal surface is more nearly *square* than is the occlusal surface of the two-cusp type because the crown is broad on the lingual side. When the lingual cusps are large, the occlusal surface is broader on the lingual side than on the buccal side (Fig 6.20) which is different than the two-cusp mandibular premolars (Fig. 6.17). Three-cusp premolar teeth often have greater faciolingual bulk in the distal than mesial half of the crown (*tapering from distal to mesial*) which is an EXCEPTION to the normal taper to the distal. [This was true on 56% of 229 specimens examined, but more than one-third (38%) tapered the more conventional way (mesial to distal), like two-thirds of the two-cusp type.] Examples of these types of crown taper are seen in Figure 6.16. The mesiolingual cusp is usually larger than the distolingual cusp [90% of 818 teeth]. This difference in size may be little or great.

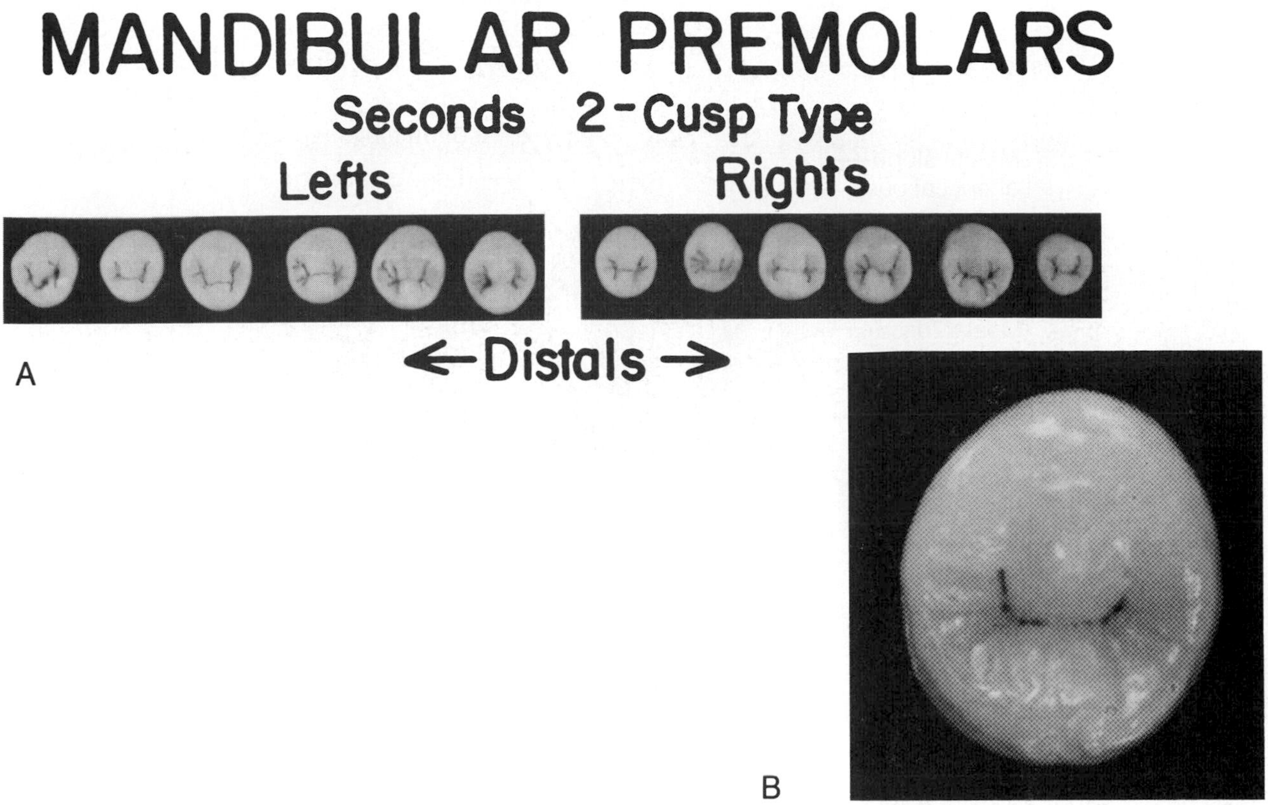

# MANDIBULAR PREMOLARS
## Seconds   2 - Cusp Type
## Lefts                    Rights

← Distals →

A

B

**Figure 6.17. A.** Occlusal view of two-cusp type of mandibular second premolars (43% occurrence). **B.** Close-up view of a mandibular left second premolar (two-cusp type); buccal *above* and mesial at *right*. The single lingual cusp is mesial to the center line. The central groove is U-shaped. Compared with the three-cusp premolar in Figure 6.11**B** view **B,** the occlusal surface of this tooth has a square shape, but is not as broad faciolingually and has a smaller lingual cusp than the maxillary second premolar. Twelve other two-cusp second premolars can be seen in Figure 6.16 (*bottom row*).

### b. Ridges and Fossae and Grooves of the Mandibular First Premolar

Due to the larger buccal cusp on the mandibular *first* premolars, the *triangular ridge of the buccal* cusp is *long* and slopes lingually from the cusp tip to where it joins the *short* triangular ridge of the lingual cusp (Fig. 6.18). Often the two triangular ridges unite smoothly near the center of the occlusal surface and from an uninterrupted pronounced *transverse ridge*, which completely separates the mesial and distal fossae (Fig. 6.11**A,** *occlusal view*).

Sometimes the pronounced transverse ridge of the first premolar is crossed near the center of the occlusal surface by a shallow *central groove*, which extends from the mesial to the distal fossa. This is rare.

The mesial and distal developmental grooves run in a nearly buccolingual direction, flaring toward the buccal. The mesial groove is continuous with the *mesiolingual groove* (when present). The grooves on the first premolars are fewer in number but may be deeper than those on the second premolars.

On the *first* premolar, there is a *mesial fossa* and a *distal fossa;* both are *circular,* not triangular; the mesial fossa is more linear. Each fossa has a pit. The distal fossa is usually larger or deeper [largest of 82 of 100 teeth examined, with the mesial fossa largest on only eight teeth]. Whatever the arrangement of the grooves on the occlusal surface, there may be fissures and pits at the bottom of

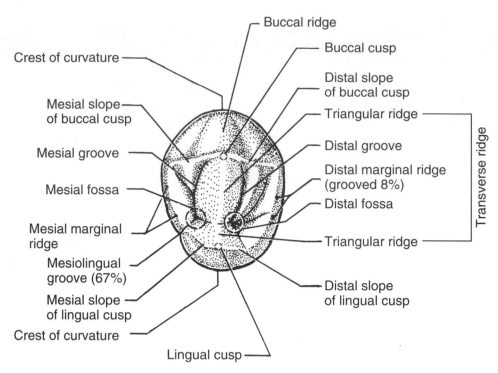

**Figure 6.18.** Occlusal surface of a mandibular right first premolar.

the grooves (Fig. 6.19**A** and **B**). Sometimes these deep pits are restored with gold, amalgam, or, more often, with a tooth-colored composite resin. The possibility of there being fissures and pits is, of course, always present wherever there are grooves on teeth. Fissures and pits are susceptible to caries (see Chapter 12).

### c. Ridges, Fossae and Grooves of the Two-Cusp Mandibular Second Premolars, Two-Cusp Type

Mandibular *second* premolars have more numerous supplemental grooves on their occlusal surfaces than do first premolars (Fig. 6.16) (4).

On the *two-cusp type mandibular second premolars,* the lingual cusp is smaller than the buccal cusp. There is a large triangular ridge on the buccal cusp and a correspondingly smaller one on the lingual cusp (Figs. 6.10**B** and 6.16, *bottom row*). These two ridges form a transverse ridge (unlike the three-cusp type). There is a curved central developmental groove but no lingual groove on the two-cusp type second mandibular premolar. The *central groove* extends mesiodistally across the occlusal surface. Sometimes this groove is short and nearly straight; sometimes it is U-shaped or like a crescent with the open end directed buccally. It may be interrupted near its center by a union of the buccal and lingual triangular ridges as they form the transverse ridge, unique to the two-cusp type (Figs. 6.10**B,** *below,* and 6.17). The central groove ends in the *circular mesial* and *circular distal fossae,* where it often joins a *mesiobuccal and distobuccal supplemental groove.* The distal fossa is generally larger than the mesial fossa (Fig. 6.16, *bottom row,* and 6.17). There may be a depression separating the distal marginal ridge from the distal slope of the lingual cusp.

### d. Ridges, Fossae and Grooves of the Three-Cusp Mandibular Second Premolar

On the three-cusp type, there is a triangular ridge on both of the lingual cusps and on the buccal cusp. These three ridges converge toward the central fossa (Fig. 6.21). There is *no transverse ridge.* The large *central fossa* unique to this three-cusp premolar is located quite distal to the center of the occlusal surface and in

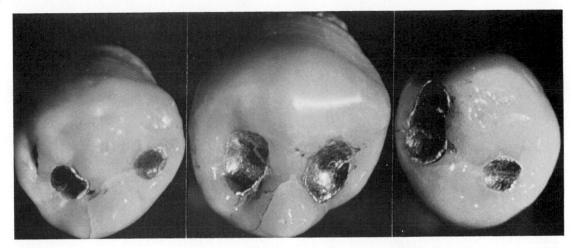

A

**Figure 6.19. A**. Two left and one right mandibular first premolars that have class I amalgam restorations in their mesial and distal fossae. These restorations are sometimes nicknamed "snake eyes." Can you find a pit that has not been restored? Two of the amalgam restorations are short of the cavosurface margins (see Chapter 12) and would most likely permit leakage. Can you find these gaps?

the middle buccolingually (Figs. 6.16, *third* and *fourth rows from top,* and 6.21). **These three-cusp types of mandibular second premolars do not have a central groove.** The *long mesial groove* extends from the central fossa to a small *mesial triangular fossa* (Fig. 6.21). The *distal triangular fossa* is so small it appears to be in the outer edge of the central fossa. The short *distal groove* extends from the central fossa to the minute distal triangular fossa (Fig. 6.21).

The *lingual groove* extends from the central fossa lingually between the mesiolingual and distolingual cusps and onto the lingual surface of the crown resulting in a Y-shaped occlusal groove pattern (Fig. 6.21).

Comparing size and depth of the mesial triangular fossa and central fossa, the central fossa was usually largest [65% of 200 teeth]. The mesial fossa was largest on only 25% of the teeth.

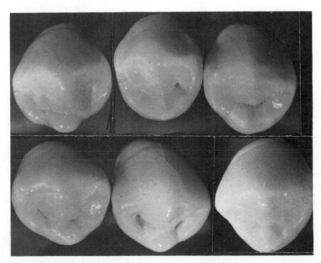

B

**Figure 6.19. B**. Occlusal aspect of several forms of mandibular first premolars. These are not the most common form, but would not be called an anomaly. Facial surfaces are *above*, lingual surfaces are *below*. With these shapes it is difficult to determine right from left premolars from this aspect.

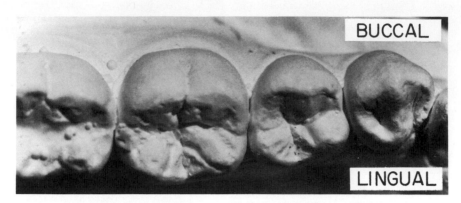

**Figure 6.20.** Mandibular second premolar (three-cusp type) and first molar (four-cusp type), which are wider lingually than buccally. Note that the distolingual cusp on the second premolar is wider than the mesiolingual cusp (found on only 7%), and that the second premolar is larger than the first premolar (a common occurrence unlike the maxillary premolars). Observe the pronounced mesiolingual groove on the first premolar.

### e. Marginal Ridge Grooves

On both the two-cusp and three-cusp second premolar types, grooves crossing the marginal ridges are not commonplace. [On the mesial marginal ridge, 24% of 200 teeth, compared to distal marginal ridge grooves on only 11%.] The first premolar is much more likely to have a mesiolingual groove.

## C. Summary of Differences Between Mandibular Premolars

Refer also to Tables 6.5 and 6.6.

### 1. USUAL DIFFERENCES BETWEEN THE MESIAL AND DISTAL ASPECTS OF MANDIBULAR FIRST PREMOLARS

The mesiolingual groove is present more often [67%] than a distolingual groove [8%].

The crown is asymmetrical with the mesiolingual portion bent or pushed distally (occlusal view).

The *mesial* marginal ridge slopes down from buccal to lingual, is in a more cervical position and is shorter than the distal (proximal view).

There is more often a deeper root depression on the distal [69%].

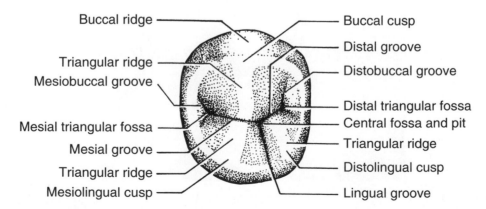

Buccal ridge — — Buccal cusp

Triangular ridge — — Distal groove

Mesiobuccal groove — — Distobuccal groove

Mesial triangular fossa — — Distal triangular fossa

Mesial groove — — Central fossa and pit

Triangular ridge — — Triangular ridge

Mesiolingual cusp — — Distolingual cusp

— Lingual groove

**Figure 6.21.** Mandibular right second premolar (three-cusp type). Occlusal surface. There is no central developmental groove.

**Table 6.6.** How to Differentiate Right from Left Mandibular Premolars

| View | First Premolars | Second Premolars |
|---|---|---|
| Buccal (Figs. 6.10**A** and **B,** and 6.12 Below) | Shorter mesial cusp arm<br>Notch on mesial cusp arm (65%)<br>Depression occlusal third below mesial cusp arm (17%) | Shorter mesial cusp arm<br>Notch on distal cusp arm (66%)<br>Depression occlusal third distal cusp arm (25%) |
| Lingual (Fig. 6.14) | Mesial marginal ridge lower than distal<br>Mesiolingual groove (only 67%)<br>More occlusal visible in mesial half | Distal marginal ridge lower than mesial<br>Mesiolingual cusp larger (90%)<br>More occlusal visible in distal half |
| Proximal (Fig. 6.15) | Mesial marginal ridge is more cervical than distal<br>Deeper distal than mesial root depression (69%)<br><br>Mesial marginal ridge parallel to buccal triangular ridge<br>More occlusal is visible from mesial | Distal marginal ridge is more cervical than on mesial side<br>No mesial root depression in middle third (81%)<br>Distal root depression (73%)<br>More occlusal is visible from distal<br><br>Mesiolingual cusp larger (90%) |
| Occlusal (Figs. 6.16, 6.18, and 6.21) | Asymmetrical crown outline: convex on distal but with mesial side flat (chopped off)<br>Acute angle of mesial marginal ridge with mesial cusp ridge<br>Mesiolingual groove (only 67%)<br>Distal fossa slightly larger and deeper than mesial fossa<br>Shorter mesiobuccal cusp arm | More faciolingual bulk in distal half of crown than on mesial<br><br>Mesial groove runs distolingually<br>Larger mesiolingual cusp (90%)<br>Central fossa (distal half) is larger than mesial triangular fossa mesial triangular fossa<br>Shorter mesiobuccal cusp arm |

## 2. HOW TO DISTINGUISH THE MESIAL SIDE FROM THE DISTAL SIDE OF MANDIBULAR SECOND PREMOLARS (DIFFERENTIATING RIGHTS FROM LEFTS)

### a. Two-Cusp Type

Differentiation of sides is often difficult because of the variability of this tooth.

1. The occlusal outline is rounded and somewhat oval, tapering toward the lingual and often from mesial to distal [62% on 138 teeth].

2. The mesial cusp arm of the buccal cusp is shorter than the distal cusp arm. There is often a depression separating the distal marginal ridge from the single lingual cusp.

3. The distal marginal ridge is usually noticeably more cervical in position than the mesial marginal ridge (proximal view). Rotate a tooth from mesial to distal and compare.

4. The distal fossa is often larger and deeper than the mesial fossa.

5. The tip of the root is often bent distally [62%].

6. There is usually a deeper depression on the distal side of the root in the middle third [76%]. Most [81%] had *no* depression on the mesial root surface.

7. The cervical line is slightly more curved on the mesial surface than on the distal surface.

### b. Three-Cusp Type

1. These share the same features as shown above in numbers 2–5 for the two-cusp type.

2. The occlusal outline is more square or angular, wider on the lingual than the buccal and often tapering from distal to mesial [56%].

3. The distolingual cusp is usually smaller than the mesiolingual cusp [90%].

4. The distal groove is shorter than the mesial groove.

5. The *distal* marginal ridge is concave, shorter, and more cervically located than the mesial marginal ridge (proximal view) (see Fig. 6.15, *lower row*).

6. The central fossa is distal to the center of the occlusal surface and is larger than the mesial triangular fossa [65%].

## LEARNING EXERCISES

Refer to Figures 6.22 through 6.25 for unusually shaped premolars and unusual alignment within the arch.

*Identify the ridges in Figure 6.26A and **B.***
*Review the summary of characteristics that differentiates the mandibular first and second premolar (Table 6.5) and mandibular right and left premolar (Table 6.6).*
***BEFORE READING ABOUT THE MOLARS, TEST YOUR COMPREHENSION ABOUT THE MAXILLARY AND MANDIBULAR PREMOLARS BY ANSWERING THE FOLLOWING QUESTIONS.***
*Questions on Maxillary and Mandibular First and Second Premolars*

1. Which one has the mesial slope of the buccal cusp longer than the distal cusp slope?

2. Which one has a nonfunctioning lingual cusp?

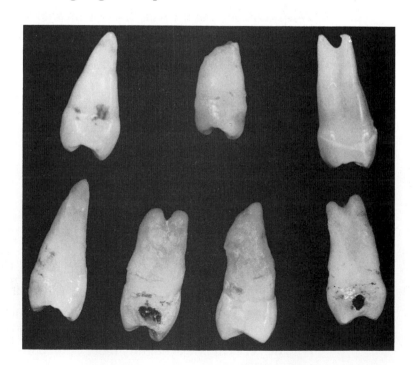

**Figure 6.22.** Proximal view of seven somewhat unusually shaped maxillary second premolars. Buccal surfaces face *right*, lingual surfaces fact *left*. Notice that three teeth have a root division in their apical fifth and would necessarily have two root canals.

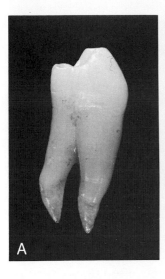
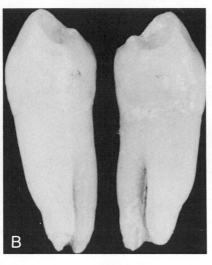

**Figure 6.23. A.** Mandibular right first premolar; distal surface. Notice that the distal marginal ridge is typically in a horizontal plane buccolingually. This tooth has a widely bifurcated root, a condition that is less common for this tooth than in mandibular canines. A Japanese study of 500 mandibular first premolars found this type of bifurcation occurred in 1.6% of their teeth. The researchers also found one very rare specimen with two buccal and one lingual root (5). Notice the heavy attrition on the buccal cusp. **B.** Two more right first premolars, each with a bifurcated root but no attrition on the buccal cusps. The tooth on the *left* is viewed from the mesial aspect; note how its mesial marginal ridge is typically parallel to the triangular ridge of the buccal cusp (type trait).

3. Which two must frequently have a groove crossing the mesial marginal ridge or one groove just lingual to it?

4. Which premolar has a depression in the cervical one-third of the mesial side of the crown and root?

5. Which maxillary premolar has the longer sharper buccal cusp?

6. Which maxillary premolar is usually the largest?

7. Which mandibular premolar has the longest and sharpest buccal cusp?

8. Which mandibular premolar is the smallest ?

# Mandibular Second Premolars

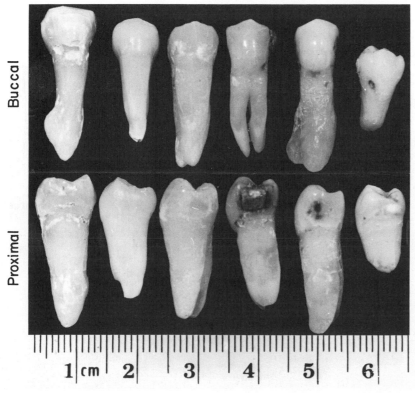

**Figure 6.24.** Unusual mandibular second premolars; two have severe hypercementosis, one has a dwarf root, and one has a mesial and distal root (*upper row*). *Lower row:* A proximal view of these same teeth is shown with their buccal sides on the *left*. In Figure 11.15, another second premolar is seen with a mesial and distal root.

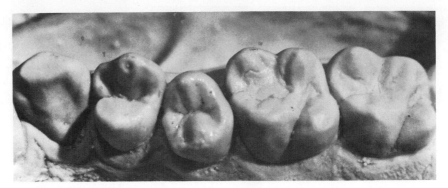

**Figure 6.25.** What is wrong? If you can't figure this out, refer to Secion III, Part 5 under "Additional Anomalies" in Chapter 11.

9. Which maxillary premolar is most symmetrical (occlusal view)?

10. Which premolar has three cusps? Can you name them? How often does this type occur?

11. Which premolars have their crowns tipped lingually with respect to the root axis line (proximal view)?

12. From the buccal view, which premolar has its crown tipped distally from the root axis?

13. Does one premolar have its mesial marginal ridge more cervically located than its distal marginal ridge? If so, which one?

14. Which premolars have the greatest curvature of the cervical lines on the proximal? How much on the mesial and distal? Is the cervical line more occlusal on the lingual?

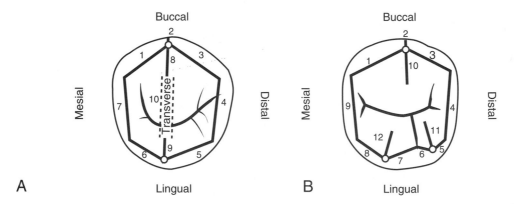

**Figure 6.26. A.** Mandibular second premolar, two-cusp type. **B.** Mandibular second premolar, three-cusp type.

A. Name the Ridges

| Ridges | Name |
|--------|------|
| 1. | |
| 2. | |
| 3. | |
| 4. | |
| 5. | |
| 6. | |
| 7. | |
| 8. | |
| 9. | |
| 10. | |

B. Name the Ridges

| Ridges | Name |
|--------|------|
| 1. | |
| 2. | |
| 3. | |
| 4. | |
| 5. | |
| 6. | |
| 7. | |
| 8. | |
| 9. | |
| 10. | |
| 11. | |
| 12. | |

15. Which maxillary premolar has the longer central groove?

16. Which premolar has two major cusps almost the same size and length?

17. Which premolars have a central fossa?

18. Which premolars have two circular fossae? Two kinds have them.

19. Which premolars have two triangular fossae?

20. Which premolar has a central fossa and two small triangular fossae?

21. Is there a type of premolar that has a lingual groove?

22. Name the two premolars that have no central groove.

23. Which premolar has no transverse ridge?

24. On the outlines in Figures 6.26**A** and **B,** name the ridges that make up each of the short straight lines (OCCLUSAL VIEW). The circles represent the cusp tips.

25. Have you ground off one side of some single-rooted maxillary first premolars to find out how many root canals there are?

26. What is the clinical significance of the depression on the mesial side of the crown of the maxillary first premolars?

27. Which teeth precede the maxillary premolars?

28. In Figure 6.25, what is wrong?:

    a.  Are both premolars from the same side?

    b.  On which side of the mouth do these teeth belong?

    c.  Why is one premolar widest on the lingual?

    d.  Is this a deciduous tooth?

    e.  Do any of these teeth have restorations in them?

    f.  Why does the canine have a flat spot on its cusp tip?

    g.  What is the name for this flat spot?

    h.  How many fossae has the canine, the first premolar, the mystery tooth, and the first molar?

    i.  What would be the minimum possible age of this person?

    j.  Is the illustration upside down?

# References

1. Morris DH. Maxillary premolar variations among Papago Indians. J Dent Res 1967;46:736–738.
2. Kraus BS, Furr ML. Lower first premolars. Part I. A definition and classification of discrete morphologic traits. J Dent Res 1953;32:554.
3. Ludwig FJ. The mandibular second premolar: morphologic variations and inheritance. J Dent Res 1957;36:263–273.
4. Brand RW, Isselhard DE. Anatomy of orofacial structures. St. Louis: C.V. Mosby, 1982.
5. Takeda Y. A rare occurrence of a three-root mandibular premolar. Ann Dent 1988;44:43–44.
6. Osborn JR, ed. Dental anatomy and embryology. Oxford: Blackwell Scientific Publications, 1981:133.
7. Palmer RS. Elephants. In: World Book Encyclopedia. Vol. 6. 1979:178c.
8. Brant D. Beaver. In: World Book Encyclopedia. Vol. 2. 1979:147.
9. Zoo Books: Elephants. Wildlife Education Ltd. San Diego: Frye & Smith, 1980:14.

## General References

Grundler H. The study of tooth shapes: a systematic procedure. (Weber L, trans.) Berlin: Buch-und Zeitschriften-Verlag "Die Quintessenz," 1976.

Oregon State System of Higher Education. Dental anatomy: a self-instructional program. 9th ed. East Norwalk: Appleton-Century-Crofts, 1982.

Renner RP. An introduction to dental anatomy and esthetics. Chicago: Quintessence Publishing, 1985.

# Morphology of
# Permanent Molars

(blank note lines)

## LEARNING EXERCISE

*Using the mandibular right second molar as a representative example for all molars, refer to the Appendix, page 7 while reading Section I of this chapter. Throughout this chapter, "Appendix" followed by a number and letter (e.g., Appendix 7a) is used within the text to denote reference to the page (number 7) and item (letter a) being referred to on that appendix page. The appendix pages are designed to be torn out to facilitate study and minimize page turns. Other appendix pages will be referred to throughout this chapter.*

## SECTION I: OVERVIEW OF MOLARS

### A. General Description

There are 12 permanent molars—six maxillary and six mandibular. The six permanent molars in each arch are the first, second, and third molars on either side of the arch. They are the sixth, seventh, and eighth teeth from the midline. Using the Universal Numbering System, the maxillary molars are #1, #2, and #3 for the right third, second, and first molars, and #14, #15, and #16 for the left first, second, and third molars, respectively. The mandibular molars are #17, #18, and #19 for the left third, second, and first molar, and #30, #31, and #32 for the right first, second, and third molars, respectively.

In the adult dentition, the *first* molars are distal to second premolars. The permanent first molars are located near the *center of the arch*, anteroposteriorly. This is one reason that their loss is so devastating to arch continuity (allowing drift of the teeth on either side). They are the largest and strongest teeth in each arch. The *second* molars are distal to the first molars, and the *third* molars are distal to the second molars. Said another way, in adult dentition the mesial surface of the *first* molar contacts the distal surface of the second premolar. (The relationship with primary teeth is discussed in the chapter on Primary Teeth.) The mesial surface of the *second* molar contacts the distal of the first molar, and the mesial of the *third* molar contacts the distal of the second molar.

The *third* molar is the last tooth in the arch, and its distal surface is not in contact with any other tooth. Unfortunately, this tooth's nickname is "wisdom tooth." It also has unfairly been given a bad reputation for having soft enamel, not serving any function, readily decaying, causing crowding of the anterior teeth, and other dental problems. The reason for this bad reputation is probably its posterior location that makes it difficult to keep clean. Frequently, one or more of the third molars is congenitally missing (never develop); this occurs in nearly 20% of the population.

The combined mesiodistal width of the three *mandibular* molars on one side make up over half (51%) of the mesiodistal dimension of their quadrant. The *maxillary* molars constitute 44% of their quadrant's mesiodistal dimension, still a significant portion (Table 3.2).

## B. Functions

The permanent molars (a) play a major role in the mastication of food (chewing and grinding to pulverize), and (b) are most important in maintaining the vertical dimension of the face (preventing a closing of the bite or vertical dimension, protruding chin, and a prematurely aged appearance). They are also (c) important in maintaining continuity within the dental arches, thus keeping other teeth in proper alignment. You have probably seen someone who has lost all 12 molars (six upper and six lower) and has sunken cheeks. The molars, therefore, have (d) at least a minor role in esthetics or keeping the cheeks normally full or supported as well as keeping the chin a proper distance from our nose.

The loss of a first molar is really noticed by most people when it has been extracted. More than 80 mm² of efficient chewing surface is gone, the tongue feels the huge space between the remaining teeth, and during mastication of coarse or brittle foods, the attached gingiva in the region of the missing molar often becomes abraded and uncomfortable. Loss of six or more molars would also predispose problems in the craniomandibular joints.

## C. Class Traits of All Molars

### 1. CROWN SIZE AND SHAPE

Molars have an occlusal (chewing) surface with three to five cusps. Molars are larger than the other teeth in their respective arches. All molars have broader occlusal surfaces than other posterior teeth (i.e., the premolars). The crowns of molars are much larger both faciolingually and mesiodistally than are the crowns of the premolars [ave. 2.2 mm and 3.0 mm respectively in maxillary molars and averaging 2.1 mm and 3.2 mm respectively in mandibular molars]. The crowns of *mandibular* and *maxillary* molars are wider mesiodistally than long cervico-occlusally (Appendix 7a). Also, molar crowns are shorter cervico-occlusally than all other crowns.

**Refer to Tables 7.1 and 7.2 for the average and range in size of molars in all dimensions.**

**Table 7.1.** Size of Maxillary Molars (Millimeters) (Measured by Dr. Woelfel and his dental hygiene students 1974–1979)

| Dimension Measured | 308 First Molars Average | Range | 309 Second Molars Average | Range | 303 Third Molars Average | Range |
|---|---|---|---|---|---|---|
| Crown length* | 7.5 | 6.3–9.6 | 7.6 | 6.1–9.4 | 7.2 | 5.7–9.0 |
| Root length | | | | | | |
|   Mesiobuccal* | 12.9 | 8.5–18.8 | 12.9 | 9.0–18.2 | 10.8 | 7.1–15.5 |
|   Distobuccal | 12.2 | 8.9–15.5 | 12.1 | 9.0–16.3 | 10.1 | 6.9–14.5 |
|   Lingual | 13.7 | 10.6–17.5 | 13.5 | 9.8–18.8 | 11.2 | 7.4–15.8 |
| Overall length* | 20.1 | 17.0–27.4 | 20.0 | 16.0–26.2 | 17.5 | 14.0–22.5 |
| Crown width (M-D) | 10.4 | 8.8–13.3 | 9.8 | 8.5–11.7 | 9.2 | 7.0–11.1 |
| Root width (cervix) | 7.9 | 6.4–10.9 | 7.6 | 6.2–8.4 | 7.2 | 5.3–9.4 |
| Faciolingual crown size | 11.5 | 9.8–14.1 | 11.4 | 9.9–14.3 | 11.1 | 8.9–13.2 |
| Faciolingual root (cervix) | 10.7 | 7.4–14.0 | 10.7 | 8.9–12.7 | 10.4 | 7.5–12.5 |
| Mesial cervical curvature | 0.7 | 0.0–2.1 | 0.6 | 0.0–2.2 | 0.5 | 0.0–2.0 |
| Distal cervical curvature | 0.3 | 0.0–1.4 | 0.2 | 0.0–1.0 | 0.2 | 0.0–1.7 |

*Overall length from mesiobuccal root apex to tip of mesiobuccal cusp. Root length is from cervical line to root apex. Crown length is from cervical line to tip of mesiobuccal cusp (slanted).

## 2. TAPER FROM BUCCAL TO LINGUAL

Molar crowns taper (get narrower) from the buccal to the lingual (that is, the mesiodistal width on the buccal half is wider than on the lingual half, see Appendix 7b) EXCEPT some maxillary first molars with large distolingual cusps where crowns actually taper toward the buccal.

## 3. TAPER TO THE DISTAL

For both arches, molar crowns from the occlusal taper distally so that the distal side is narrower buccolingually than the mesial side (Appendix 7c). Also, all molar occlusal surfaces slope toward the cervix from mesial to distal. This makes more of the occlusal surface visible from the distal aspect than from the mesial aspect (Appendix 7d; compare mesial to distal views in Fig. 7.10).

As with premolars, the *crest of curvature* viewed from the proximal on the buccal of molars is in the cervical third; on the lingual, it is in the middle third (Appendix 7e).

**Table 7.2.** Size of Mandibular Molars (Millimeters) (Measured by Dr. Woelfel and his dental hygiene students 1974–1979)

| Dimension Measured | 281 First Molars Average | Range | 296 Second Molars Average | Range | 262 Third Molars Average | Range |
|---|---|---|---|---|---|---|
| Crown length* | 7.7 | 6.1–9.6 | 7.7 | 6.1–9.8 | 7.5 | 6.1–9.2 |
| Root length | | | | | | |
|   Mesial* | 14.0 | 10.6–20.0 | 13.9 | 9.3–18.3 | 11.8 | 7.3–14.6 |
|   Distal | 13.0 | 8.1–17.7 | 13.0 | 8.5–18.3 | 10.8 | 5.2–14.0 |
| Overall length* | 20.9 | 17.0–27.7 | 20.6 | 15.0–25.5 | 18.2 | 14.8–22.0 |
| Crown width (M-D) | 11.4 | 9.8–14.5 | 10.8 | 9.6–13.0 | 11.3 | 8.5–14.2 |
| Root width (cervix) | 9.2 | 7.7–12.4 | 9.1 | 7.4–10.6 | 9.2 | 6.4–10.7 |
| Faciolingual crown size | 10.2 | 8.9–13.7 | 9.9 | 7.6–11.8 | 10.1 | 8.2–13.2 |
| Faciolingual root (cervix) | 9.0 | 7.3–11.6 | 8.8 | 7.1–10.9 | 8.9 | 7.0–11.5 |
| Mesial cervical curvature | 0.5 | 0.0–1.6 | 0.5 | 0.0–1.4 | 0.4 | 0.0–1.4 |
| Distal cervical curvature | 0.2 | 0.0–1.2 | 0.2 | 0.0–1.2 | 0.2 | 0.0–1.0 |

*Overall length from mesial root apex to tip of mesiobuccal cusp. Root length is from cervical line to root apex. Crown length is from cervical line to tip of mesiobuccal cusp.

## 4. CONTACT AREAS

The contact areas (Appendix 7f) of all molars are at or near the junction of the occlusal and middle thirds *mesially,* and are more cervical on the *distal,* near the middle of the tooth.

## D. Arch Traits That Differentiate Maxillary From Mandibular Molars

### LEARNING EXERCISE

*Compare extracted maxillary and mandibular molars and/or tooth models while reading about these differentiating traits. Also refer to study pages 7 and 8 in the Appendix.*

## 1. CROWN SHAPE

From the occlusal view, the crowns of *mandibular* molars are oblong: they are characteristically much wider mesiodistally than faciolingually (by 1.2 mm on 839 teeth). This is just the opposite of the *maxillary* molars, which have their greater dimension faciolingually (by 1.2 mm on 920 teeth). From the occlusal, *maxillary* molars have a more square or parallelogram shape; *mandibular* molars have a rectangular or pentagon crown shape. See Appendix 8a and 8k.

## 2. NUMBER AND RELATIVE SIZE OF CUSPS

*Mandibular* molar crowns have four major cusps, two buccal and two lingual, often with a fifth minor one (the minor cusp is distal and found on the first, and sometimes the third, molar). The two lingual cusps are of nearly equal size (much different than the maxillary molars). The crowns of *maxillary* molars are centered over the roots and have three large cusps (two buccal and one mesiolingual) with a fourth cusp of lesser size (distolingual). The longest and largest mesiolingual cusp is connected by an *oblique ridge* to the distobuccal cusp (unique to maxillary molars) (Appendix 8d). A fifth minor cusp (of Carabelli) is often found on the mesiolingual cusps of maxillary first molars (Appendix 8i and compare occlusal views).

## 3. LINGUAL AND DISTAL TILT

When examined from the mesial or distal sides, mandibular molar crowns appear to be tilted lingually (an arch trait; true for all mandibular teeth) (Appendix 8b; Fig. 7.10). This is not apparent on maxillary molars (Fig. 7.28). Mandibular molar crowns also tip distally relative to the long axis of the root (Fig. 7.9).

## 4. ROOTS (APPENDIX 8C)

*Maxillary* molars have *three* roots of generous size that are nearly twice as long as the crown: mesiobuccal, distobuccal, and lingual (palatal). The lingual root is usually the longest; the distobuccal root the shortest. The roots converge into a broad cervical root base called the *root trunk. Mandibular* molars have only *two* roots: a mesial root and a distal root [mesial roots averaged 1 mm longer than the distal roots for 839 mandibular molars]. The root furcation is usually close to the cervical line; making the root trunk short (shorter than on the maxillary molars, especially on first molars). See Appendix 8c and Table 7.3.

**Table 7.3.** How to Distinguish Maxillary from Mandibular Molars (Arch Trait)

| Maxillary Molars (Figs. 7.25, 7.26, and 7.27) | Mandibular Molars (Figs. 7.5, 7.9, 7.10, and 7.12) |
|---|---|
| Three or four cusps and three roots (two buccal, one lingual) | Four or five cusps and two roots (mesial and distal) |
| Crowns wider faciolingually than mesiodistally | Crowns wider mesiodistally than faciolingually |
| Buccal surface of crown relatively vertical and flat on buccal | Buccal crown surface covex and tipped lingually |
| Large and small lingual cusps | Two nearly equal-sized lingual cusps |
| Square or parallelogram shape (twisted on second molar) | Rectangular or pentagonal crown shape |
| First molars wider on lingual than buccal | First molars taper from buccal to lingual |
| First molars have tubercles on mesial marginal ridge (86%) and mesial ridge grooves (78%) | First molars have mesial marginal ridge grooves (68%), second molars (57%), usually no tubercles on ridges |
| Carabelli cusp on first molar (not always) | No Carabelli formation on mesiolingual cusps |
| One buccal groove | First molar usually has three buccal cusps (two buccal grooves on first and some thirds) |
| Oblique ridge (mesiolingual to distobuccal) | No oblique ridge but have two transverse ridges |
| Four fossae including large distal fossa | Three fossae (large central fossae) |
| Second molar has more taper buccal to lingual than the first molar | Second molar has less taper buccal to lingual than the first molar |
| Third molar occlusal is small and often heart-shaped or triangular (flat buccal side, lingual is apex) | Third molar resembles first or second molar (five or four cusps), large bulbous rectangular crown |
| Crowns much narrower on lingual near cervix | Shorter root trunk |
| | Y or + groove pattern (five-cusp or four-cusp type) |

# SECTION II. TYPE TRAITS THAT DIFFERENTIATE MANDIBULAR *SECOND* MOLARS FROM MANDIBULAR *FIRST* MOLARS

## LEARNING EXERCISE

*For this exercise, hold a mandibular first and second molar in front of you (with crowns up, roots down) and make the following comparisons:*

*General characteristics:*
First and second mandibular molars have specific characteristics that can be used to distinguish one from the other. The third molars vary considerably, often resembling a first or a second molar while still having unique characteristics that are discussed later.

*Cusp number and size* (described on the back of Appendix page 8 under e):
Mandibular *first* molars have *five* cusps, in order from longest to shortest: mesiolingual, distolingual, mesiobuccal, distobuccal, plus a smaller distal cusp. Mandibular *second* molars have *four* cusps, in order from longest to shortest: mesiolingual, distolingual, mesiobuccal, and distobuccal.

*Relative crown size:*
The crown of the mandibular second molar is usually smaller than the crown of the first molar in the same mouth.

*Roots* (Appendix 8f):

The roots of mandibular *second* molars are as long, but less broad buccolingually, than on the first molar (Fig. 7.10), and are less widely separated or more parallel. The root trunk is slightly longer on second molars (Fig. 7.5).

## A. Buccal Aspect of Mandibular Molars

Refer to Figures 7.1 through 7.4, *left tooth,* and 7.5 for similarities and differences of mandibular first and second molars.

### 1. CROWN SHAPE FROM THE BUCCAL: WIDER MESIODISTALLY THAN CERVICO-OCCLUSALLY OR BUCCOLINGUALLY

For both mandibular molars, the crowns are wider mesiodistally than high cervico-occlusally, but more so on first molars [3.7 mm larger on first molars versus 3.1 mm for second molars].

#### a. First Molar Cusps

The mesiolingual cusp is highest and widest (see Fig. 7.1). The mandibular first molar has the *largest mesiodistal dimension (11.4 mm) of any tooth* [includes measurements of 2392 maxillary and 2180 mandibular teeth; see Table 3.2].

The mandibular *first* molar usually has three buccal cusps [81% of the time]: mesiobuccal, distobuccal (in center), and distal. The *mesiobuccal cusp is the largest, widest, and highest cusp on the buccal side.* [The mesiobuccal cusp was widest in 61%, compared to only 17% for the distobuccal cusp, for 1367 mandibular first molars.] The *distobuccal cusp* is slightly smaller, shorter, and may be sharper than the mesiobuccal cusp. [After examination of 430 teeth, it was considered to be sharper than the mesiobuccal cusp 55% of the time, compared to only 17% for the mesiobuccal cusp. The rest were equally sharp.] The *distal cusp* (minor cusp), which is on the distobuccal angle of the crown, is the smallest of the five cusps. [In Mongoloid peoples this cusp is often placed lingually. It may also be split into two parts by a fissure (1).] The *mesiolingual cusp,* which is the highest or longest *of all the cusps,* is visible behind the mesiobuccal cusp even from the buccal view. The *distolingual cusp* is visible behind the distobuccal cusp and is usually the second highest cusp when the tooth is oriented

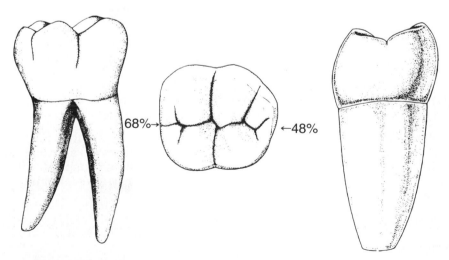

**Figure 7.1.** *Mandibular* right *first* molar: buccal, occlusal, and mesial views. Percentages give the frequency of occurrence of marginal ridge grooves on 215 unrestored first molars examined by Dr. Woelfel.

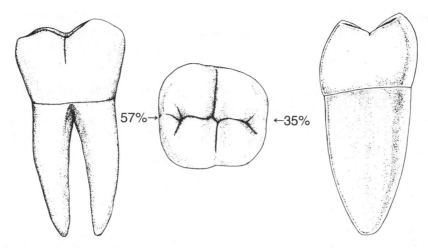

**Figure 7.2.** *Mandibular* right *second* molar: buccal, occlusal, and mesial views. Percentages give the frequency of occurrence of marginal ridge grooves on 233 unrestored teeth examined by Dr. Woelfel.

vertically. Even though the lingual cusps are higher than buccal cusps, in the mouth their lingual cusp tips are at a lower level than the buccal cusps due to the lingual tilt of the root axis in the mandible (refer to the curve of Wilson shown in Fig. 10.8c).

### b. Grooves of First Molar: Two Buccal Grooves; Mesiobuccal Groove Is Longer

The *mesiobuccal groove* on the buccal surface separates the mesiobuccal cusp from the distobuccal cusp. There may be a deep pit at the cervical end of the mesiobuccal groove. This pit is sometimes a site of caries. (This pit is common in the teeth of Mongoloid persons.) Six of the teeth in Figure 7.5 have pits at the end of this groove, and a seventh has an amalgam restoration. The *distobuccal groove* separates the distobuccal cusp from the distal cusp. It is shorter [70% of the time on 720 molars] than the mesial buccal groove and is not frequently pitted. One of the teeth in Figure 7.5 upper row has this pit; can you find it?

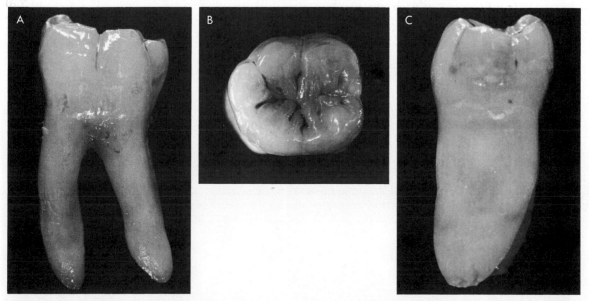

**Figure 7.3.** *Mandibular* left *first* molar. **A.** Buccal surface. **B.** Occlusal surface. Buccal side at top; mesial side at right. Compare this with the drawing of a right first molar (Fig. 7.11). **C.** Distal surface. Buccal side at *left*. Notice the curvatures of the buccal and lingual surfaces, and the height of the lingual cusps compared to the buccal cusps. There is some attrition on the tip of the mesiobuccal cusp.

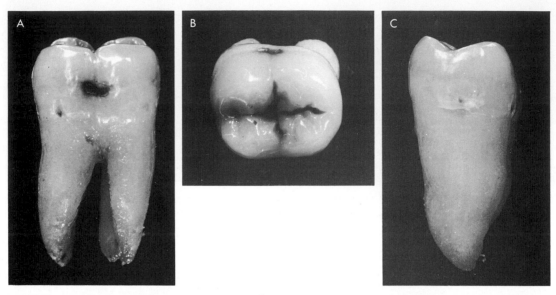

**Figure 7.4.** *Mandibular* right *second* molar. **A.** Buccal surface. Mesial side on *right*. The pit at the end of the buccal groove appears to be carious. **B.** Occlusal surface. Buccal side at *top*, mesial at *left*. This would be an interesting tooth to grind down in order to examine the deeply fissured grooves for underlying caries. **C.** Distal surface. Buccal side at *right*. Due to the low camera angle, the distal marginal ridge appears high preventing the normal view of the occlusal surface (Fig. 7.10, *lower right*).

### c. Second Molar Cusps: Two Buccal Cusps, Mesiobuccal Wider than Distobuccal

The mandibular *second* molar has four cusps: mesiobuccal, distobuccal, mesiolingual, and distolingual. The crown of the second molar appears to be wider at the cervix than the first molar because of the absence of a distal cusp (less taper toward the cervix below the contact points). As on the first molar, the *mesiobuccal cusp* is usually wider mesiodistally than the *distobuccal cusp*. [The mesiobuccal cusp was considered widest on 66%, compared to only 19% with a wider distobuccal cusp, for 1514 mandibular second molars examined on dental stone casts.] As on the first molar, the lingual cusp tips are visible from the buccal side. The tips of the slightly longer *mesiolingual* and *distolingual cusps* are seen behind the mesiobuccal and distobuccal cusps (Figs. 7.5, *lower row*, and 7.4**A**).

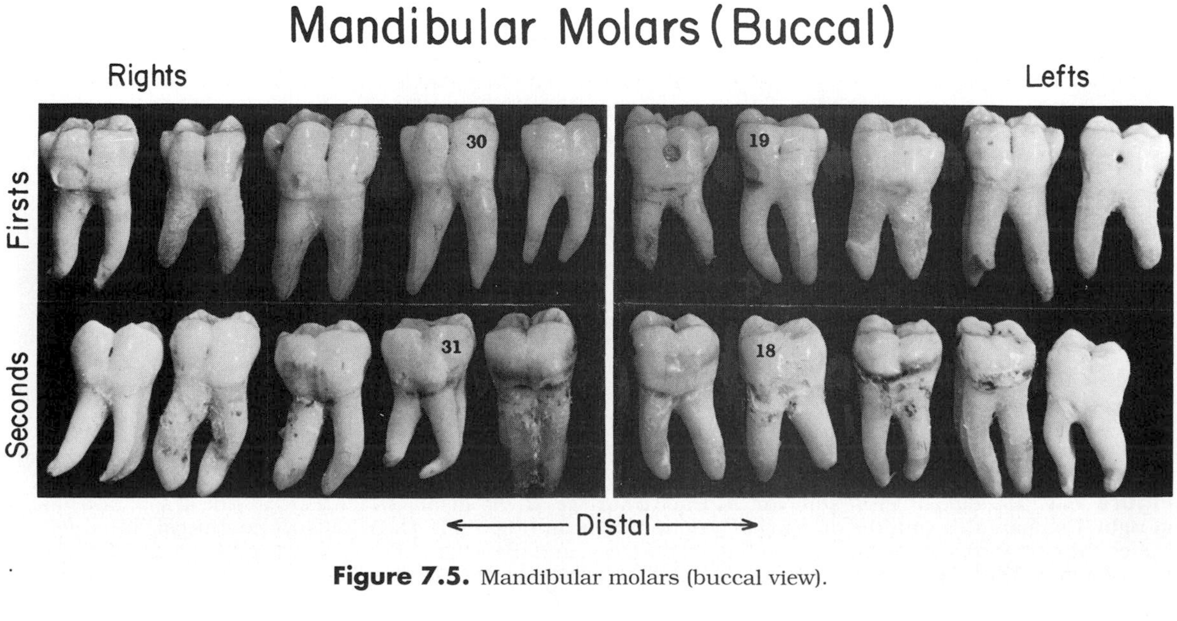

# Mandibular Molars (Buccal)

**Figure 7.5.** Mandibular molars (buccal view).

### d. Grooves of Second Molar (Only One Buccal Groove)

On mandibular *second* molars, the *buccal groove* separates the mesiobuccal and the distobuccal cusps, and it may end on the middle of the buccal surface in a pit (Fig. 7.4**A,** and two of the 10 second molars in Fig. 7.5). There is no distobuccal groove as on the first molar.

### e. Contacts: Same as for All Molars

*Mesial*—junction of middle and occlusal thirds.
*Distal*—middle of tooth.

### f. Cervical Line

The cervical line of both mandibular first and second molars is often nearly straight across the buccal surface. Sometimes there is a point of enamel that dips down nearly into the root bifurcation (Fig. 8.14**B**). (This point of enamel is reported to occur in 90% of Mongoloid peoples studied.) Sometimes there is dipping down of enamel on both the buccal and the lingual surfaces, and these extensions may meet in the root bifurcation (1, 2). Such enamel extensions may cause periodontal problems because of the deep gingival sulcus in these regions.

### g. Taper to the Cervical and to the Distal

There is proportionally more tapering of the crown from the contact areas to the cervical line on mandibular *first* molars than on second molars because of the bulge of the distal cusp (Appendix 8g; Fig. 7.5). The mesial sides of the mandibular molar crowns is nearly straight, *or slightly concave,* from the cervical line to the convex contact area (Figs. 7.1 and 7.3**A**). The distal sides are straight, or slightly convex, from the cervical line to the contact areas, where it is convex.

The occlusal surface slopes cervically from mesial to distal because the crown is tipped distally on its two roots (somewhat less so on first molars, again due partly to the shorter distal cusp). (See Figs. 7.1 and 7.2.)

### h. Variations in Mandibular Molar Crowns

The mandibular *first* molar sometimes has an extra cusp on the buccal surface of the mesiobuccal cusp, about in the middle third of the crown. Studies have shown this to occur frequently in the Pima Indians of Arizona (3) and in Indian (Asian) populations (4, 5). An extra cusp in the same location has also been found on second, and especially on third, molars (see Fig. 7.17).

The distal cusp of first molars is absent about a fifth of the time (Fig. 7.6). [Among 874 dental hygiene students at the Ohio State University College of Dentistry (1971–1983), dental stone casts revealed that 81% of 1327 nonrestored first molars had five cusps and 19% had only four cusps. Seventy-seven percent of the females had five-cusp first molars on both sides, 16% had four-cusp first molars on both sides, and 3% had one four-cusp and one five-cusp mandibular first molar]. Consequently, not all four-cusp molars are second molars. Almost one-fifth may be mandibular first molars.

## 2. ROOTS OF MANDIBULAR MOLARS: ONE MESIAL (SLIGHTLY LONGER) AND ONE DISTAL

Both mandibular first and second molars have *two* roots, a *mesial* root and a *distal* root, approximately the same length. [For first molars, the mesial root averaged 1 mm longer than the distal root on 281 teeth.] Both roots are nearly twice as long as the crown [root to crown ratio for first molars is 1.83:1, the highest of any tooth as shown in Table 3.2]. The *root bifurcation* of the mandibular *first* molar is near the cervical line with a depression existing between the bifurcation and cervical line, and the *root trunk* is relatively short (*shorter than on second molars*) (Fig. 7.1, *left*). On sec-

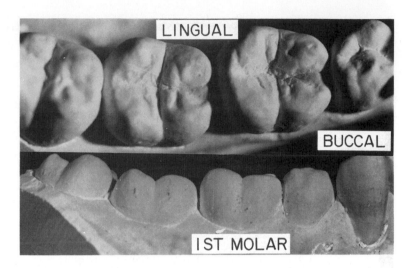

**Figure 7.6.** Buccal view (*below*) and occlusal view (*above*) of three mandibular molars, each with only four cusps. This occurrence on mandibular first molars was found in 19% of 874 dental hygiene students. These four-cusp molars do not taper as much from buccal to lingual as do the five-cusp types. Also note that their distal two cusps (to the *left* side in the *top* photograph) are wider faciolingually than the two mesial cusps. This makes these molars taper from distal (widest) to mesial.

ond molars, there is also a depression on the root trunk from the cervical line to the root bifurcation (Fig. 7.2, *left*).

The roots of the *first* molar are *widely separated* (Fig. 7.5, *upper row*), *more so than on the second where they are more parallel* (Fig. 7.5, *lower row*), and much more than on the third molars (Fig. 7.19). The apical half of the roots curve distally. The crest of curvature of the mesial side of the *mesial root may extend mesial* to the mesial surface of the first molar crown. From the buccal aspect, it is possible to see the distal surface of the mesial root because of the way it is twisted on the trunk. The distal root is straighter than the mesial root and may have a more pointed apex. The curvature and direction of the roots is enough that the apex of the mesial root may be in line with the mesiobuccal groove of the crown, and the apex of the distal root often lies distal to the distal surface of the crown (Fig. 7.5, *upper row*).

The roots of the mandibular *second* molar taper apically. Both roots are more pointed than the roots of the first molar. Often the apex of both roots is directed toward the center line of the tooth (two of the 10 teeth in Fig. 7.5, *lower row*; see if you can find them). Both roots may curve distally, and the mesial root is slightly longer than the distal [averaging 0.9 mm longer on 296 teeth measured].

### a. Variations in Roots

Extreme distal root curvature is seen for one tooth in Figure 7.7, *lower row*, center tooth. This condition is called flexion.

In Mongoloid peoples, there is usually a longer root trunk (1).

In the mandibular first molar, there is often a ridge of cementum crossing the space in the root bifurcation in a mesiodistal direction (6).

Occasionally, the mesial root is divided into a mesiobuccal and a mesiolingual root, making three roots on the mandibular first molar. It is reported that this condition is found in 10–20% of the mandibular first permanent molars in Eskimos (7). In Mongoloid peoples, 10% of the mandibular first molars have an additional distolingual root, and sometimes the mesial root is bifurcated, giving a four-rooted first molar (8). It is reported that in both deciduous and permanent dentitions, three-rooted mandibular molars occur frequently in Mongoloid (Chinese) peoples, but rarely in European groups (1, 9). A small, third buccal root can be seen in Figure 7.8.

## B. Lingual Aspect of Mandibular Molars

Refer to Figure 7.9 for similarities and differences.

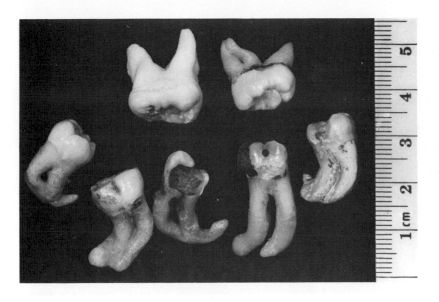

**Figure 7.7.** Buccal aspect of unusual maxillary third molars (*top row*) and mandibular molars (*below*). *Left to right:* third, second, two firsts, and third molar. Observe the wide variation in form from the so-called normal.

## 1. CROWN SHAPE FROM THE LINGUAL

### a. Taper or Convergence from Buccal to Lingual and from Proximal Contacts to Cervix

As with most teeth, mandibular first and second molar crowns are narrower on the lingual side, more so on *first* molars where much of the taper is on the distal surface lingual to the distal cusp. (There are exceptions; see wide lingual sides in Fig. 7.6.)

### b. Cusps: Mesiolingual Longest; Wider than Distolingual Cusp; Lingual Cusps More Pointed

The lingual cusps of mandibular molars are both slightly *longer* and more *pointed* or conical than the buccal cusps, which are hidden behind them. Therefore, in most cases, only the *mesiolingual* and *distolingual* cusps of mandibular

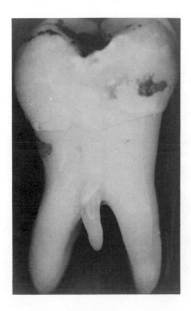

**Figure 7.8.** Buccal view of a mandibular left second molar with peduncular-shaped extra root (approximately 6 mm long) on the buccal side. There is a very large occlusal decay area that has caused some of the buccal enamel to chip off between the two cusps (mesial side is on the *left*). (Tooth courtesy of Dr. John A. Pike and photograph by Dr. Lewis J. Claman.)

# Mandibular Molars (Lingual)

**Lefts**

**Rights**

Firsts

Seconds

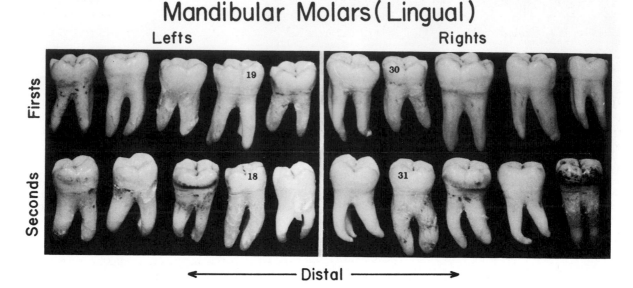

← Distal →

**Figure 7.9.** Mandibular molars (lingual view).

molars are visible from the lingual aspect (not true in Fig. 7.9, because of the camera angle). The mesiolingual cusp is often the slightly wider and longer of the two (noticeably wider on first molars). [On mandibular first molars, the mesiolingual cusp was wider on 58% of 256 teeth, while on 33% the distolingual cusp was wider. On second molars, the mesiolingual cusp was wider on 65% of 263 of these teeth, compared to only 30% with a wider distolingual cusp.] On sharpness, the lingual cusps were rated about even. [On first molars, 48% of the mesiolingual cusps were more pointed versus 47% distolingual cusps; on second molars, it was 44% versus 51%, respectively.]

### c. Grooves

The *lingual groove* separates the mesiolingual from the distolingual cusp. It terminates on the lingual surface (usually occlusal third) with no pit.

### d. Cervical Line

The *cervical line* is *relatively flat* (mesiodistally) or irregular, and may dip cervically between the roots over the bifurcation as it often does on the buccal side of the crown. (Fig. 7.9, left-most second molar). On *first* and *second* molars, the short root trunk has a depression between the cervical line and the bifurcation.

## 2. ROOTS OF MANDIBULAR MOLARS FROM THE LINGUAL

On *first* molars, the *root trunk appears longer on the lingual side* than on the buccal because the cervical line is more occlusal in position on the lingual than on the buccal surface. The roots are narrower on the lingual side than they are on the buccal side (compare Fig. 7.5 with Fig. 7.9). From the lingual aspect, it is often possible to see the mesial surface of the mesial root owing to the way it is twisted on the trunk. One can also see the distal side of the distal root because of its taper toward the lingual.

## C. Proximal Aspect of Mandibular Molars

Refer to Figure 7.1 through 7.4, *right side*, and 7.10 for similarities and differences.

## 1. CROWN SHAPE FROM THE PROXIMAL

### LEARNING EXERCISE

*For proper orientation, as you study each trait, hold the crown so that the root axis line is in a vertical position as seen in Figure 7.10.*

#### a. Wide and Short

Mandibular molar crowns are relatively shorter cervico-occlusally compared to faciolingually.

#### b. Lingual Tilt

The crowns of both mandibular molars are tilted lingually from the root base. Remember that this slant is an arch trait characteristic of all mandibular teeth and is nature's way of shaping them to fit beneath and lingual to the maxillary buccal cusps. Because of this lingual inclination in the mouth, the tip of the buccal cusps viewed from the mesial are usually lingual to the buccal side of the wider mesial root, and the crest of curvature of the lingual crown surface is lingual to the lingual root surface (Fig. 7.10). The buccal outline is convex in the cervical third, then slightly curved and tapered occlusally in the middle and occlusal thirds.

#### c. Crest of Curvature: Buccal Cervical Ridge (More Prominent on Second Molars)

As with all molars, the crest of curvature or bulge of the *buccal* surface is in the cervical third, close to the cervical line for second molars. It is called the *buccal cervical ridge* (sometimes called buccal cingulum). This ridge runs in a mesiodistal

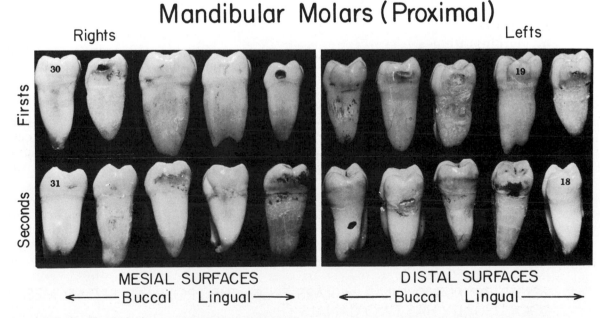

**Figure 7.10.** Mandibular molars (proximal view). Make note of the considerably different heights of the marginal ridges when comparing mesial and distal views.

direction on the buccal surface of the crown. It is *not* as prominent on mandibular first molars as on second molars (Fig. 7.10).

The *lingual* outline of the crown of both molars appears nearly straight in the cervical third with its crest of curvature in the *middle third*.

### d. Cusp Height

In review, the cusp length for mandibular molars is, from longest to shortest, mesiolingual, distolingual, mesiobuccal, distobuccal, and, when present, the smallest cusp found on most first molars is the distal cusp. In general, the lingual cusps are more conical or pointed than the buccal.

### e. Distal Tilt

Due to the distal tilt to the crown and the sloping of the occlusal surface (Fig. 7.3**A**), much of the occlusal surface and all cusps can be seen from the distal aspect (Fig. 7.3**C**). Subsequently, on both first and second molars, from the distal aspect the tips of the mesiobuccal and mesiolingual cusps can be seen behind the distobuccal and distolingual cusps. On the first molar, the distobuccal cusp is seen above and somewhat buccal to the smaller, shorter distal cusp (Fig. 7.3**C**).

### f. Taper to Distal

On both molars, the crown is more narrow on the distal side than on the mesial side. Therefore, from the distal aspect, some of the lingual and the buccal surfaces can be seen (Figs. 7.3**C** and 7.10, *right side*). The distal contact is centered on the distal surface cervical to the distal cusp on *first* molars. There may be a wear facet here from proximal wear due to functional movement.

### g. Cervical Line

The *mesial cervical line* of both first and second molars slopes occlusally from buccal to lingual and are convex toward the occlusal surface [0.5 mm on first molars, 0.2 mm on second molars]. The *distal cervical line* is nearly straight but also slants occlusally from buccal to lingual. It is less occlusal in position than on the mesial surface.

### h. Marginal Ridges

The *mesial marginal ridge* is concave buccolingually; usually longer on the first molar and often sharply V-shaped on the second molar. It is occlusally positioned so that not much of the triangular ridges are visible from this aspect. The *distal marginal ridge* is more cervically located than the mesial marginal ridge (like most posterior teeth), and it may have a groove crossing it [4 of 10 first molars in Figure 7.12]. To grasp the concept of this marginal ridge height phenomenon, compare the five *mesial* side views with the five *distal* side views of mandibular second molars shown in Figure 7.10.

The mesial marginal ridge is often crossed by a marginal ridge groove [68% of 209 first molars and 57% of 233 second molars]. On the *first* molar, the *distal marginal ridge* is short and V-shaped, located just lingual and distal to the distal cusp. The distal marginal ridge of the *second* molar is less likely to have a ridge groove [35% of 233 teeth compared to 48% of 215 first molars].

## 2. ROOTS OF MANDIBULAR MOLARS FROM THE PROXIMAL: BROAD MESIAL ROOT USUALLY HAS TWO CANALS

From the mesial aspect, the *mesial* root of the *first* molar is broad buccolingually, hiding the distal root. It has a blunt apex (Figs. 7.1 and 7.10, *upper row*). It is less broad buccolingually on *second* molars, narrower in the cervical third, and more pointed at the apex. There is usually a *deep depression on the mesial surface* of the mesial root extending from the cervical line to the apex, indicating the likelihood of two root canals in this broad root, as vividly seen in Fig. 8.7. The furcal depressions (between the roots) are often deeper than the ones on the outer surface of the mesial and distal roots. The mesial root always has two root canals; one buccal and one lingual. Sometimes this root is divided into a buccal and lingual part (8).

The *distal* root is not quite as broad (buccolingually) nor as long as the mesial root, and it is more pointed at the apex. On some teeth the distal surface of the distal root is convex; on other teeth, there may be a shallow longitudinal depression (Fig. 8.7). Such a depression may indicate two root canals rather than the single canal usually found in this root (Fig. 7.10, *tooth labeled 19*).

## D. Occlusal Aspect of Mandibular Molars

Refer to Figures 7.1, *center,* 7.2, *center,* 7.3**B,** 7.4**B,** 7.6, and 7.11 through 7.14 for similarities and differences.

### LEARNING EXERCISE

*To follow this description the tooth should be held in such a position that the observer is looking exactly parallel to the axis line of the root.*

### 1. LINGUAL INCLINATION

Because of the inclination lingually of the crown, a considerable portion of the buccal surface is visible when the tooth is in this position. As stated previously, both

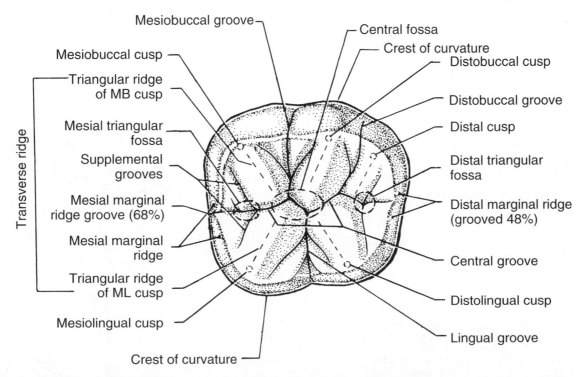

**Figure 7.11.** Occlusal surface of mandibular right first molar. After studying these landmarks, cover up the names with a couple of index cards and see how many of the structures at the inner ends of the lines you are able to identify and name. Observe the buccal and lingual crests of curvature.

# Mandibular Molars (Occlusal)

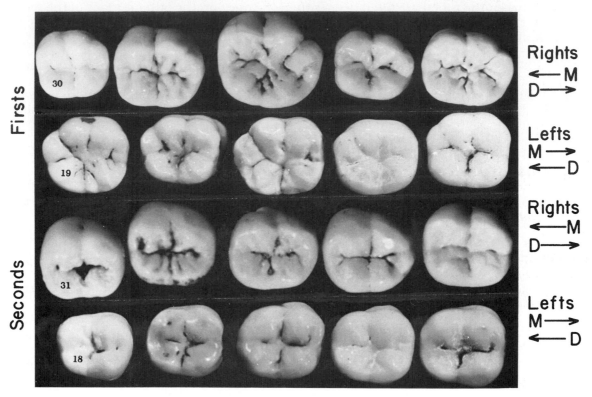

**Figure 7.12.** Mandibular molars (occlusal view). *M* denotes the direction of mesial surfaces; *D* denotes the direction of distal surfaces. Buccal surfaces are *above*, lingual surfaces are *below*. Count the pits.

molars are wider mesiodistally than faciolingually [by 1.2 mm for 281 first molars; 0.9 mm wider for 296 second molars].

## 2. SHAPE: RECTANGULAR OR PENTAGON SHAPE

The *second* molar shape is roughly rectangular, whereas the first molar, with the distal cusp, is more like a pentagon. The two mesial cusps (mesiobuccal and mesiolingual) are larger than the two major distal cusps (Fig. 7.12). (Recall, the first mo-

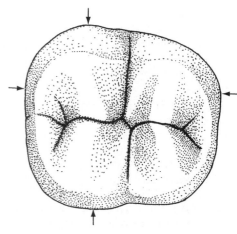

**Figure 7.13.** Mandibular right second molar. The buccal surface is at the *top* and the distal surface is on the *right*. Can you identify the four major cusps and the three major grooves? Can you locate the three fossae? Notice the bulge caused by the buccal cervical ridge beneath the mesiobuccal cusp. Crests of curvature are indicated by *arrows*. The mesial and distal crests of curvature would also be the contact areas.

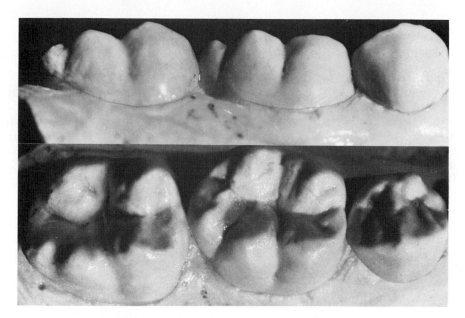

**Figure 7.14.** Mandibular second molar with three buccal cusps (buccal view *above;* occlusal view *below* with buccal side *down*).

lar also has a minor distal cusp.) There are a couple of exceptions to this among the 10 first molars in Figure 7.12. Can you locate them?

## 3. TAPER TO DISTAL AND LINGUAL

The crown tapers two ways so that it is narrower buccolingually on the distal than mesial side and is narrower mesiodistally on the lingual than on the buccal side (Fig. 7.13). This is helpful in determining mesial from distal, and rights from lefts. On the buccal surface of the *second* molar below the mesiobuccal cusp, there is a prominent bulge (buccal cervical ridge). The widest buccolingual dimension of the crown is at this bulge, and spotting it should help you locate the mesial side on mandibular second molars (Figs. 7.12, *lower two rows,* and 7.13). However, the widest portion of the crown of the *first* molar (buccolingually) is at the distobuccal cusp, which is different than on second molars (see crests of curvature in Fig. 7.11).

The outline of the crown on the *first* molar is convex on the buccal, lingual, mesial, and distal (more so on the buccal). On the *second* molar, the mesial side outline is nearly straight; the distal shorter side is more convex.

## 4. RIDGES

On both first and second molars, the triangular ridges of the mesiobuccal and mesiolingual cusps meet to form a transverse ridge, and the triangular ridges of the distobuccal and distolingual cusps form a second transverse ridge (Fig. 7.11). Since lingual cusps are higher, the *triangular ridges* of the lingual cusps of first molars are longer than the triangular ridges of the buccal cusps.

## 5. FOSSAE: THREE

There are three fossae (Fig. 7.11) on mandibular molars: the large *central fossa* (approximately in the center of the tooth), a smaller *mesial triangular fossa* (just inside the mesial marginal ridge), and the smallest *distal triangular fossa* (just inside the distal marginal ridge; it is minute on second molars). There may be a pit at the bottom of any of these fossae.

## 6. GROOVES

### a. Mandibular Second Molar Grooves: Grooves in "+" Shape with One Buccal Groove

The typical groove pattern on second molars is simpler than that of the first molars. It resembles a cross (Appendix 8, occlusal views). The *central groove* extends through the central fossa from the mesial triangular fossa to the distal triangular fossa. Its mesiodistal course is straighter than on mandibular first molars (type trait). Compare the central grooves in Figs. 7.11 and 7.13. The *buccal groove* separates the mesiobuccal and distobuccal cusps (often extending onto the buccal surface), and is usually continuous with the *lingual groove* that separates the mesiolingual and the distolingual cusps.

Developmental marginal ridge grooves occur more frequently on the mesial than the distal [57% and 35%, respectively, on 233 teeth]. There are sometimes supplemental grooves named according to their location and direction (mesiobuccal supplemental groove, distolingual supplemental groove, etc.). One author says that mandibular second molars have more secondary grooves and a more rectangular shape than first molars (10). *Supplemental ridges* are located between supplemental and major grooves and serve as additional cutting blades. All grooves provide important escapeways for food as it is crushed. Without these ridges and grooves the teeth would be subject to unfavorable loading and lateral forces during mastication, as well as being inefficient crushers.

### b. Mandibular First Molar Grooves: "Zigzag" Shape with Two Buccal Grooves

The grooves on the mandibular *first* molar separate the five cusps instead of four, so the pattern is slightly more complicated (Appendix 8, occlusal views; Fig. 7.11). As in the second molars, there are several principal grooves: the *central groove* extends through the central fossa from the mesial triangular to the distal triangular fossa. The central groove is more *zigzag* or crooked in its mesiodistal course. The *lingual groove* starts in the central fossa and extends lingually between the mesiolingual and the distolingual cusps onto the lingual surface.

Instead of one buccal groove, the mandibular first molar has two. The *mesiobuccal groove,* like the buccal groove of the second molar, starts from the central groove at or just mesial to the central fossa and extends between the mesiobuccal and the distobuccal cusps onto the buccal surface. This groove may be nearly continuous with the lingual groove. (Compare this location to the buccal groove of the second molar.) The *distobuccal groove,* unique to the first molar, starts from the central groove between the central fossa and the distal triangular fossa and extends between the distobuccal and the distal cusps onto the buccal surface.

There are numerous minor supplemental ridges and grooves (named according to their direction and cusp).

The *mesial* marginal ridge is often crossed by a groove [68% of 209 first molars]. Seven of the 10 first molars in Figure 7.12 have marginal grooves on the mesial, but only four have them on the distal ridge. The *distal* marginal ridge is less often crossed by a marginal ridge groove [48% of 215 first molars].

## 7. CONTACT AREAS

The *mesial* contact area of the *first* molar is about in the center buccolingually, whereas on the *second* molar it is near the junction of the middle and buccal thirds.

The *distal* contact of the *first* molar is just lingual to the distal cusp, whereas on the *second* molar, it is centered buccolingually.

## 8. VARIATIONS

As mentioned, on 874 casts of dental hygienists' dentitions at Ohio State University, 19% of the 1327 mandibular first molars had only four cusps (no distal cusp). This four-cusp type of first molar does not taper as much from buccal to lingual as a four-cusp mandibular second molar (occlusal aspect), it often tapers from distal to mesial (Fig. 7.6), which is unusual, and, of course, has only one buccal groove, called the *buccal groove*.

Some mandibular first molars have a sixth cusp, which is named *tuberculum sextum* when located on the distal marginal ridge between the distal cusp and distolingual cusp; it is named *tuberculum intermedium* (Figs. 7.16 and 2.8) when located between the two lingual cusps (11). The sixth cusp and a third root on the lingual aspect are common among the Chinese people.

Two of the specimens in Figure 7.7 (*lower row*) are first molars, one with extremely long roots, the other with a large buccal cavity that has both roots bent at a right angle (flexion).

The pattern of the grooves on the occlusal surface of the mandibular molars shows considerable variation. Studies have been made of the occlusal anatomy of these teeth, both in ancient and in modern man. Three principal types of occlusal groove patterns have been described: type Y, in which the central groove forms a Y figure with the lingual groove; type +, in which the central groove forms a + figure with the buccal and the lingual grooves (common in four-cusp type of first molars); and type X, in which the occlusal grooves are somewhat in the form of an X (12). If you examine a collection of extracted mandibular molar teeth, you will see some of these variations (Fig. 7.12).

It is reported that in the Bantu people in Africa, and sometimes in Eskimos, the mandibular molars often increase in size from first to third so that the third molar is the largest and the first molar is the smallest. This is reported to occur also in Pima Indians (13). This is not the most frequent order of size found in American and European peoples.

In Mongolians, the root trunk may be long, or the roots may be completely fused (1). Some unusual root curvatures are seen among the lower five teeth in Figure 7.7 (one is a second molar; can you spot it?).

Five cusp mandibular second molars (shaped just like five-cusp first molars with a distal cusp) are not uncommon among the Chinese and Negroid populations (11). In Figure 7.14, one is shown from a Caucasian mouth or dentition.

### LEARNING EXERCISE

*Name all of the ridges that can be seen from the occlusal aspect of a mandibular first or second molar as shown in the two line drawings (Fig. 7.15**A** and **B**). In case you wondered, ridge 17 on the second molar is the buccal cervical ridge (sometimes evident, sometimes not).*

*Review how to distinguish mandibular second molars from first molars (Table 7.4).*

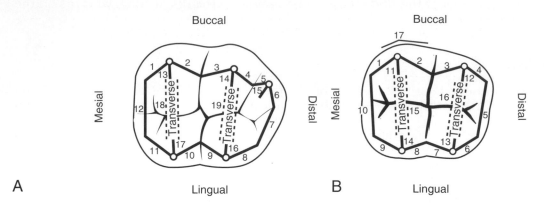

**Figure 7.15. A.** Ridges on mandibular first molar (*circles* indicate cusps). Name all 19 ridges. **B.** Ridges on mandibular second molar and four-cusp first molars. Name all 17 ridges.

A. Name the Ridges

| Ridges | Name |
|--------|------|
| 1. | _____ |
| 2. | _____ |
| 3. | _____ |
| 4. | _____ |
| 5. | _____ |
| 6. | _____ |
| 7. | _____ |
| 8. | _____ |
| 9. | _____ |
| 10. | _____ |
| 11. | _____ |
| 12. | _____ |
| 13. | _____ |
| 14. | _____ |
| 15. | _____ |
| 16. | _____ |
| 17. | _____ |
| 18. | _____ |
| 19. | _____ |

B. Name the Ridges

| Ridges | Name |
|--------|------|
| 1. | _____ |
| 2. | _____ |
| 3. | _____ |
| 4. | _____ |
| 5. | _____ |
| 6. | _____ |
| 7. | _____ |
| 8. | _____ |
| 9. | _____ |
| 10. | _____ |
| 11. | _____ |
| 12. | _____ |
| 13. | _____ |
| 14. | _____ |
| 15. | _____ |
| 16. | _____ |
| 17. | _____ |

**Table 7.4.** How to Distinguish Mandibular Second Molars from First Molars

| SECOND MOLARS CHARACTERISTICS (VERSUS FIRST MOLARS) | |
|---|---|
| All Views | Four cusps and crowns are more symmetrical from all aspects |
| Buccal (Fig. 7.5) | Less cervical convergence of crown and only one buccal groove which is usually shorter and without a pit<br>More cervically located contact areas<br>Longer root trunk and straighter roots, which are closer together mesiodistally<br>Crowns appear to be tipped distally more on their roots |
| Mesial (Fig. 7.10, *left side*) | Less broad mesial root (faciolingually)<br>Less wide root apex |
| Occlusal (Fig. 7.12) | Their distal contact is located in the middle of the crown buccolingually and cervico-occlusally<br>A more prominent buccal cervical ridge (toward mesial)<br>A more rectangular outline (not like pentagon firsts)<br>A cross-shaped groove pattern<br>Widest portion of crown opposite the mesiobuccal cusp (Fig. 7.13)<br>Less crown taper from buccal to lingual [sometimes none (10)], see (Fig. 7.6)<br>More secondary developmental grooves<br>Less frequent marginal ridge grooves (mesial 57%, distal 35%)<br>Central groove is straight (not zig zag as on first molar) |

# SECTION III. MANDIBULAR THIRD MOLAR CHARACTERISTICS

## A. Crowns

Refer to Figures 7.17 through 7.20 for similarities and differences.

### 1. SHAPE AND RELATIVE SIZE: BULBOUS; RESEMBLING FIRST OR SECOND MOLARS BUT EXTREMELY VARIABLE

This tooth is the shortest of the mandibular teeth [averaging 18.2 mm]. This tooth is extremely variable and can be either large or small (Fig. 7.18). The crown of the mandibular third molar sometimes *resembles* the crown of the mandibular second molar (four cusps) and sometimes the crown of the mandibular first molar (five cusps). Again, it may bear little resemblance to either. There may even be a small or large supernumerary tooth fused to it.

Mandibular third molars are generally characterized by their bulbous crowns (very convex on buccal and lingual) and short roots (Fig. 7.17, and the *lower rows* in Figs. 7.19 and 7.20).

### 2. DISTAL TIP

Like mandibular first and second molars, third molars are tipped distally on their root base so, from the buccal aspect, the distal half of the crown is usually noticeably shorter than the mesial half (Fig. 7.19, *lower row*).

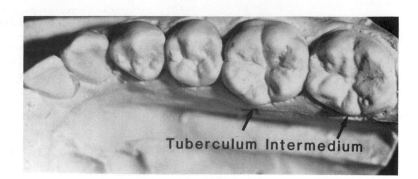

**Figure 7.16.** Mandibular first and second molars with three lingual cusps (tuberculum intermedium). When an extra cusp is found on the distal marginal ridge, it is called tuberculum sextum.

### 3. CUSP SIZE

The lingual cusps are larger and longer than the buccal cusps, with the mesiolingual being the largest of all. The mesiobuccal cusp is the widest and usually highest of the two or three buccal cusps. This is an aid in determining mesial from distal sides and rights from lefts.

### 4. GROOVES: WRINKLED SURFACE WITH MANY SUPPLEMENTAL GROOVES AND RIDGES

Unique to the third molar is its likelihood of having an irregular groove pattern with numerous supplemental grooves and pits on the occlusal surface that produce a wrinkled appearance (Fig. 7.20, *lower row*).

### 5. OCCLUSAL SHAPE: RECTANGULAR OR OVAL

The occlusal outline of a mandibular third molar crown is rectangular or oval mesiodistally (Fig. 7.20, *lower row*), and third molars have a small occlusal table (the buccal cusp tips are closer to the lingual cusp tips than on first and second mandibular molars).

### 6. TAPER TO DISTAL

The crown of the four-cusp type tapers from mesial to distal, but only slightly from buccal to lingual (occlusal aspect) (Fig. 7.20). [It was wider mesiodistally than faciolingually by 1.2 mm on 262 teeth.] The buccal crown outline is often relatively flat compared to the lingual side (occlusal view).

**Figure 7.17. A**. Four-cusp mandibular right third molar. Buccal surface. Note the bulbous crown and the short, fused roots. An extra cusplet is on the buccal surface of the mesiobuccal cusp. This extra cusp or cusplet is *not* called a Carabelli cusp. **B.** Five-cusp mandibular left third molar. Buccal surface. There is an extra cusplet (not Carabelli) on the mesial surface of the mesiobuccal cusp and a tubercle on the mesial marginal ridge. The crown is very large and the roots are barely longer than the crown. The distal root (*right* side) is not quite complete.

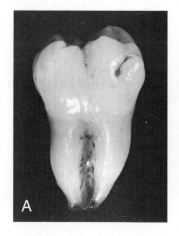
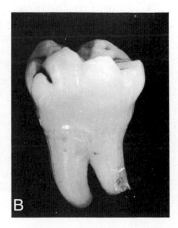

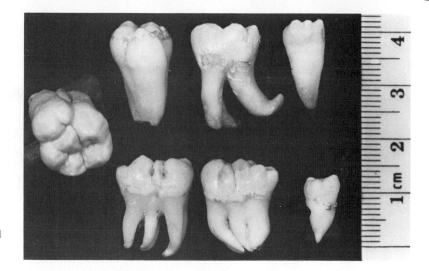

**Figure 7.18.** Buccal view of six unusual mandibular third molars and occlusal view (*left* side) of one with a paramolar fused to its buccal surface. Two in the *lower row* are double or fused teeth (Fig. 11.13).

## 7. RELATIVE SIZE

In Caucasians, the third molar is usually the smallest of the mandibular molars. A common exception is the five-cusp third molar, which may have a crown somewhat larger and more bulbous than the second molar.

## B. Roots of Mandibular Third Molars: Short and Fused

As with first and second mandibular molars, there are two roots, mesial and distal, but often these are *fused* together. If the roots are separate, the *root trunk is long* and the roots are usually more pointed at the apex than on the other molars (Fig. 7.19). Often they curve more distally than the roots of first and second molars. They may have one or more extra roots.

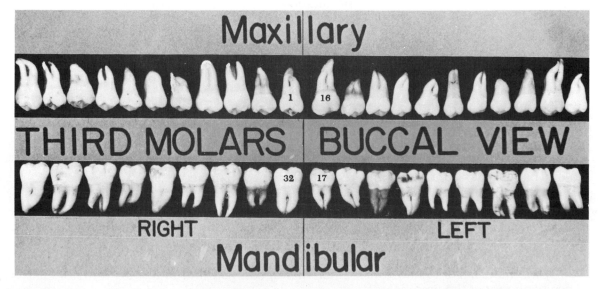

**Figure 7.19.** Buccal views of maxillary and mandibular third molars. Notice the tremendous variation among the maxillary third molars. They are still characteristically different in morphology than the mandibular third molars in the *lower row*, however. The occlusal view of these 40 teeth is shown in Figure 7.20. The mesial surfaces all face toward the center line. (Method of comparison and teeth furnished by Kelli Whapham, first-year O.S.U. dental hygiene student, 1978.)

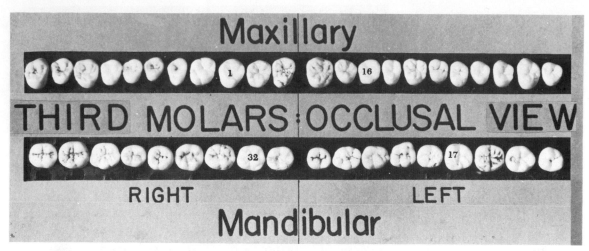

**Figure 7.20.** Occlusal views of maxillary and mandibular third molars. The lingual surfaces of the maxillary teeth *face down* and those of the mandibular teeth *face up*. All mesial surfaces face the center line. Most of the maxillary third molars are largest faciolingually in contrast to the mandibular third molars whose greater dimension is mesiodistally. Observe the wrinkled occlusal designs in both and try to recognize the characteristic appearance of mandibular as opposed to maxillary third molars. The buccal view of these same 40 teeth is shown in Figure 7.19. Several of the mandibular molars have six cusps. Can you find them?

The third molar roots are normally significantly shorter than those on the second molar [averaging over 2 mm shorter on 839 mandibular molars]. Extreme root curvature is seen on the two third molars in Figure 7.7 and the center one in the *upper row* in Figure 7.18. The roots on mandibular third molars are only about half again as long as the crown, and the root-to-crown ratio is noticeably different from that of mandibular first and second molars [1.6:1 compared to 1.8:1 on 839 teeth].

## C. In Summary: Mandibular Third Molar Characteristics

1. Bulbous crowns—convex on buccal and more so on the lingual.

2. Short roots, close together with long root trunks, roots frequently fused; apical third of both curved distally and pointed.

3. Small or narrow wrinkled occlusal surfaces (chewing areas).

4. Four or five cusps—resembling first or second molars; mesiolingual is largest.

5. Mesiobuccal cusps that are usually wider and longer than distobuccal cusps.

6. Crowns that usually taper from mesial to distal.

7. Small root-to-crown ratios.

8. Oblong crowns mesiodistally (rectangular or oval mesiodistally).

### LEARNING EXERCISES

*Examine the mouth of a number of your associates and see how many still have third molars.*

*Of the third molars you examine, how many can you find that have a distal cusp resembling that of the first molar?*

*Of the individuals you examine, what proportion of those over age 18 have lost one or both mandibular first molars?*

*How many of your classmates have had one or more third molars that never formed?*

*Can you find a classmate who has four-cusp mandibular first molars or one who has five-cusp second molars?*

## TEST YOUR KNOWLEDGE OF THE MANDIBULAR MOLARS BY ANSWERING THESE QUESTIONS:

*Name the grooves that radiate out from the central fossa in a mandibular first molar.*

*Which cusp has two triangular ridges in the mandibular first molar? (Watch out, this might be a trick question.)*

*Draw an occlusal view of a mandibular second molar and make up a list of all the ridges that can be seen from this view. If you can do this easily, then name the 19 ridges on the mandibular first molar listed in Figure 7.15A. Most of this you should find easy and somewhat repetitive.*

*Which cusp is the largest and longest on a mandibular second molar?*

*Which cusp is the largest in area from the occlusal view on a mandibular second molar?*

*Which cusp may be absent on a mandibular first or third molar?*

*Name the fossae on a mandibular first molar.*

*Which developmental groove connects with the lingual groove running in the same direction on a mandibular second molar?*

*From which aspect is only one root visible on a mandibular first molar?*

*Which root may occasionally be divided or bifurcated on a mandibular first molar?*

*Can you list six ways that mandibular second molars differ from mandibular first molars?*

*List in sequential order the longest to shortest cusps on the mandibular first molar.*

*List in sequential order the largest to smallest cusp area on the mandibular first molar (occlusal view).*

*Which cusp is most likely to be absent on some third molars? When this occurs, which groove would not be present? What is the same groove called when the tooth has three buccal cusps?*

*Describe those characteristics of a mandibular third molar that would distinguish it from other mandibular molars.*

*Name the grooves that radiate out of the mesial triangular fossa on the mandibular first molar.*

*Name the grooves that radiate out of the distal triangular fossa on a mandibular second molar.*

*Which is the largest fossa on a mandibular first molar? Which ridges form its boundaries?*

*Can you list ALL of the ridges that circumscribe or make up the boundary of the occlusal surface of a mandibular first molar? Check your answer with Figure 7.15A.*

*Which two pairs of cusp triangular ridges make up or join to form the two transverse ridges on a mandibular second molar?*

*Which cusp triangular ridge does not meet to form a transverse ridge on a five-cusp third molar?*

*Have you ever seen a six-cusp mandibular molar? The answer had better be yes because there is one in this chapter (Fig. 7.16) (14).*

*What is the frequency of developmental marginal ridge grooves on mandibular first and second molars? Is there a difference on the mesial and distal ridges? The percentages are not as important as the relative frequency.*

*Can you find any third molars that have part of another tooth fused to them (Fig. 7.18)?*

# SECTION IV. TYPE TRAITS OF MAXILLARY FIRST AND SECOND MOLARS

## A. Buccal Aspect of Maxillary First and Second Molars

### LEARNING EXERCISE

*Examine a maxillary first and second molar as you read. Hold the roots up and the crowns down, with the two somewhat parallel roots toward you.*

## 1. CROWN FROM THE BUCCAL

Refer to Figures 7.21, *left*, 7.22, *left*, 7.23**A** and **B**, *left sides*, 7.24, *left*, and 7.25 for similarities and differences.

### a. Shape

#### (1) Relative Size

Maxillary molars are the largest maxillary teeth.

The second molar is smaller than the first molar in the same mouth (Fig. 7.31) especially mesiodistally. (Third molars are generally the smallest.)

#### (2) Taper Cervically from Contact Areas

From the buccal aspect, the crown of both maxillary molars are broad near the junction of the occlusal and middle thirds and narrower near the cervical line. However, the *second* molar is less broad mesiodistally than the first molar, and is often tipped distally on the root base or trunk.

### b. Number and Size of Cusps: Mesiobuccal Longer and Wider than Distobuccal

On both maxillary molars, there are two cusps on the buccal side: a *mesiobuccal cusp* and a *distobuccal cusp*. Of the two buccal cusps, the mesiobuccal cusp is usually longer and wider than the distobuccal cusp, but not necessarily sharper. [Of 1539 maxillary *first* molars, the mesiobuccal cusp was wider 64% of the time; on 1545 *second* molars, this cusp was wider 92% of the time. On 468 *first* molars, the distobuccal cusp was sharper 72% of the time; whereas, on 447 *second* molars, the sharpness of buccal cusps was equal.]

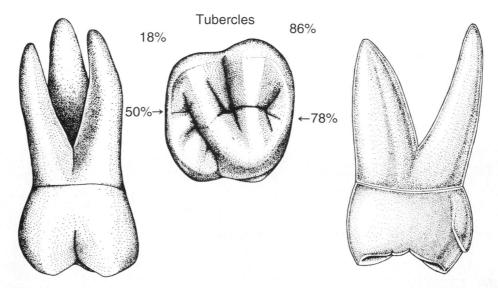

**Figure 7.21.** Maxillary right first molar: buccal, occlusal, and mesial views. Percentages give the frequency of marginal ridge tubercles (*above*), and of marginal ridge grooves (*arrows below*).

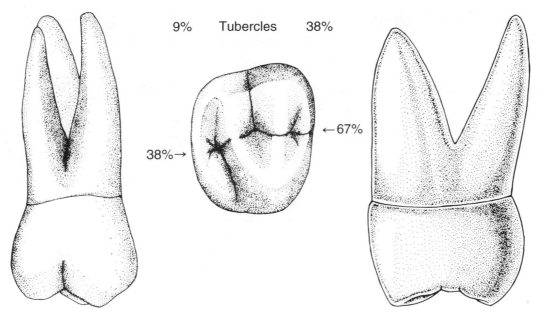

9%     Tubercles     38%

38%→     ←67%

**Figure 7.22.** Maxillary right second molar: buccal, occlusal, and mesial views. Percentages give the frequency of marginal ridge tubercles (*above*), and of marginal ridge grooves (*arrows below*).

### c. Buccal Groove: May End in Pit on Buccal Surface

The *buccal groove* lies between the buccal cusps and extends cervically on the buccal surface to the middle third of the crown (shorter on second molars). At the end of the buccal groove there is sometimes a pit that can become the site of dental caries (less often on second molars).

### d. Proximal Contacts (Same as for All Molars)

*Mesial*—junction of occlusal and middle thirds.

*Distal*—middle of tooth.

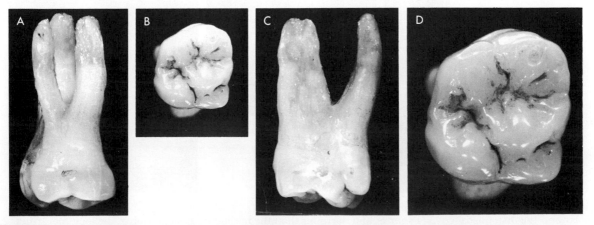

**Figure 7.23. A**. *Maxillary* right *first* molar. **1.** Buccal surface. **2.** Occlusal surface. Buccal side at *top;* mesial at *right*. This specimen has an unusually large cusp of Carabelli. **3.** Mesial surface. The wide mesiobuccal root hides the narrower distobuccal root. **4.** An enlargement of view 2. Notice that this tooth is wider on the lingual than on the buccal surface. Compare the surface morphology with the labeled diagram in Figure 7.30 and with the photograph of the occlusal surface of another maxillary right first molar in Figure 7.23**B** (view **D**). The groove at the place of attachment of the cusp of Carabelli to the mesiolingual cusp, such as is seen here, is sometimes the site of caries.

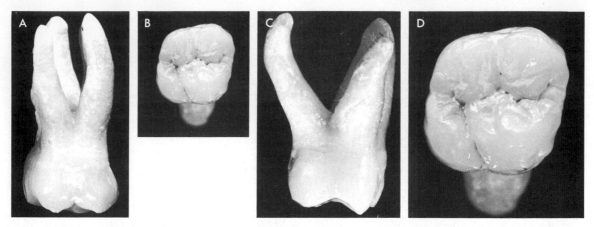

**Figure 7.23. B**. *Maxillary* right *first* molar. **A.** Buccal surface. **B.** Occlusal surface. Buccal side at *top;* mesial at *right*. **C.** Distal surface. **D.** An enlargement of **B** in this figure. That somewhat wrinkled enamel surface and the relatively shallow fossae and grooves are more easily seen in the enlargement: notice the two tubercles on the mesial (*right*) marginal ridge. The characteristically nearly square shape is apparent. The cusp of Carabelli is absent. This is not uncommon. Thirty percent of 1558 first molars examined had no Carabelli cusp.

### e. Outline Shape: Occlusocervical Dimension of Crown Tapers to the Distal

On maxillary *first* molars, from the buccal aspect, the distal side of the crown is nearly flat in the cervical third. Occlusal to this flat region, the surface is convex (Figs. 7.21, *left,* and 7.23**A**, view **A** ).

On maxillary *second* molars, the crown is often tilted distally at the cervix (Fig. 7.24, *left*). The occlusal surface slants cervically from mesial to distal. This *distal tipping* of the crown and the shortness of the distobuccal cusp make the *buccal outline of the crown appear to be shorter on the distal than mesial,* which is most helpful in determining rights from lefts.

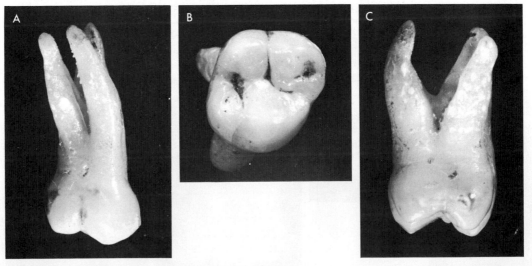

**Figure 7.24.** *Maxillary* right *second* molar. **A.** Buccal surface. The roots are less spread than those of the first molar and the distobuccal cusp is shorter and narrower than the mesiobuccal cusp. Notice the long root trunk and that the crown is tipped distally on its root base. **B.** Occlusal surface. Buccal side at *top;* mesial at *right.* The twist of the crown makes the mesiobuccal angle smaller (more acute) and the mesiolingual angle larger (more obtuse) than in the first molar. Notice the decided taper of the crown from buccal to lingual. Sometimes these differences between the shape of the first and second molars are greater than are seen here. Often in the second molar, the acute angles are smaller and the obtuse angles larger than in this tooth, and often the distolingual cusp is much smaller, or even missing. **C.** Distal surface. The roots are less spread than the first molar. The crown is noticeably shorter on the distal than mesial surface so you can see the outlines of all four cusps.

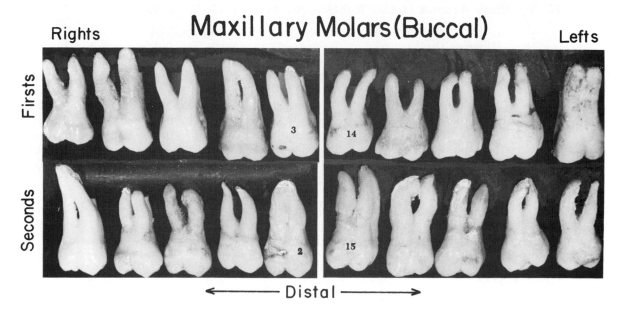

**Figure 7.25.** Maxillary molars (buccal view). The lingual roots are embedded in the black wax and do not show.

## 2. ROOTS: NORMALLY THREE (LINGUAL OR PALATAL IS LONGEST, THEN MESIOBUCCAL; DISTOBUCCAL IS SHORTEST)

At the cervical line the crown is attached to a broad, undivided base called the *root trunk* (longer on second molars). Apical to the root trunk, the root separates into three parts: the *mesiobuccal root*, the *distobuccal root*, and the *lingual root*. The point of furcation is often near the junction of the cervical and middle thirds of the roots. This furcation is called a *trifurcation* since three roots come off the trunk. The furcation between the two buccal roots is a greater distance from the cervical line on second molars than on the first molars. [In Mongoloid peoples, the maxillary first molars often have long root trunk; sometimes there is no furcation at all (1). See the last specimen on the right in Fig. 7.25, *upper row.*]

### a. Maxillary First Molar Roots

There is much variation in the shapes of the roots. On *first* molars, the mesiobuccal and distobuccal roots are often well-separated and bent in such a way that they look like the handles on a pair of pliers. This is in contrast to the roots of the *second* molar (Fig. 7.25, compare *upper row* to *lower row*), which are often close together, and more nearly parallel; and to those of the third molar (Fig. 7.19, *top row*), which are shorter and often fused (type traits).

On *first* molars, the mesiobuccal and distobuccal roots often are curved distally. The mesiobuccal root bends mesially in the cervical half before bending toward the distal (Figs. 7.21, *left;* 7.23**A**). In the first molar, the curvature of the apical third of the mesiobuccal root may be enough to place the apex of this root distal to the line of the buccal groove on the crown.

The roots are nearly the same length (within 1.5 mm); usually the mesiobuccal root is about 0.75 mm longer than the distobuccal root and 0.75 mm shorter than the lingual root [measurements from 308 teeth]. Both the mesiobuccal and distobuccal roots taper apically, with the apex of the mesiobuccal root usually more blunt. Characteristically, the spread of the middle third of the two buccal roots is nearly as wide as the crown (Figs. 7.21 and 7.23).

### b. Maxillary Second Molars Roots: Less Curved, More Parallel

On the *second* molars, the mesiobuccal and distobuccal roots are less curved than those of the first molar; they are more nearly parallel with each other, and both bend toward the distal in their apical third (not always; find the two second molars in Fig. 7.25 which are exceptions). See Appendix 8j.

[In a Japanese study of root formation on 3370 maxillary second molars, 50% had three roots, 49% were split equally between single and double roots and 1% had four roots. In the three-rooted second molars, 75% had complete separation of roots (no fusion). The tendency to fuse was higher in the roots of teeth extracted from females. Lingual roots were straight in half of the three-rooted teeth (15).]

## B. Lingual Aspect of Maxillary Molars

Refer to Figure 7.26 for similarities and differences.

### 1. CROWN: LINGUAL ASPECT

#### a. Relative Size and Taper

Due to a prominent distolingual cusp, the crown of the *first* molar may be as wide or wider on the lingual than on the buccal half, except in the cervical third. This is not as likely on *second* molars. (Compare the occlusal view in Fig. 7.21 with that in Fig. 7.22.)

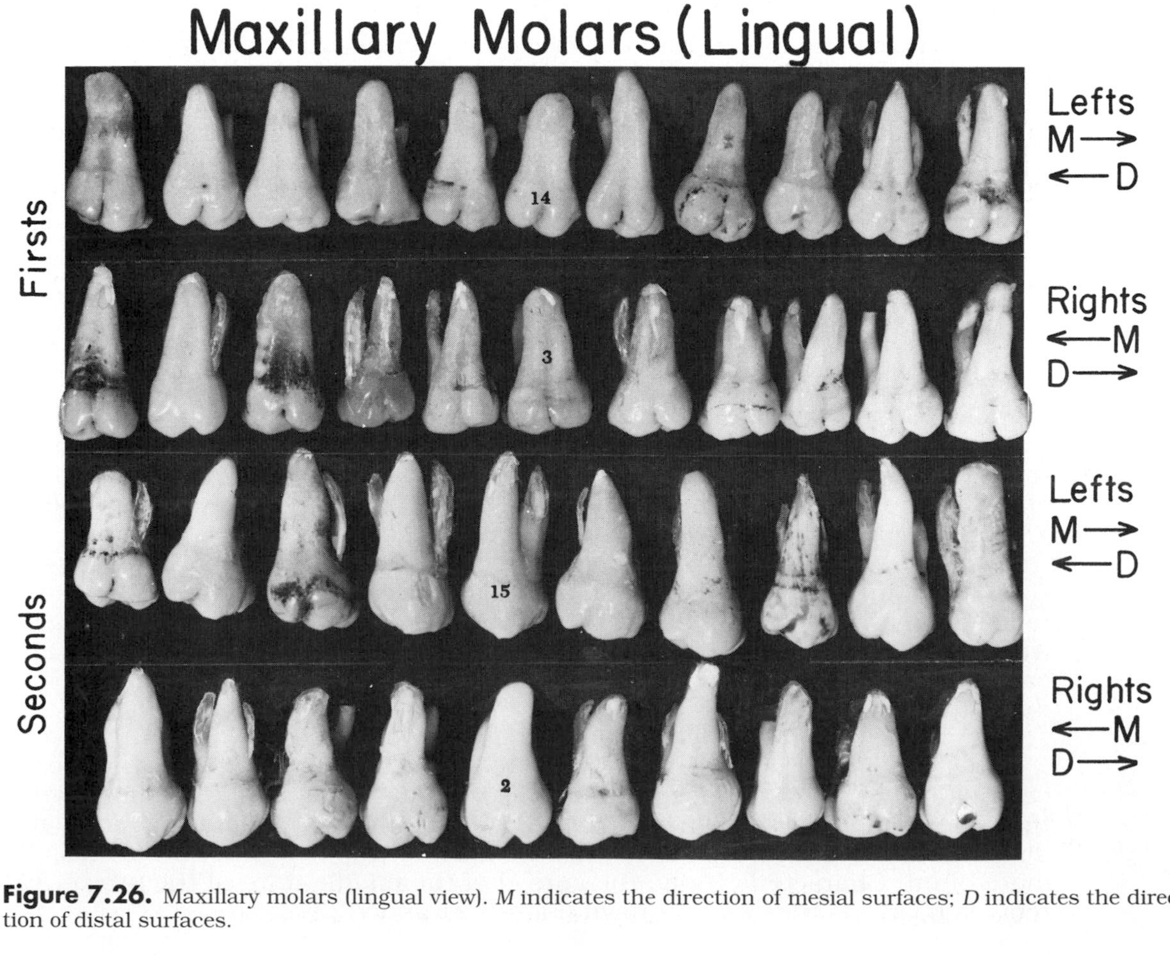

**Figure 7.26.** Maxillary molars (lingual view). *M* indicates the direction of mesial surfaces; *D* indicates the direction of distal surfaces.

The crown on the maxillary *second* molar usually appears smaller than that of the first molar in the same mouth, particularly in its width and on the lingual side which has a smaller or nonexistent distolingual cusp (Fig. 7.31). The lingual surface of both maxillary molars is narrower in the cervical third than in the middle third, since the crown tapers to join the single palatal root (Fig. 7.26).

### b. Number and Description of Lingual Cusps on a First Molar

On the *first* molar, there are two well-defined cusps on the lingual surface, the large *mesiolingual cusp* and the smaller *distolingual cusp*. The mesiolingual cusp is almost always the largest and highest cusp on any maxillary molar.

Additionally, on the *first* molar there is often a small *fifth* cusp or cusplet attached to the lingual surface of the mesiolingual cusp. It is called the *cusp of Carabelli,* or the *tubercle of Carabelli,* after the Austrian dentist (George von Carabelli) who described it in 1842 (Appendix 8i). The fifth cusp varies greatly in shape and size. It may be a conspicuous, well-formed cusp (Fig. 7.23**A**), or, at the other extreme, it may be barely discernible or absent (Fig. 7.23**B**), or there may even be a depression in this location. The presence or absence of the cusp of Carabelli seems to be a racial characteristic. It is a nonfunctioning cusp, even when large, because it is located about 2 mm short of the mesiolingual cusp tip. Some of the variations in shape and size are seen in the *upper two rows* of Figures 7.26 and 7.29. [As seen in Table 7.5, 29.5% of 1558 maxillary first molars were without any type of Carabelli formation.]

A number of studies have been done concerning the occurrence and size of the cusp of Carbelli (16–20). One investigator reports that it is extremely rare in the East Greenland Eskimo. In European people, it is usually present. The Carabelli trait was absent on 35.4% of the teeth in 489 Hindu children (21). The groove form was more common (35%) than tubercles (26%) on the first molars (21).

The cusp of Carabelli is *rarely found on second* and third maxillary molars.

### c. Number and Description of Lingual Cusps on Second Molars (Two Types)

There are two types of maxillary *second* molars based on the number of cusps (four and three). On the four-cusp second molar, there are two lingual cusps: mesiolingual cusp (which is considerably larger) and distolingual cusp. On both first and second molars with *two lingual cusps,* there is a groove extending between the mesiolingual and distolingual cusps that extends onto the lingual surface where it is called the *lingual groove.* This lingual groove may be continuous with the longitudinal depression on the lingual surface of the lingual root. It joins the *distal oblique groove* on the occlusal surface of the tooth just like the first molar (Fig. 7.30).

**Table 7.5.** Frequency of Occurrence and Type of Carabelli Cusp Formation on 1558 Maxillary First Molars*

| | | |
|---|---|---|
| Large Carabelli cusp | 19% | ⎫ 70.5% some |
| Small Carabelli cusp | 27.5% | ⎬ type of Carabelli |
| Slight depression | 24% | ⎪ formation |
| Nothing | 29.5% | ⎭ |
| Same type on right and left | 76% | |
| Different on each side | 24% | |
| (835 comparisons on casts) | | |

*Observations from dental stone casts of Ohio dental hygienists made by Dr. Woelfel and his students 1971–1983.

The *three cusp type of maxillary second molar* (tricuspid form) is one in which the distolingual cusp is absent, leaving just one lingual cusp, which is large. [The distolingual cusp was absent in 38% of 1398 second molars examined by Dr. Woelfel.] This type has no lingual groove, and no distal (cigar-shaped) fossa. See if you can find five of these in Figures 7.26 and 7.29.

## 2. FIRST AND SECOND MAXILLARY MOLAR ROOTS FROM THE LINGUAL

On the *first* molar, the longest lingual root [averaging 13.7 mm on 308 maxillary first molars] is the third longest root on any maxillary tooth, after the maxillary canine and second premolar roots. The lingual root is not curved as seen from the lingual view, but it does taper apically to a blunt or rounded apex. There is usually a longitudinal depression on the lingual side of the lingual root of the *first* molar (Fig. 7.26, *upper two rows*). The characteristically wide mesiodistal spread of the curved buccal roots on the first molar is visible from this view.

The lingual root on the *second* molar is as long as, and resembles, the lingual root of the first molar. However, the buccal roots may bend somewhat more distally and are closer together and more parallel than on first molars.

## C. Proximal Aspect of First and Second Maxillary Molars

Refer to Figures 7.21 and 7.22, *right side*, 7.27, and 7.28 for similarities and differences.

### *LEARNING EXERCISE*

*Compare important distinguishing features shown in Figure 7.27 as you also examine extracted teeth, rotating them to view the mesial, then the distal.*

## 1. CROWN: PROXIMAL ASPECT

### a. First Molar Cusps

The maxillary *first* molar crown appears short and broad faciolingually from the *mesial* view. Two (or three) cusps are seen from the mesial: the *mesiobuccal cusp* and the long and large *mesiolingual cusp.* A cusp of Carabelli, if present, would be seen 2–3 mm below the mesiolingual cusp tip. The cusps of the distal side of the tooth are shorter and usually are not seen when the tooth is examined from the mesial side. Also, the mesial marginal ridge is in a more occlusal position than the distal marginal ridge, so very little of the occlusal surface (triangular ridges) is visible from this view (Fig. 7.27, *upper row, right side*).

There is a noticeable convergence or narrowing of the crown toward the occlusal surface from the buccal and lingual crests of curvature (Fig. 7.21, *right*) resulting in a relatively narrow occlusal table.

The cusps of the first molar, in the usual order of their height, longest to shortest, are: mesiolingual, mesiobuccal, distobuccal, distolingual, and fifth cusp (cusp of Carabelli).

From the distal (Fig. 7.27, *upper left*), four cusps are clearly visible: the *distobuccal cusp;* the smallest *distolingual cusp;* part of the *mesiobuccal cusp;* and part of the largest *mesiolingual cusp.* When present on first molars, the Carabelli cusp can usually be seen on the lingual surface from this view. The distobuccal cusp is often slightly longer than the distolingual cusp.

## Maxillary Molars (Proximal)

Lefts                Rights

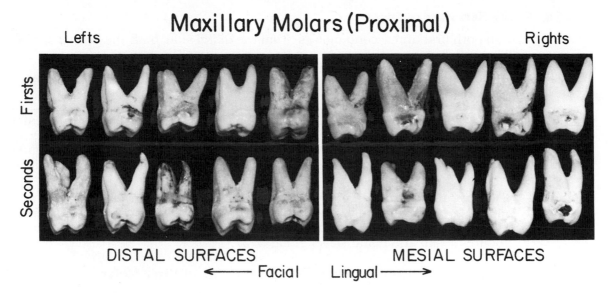

Firsts

Seconds

DISTAL SURFACES          MESIAL SURFACES

⟵ Facial     Lingual ⟶

**Figure 7.27.** Maxillary molars (proximal view). Compare heights of marginal ridges on mesial and distal sides.

### b. Second Molar Cusps

From the mesial and distal aspects, the crown of the *second* maxillary molar looks much like that of the first molar, except that there is no fifth cusp (Fig. 7.27, *lower row*). The distolingual cusp is absent on more than one-third of these teeth.

### c. Crest of Curvature (Proximal Aspects): Similar for All Molars and Premolars

As on other posterior teeth, the crest of curvature of the *buccal* side of the maxillary first molar crown is in the cervical third, usually just occlusal to the cervical line. The crest of curvature of the *lingual* side of the crown is more occlusal, in or near the middle third of the crown. On teeth in which the fifth cusp is large, the lingual crest of curvature is located more occlusally (Fig. 7.23**A,** view 3).

# Maxillary Left Second Molars
## (Mesial Surfaces)

Lingual

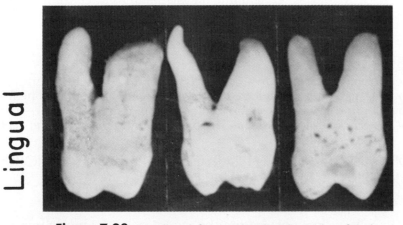

Buccal

**Figure 7.28.** Maxillary left second molars (mesial surfaces).

### d. Taper Narrower to Distal

On both first and second molars, from the *distal* side, both the buccal surface and lingual surface of the crown can be seen because the crown is narrower buccolingually on the distal side than on the mesial side (Fig. 7.27).

### e. Marginal Ridges

On both first and second maxillary molars, the concave, occlusally located *mesial marginal ridge* connects the *mesiobuccal cusp* and the *mesiolingual cusp.* It is longer buccolingually and more occlusally located than the distal marginal ridge. Consequently, little of the occlusal surface is visible from the mesial view.

Because the *distal marginal ridge* of these maxillary molars is short and concave, and is more cervically positioned than the mesial marginal ridge, more of the occlusal surface (triangular ridges) can be seen from the distal view. (Compare mesial and distal views in Fig. 7.27.)

### f. Tubercles: Most Often on Mesial Marginal Ridge of First Molar

Often on the unworn mesial marginal ridge of the maxillary *first* molar, there will be one or more projections of enamel called *tubercles* (not as common on second and third molars) (Fig. 7.29, *top rows*). [Tubercles were found on the mesial ridges on 86% of 64 first molars.]

These tubercles are seen much less frequently on the *distal* marginal ridge of *first* molars [18% of 79 teeth], or on the *mesial* or *distal* marginal ridge of the maxillary *second* molars [38% mesially and 9% distally on 79 teeth, respectively].

### g. Marginal Ridge Grooves

In general, *marginal ridge grooves* are more common on the *mesial* marginal ridge than on the distal, and are more common on *first* molars than on seconds. [On *first molars:* 78% of 69 teeth had mesial marginal grooves, but only 50% of 60 had distal marginal grooves; on *second molars,* 67% of 75 teeth had mesial marginal grooves, but only 38% of 79 teeth had marginal ridge grooves.] (See Figures 7.21 and 7.22.)

### h. Cervical Line

On maxillary molars, the mesial cervical line has slight occlusal curvature, [averaging only 0.7 mm on 308 first molars and 0.6 mm on second molars]. There is less curvature of the cervical line on the distal surface than on the mesial surface, but the difference is hardly discernible, since this cementoenamel junction is practically flat buccolingually.

### i. Contact Areas

The mesial contact arear is at the junction of the occlusal and middle third of the crown. The distal contact area of the *first* maxillary molar is near the middle of the crown both cervico-occlusally and buccolingually. Sometimes you can observe a slightly worn spot (facet) in this location where it contacted the second molar.

## 2. ROOTS OF MAXILLARY FIRST MOLARS FROM PROXIMAL: MESIOBUCCAL ROOT WIDER BUCCOLINGUALLY THAN THE DISTOBUCCAL ROOT

### a. Roots of First Molar

On maxillary *first* molars from the *mesial* view, the mesiobuccal root is broad buccolingually and is shorter than the lingual root. Its breadth (two-thirds of the faciolingual dimension) obscures the distobuccal root. The apex of this mesiobuccal root is in line with the tip of the mesiobuccal cusp, whereas the convex buccal surface of this root often *extends a little buccal* to the crown. Observe this characteristic of first molars in Figure 7.27, *upper right.* The lingual surface of the mesiobuccal root is often more convex and, in the apical third curves sharply facially toward the apex. The mesial surface of the mesiobuccal root has a *longitudinal depression* (and although they cannot be seen, this root has two root canals) (see Chapter 8).

The *lingual root* is the longest of the three roots, is "banana" shaped, and on *first* molars *extends conspicuously beyond the crown lingually* (type trait). This feature alone should help you determine maxillary first from second molars. Compare the differences in Figure 7.27. The lingual root tapers apically and usually is curved buccolingually, being concave on its buccal surface. (It has only one root canal.)

From the *distal view,* on the first molar, the *distobuccal root* is shorter and more narrow buccolingually than the mesiobuccal root. It does not extend as far buccally, and its apex is usually more pointed than the mesiobuccal root (Fig. 7.23**B,** *distal view*). The distal surface of the distobuccal root is convex, without a longitudinal depression (and it has only one root canal). See if you can find the small openings for the vessels in or near the apices of the three roots. They are minute in a fully formed tooth.

### b. Roots of Maxillary Second Molars: Roots Closer Together; Root Trunk Longer

On the maxillary *second* molars, the roots are much *less* spread apart than the roots of the first molar (Appendix 8j). The lingual root is straighter than on first molars and usually does not extend beyond the lingual surface of the crown, but there are exceptions (Fig. 7.28). Characteristically, maxillary second molar roots are more often within the confines of the crown from the proximal view, in contrast to first molars, which have the mesiobuccal and particularly the lingual roots projecting beyond the crown (Fig. 7.27). The mesiobuccal root of the maxillary second molar only rarely extends buccally beyond the buccal surface of the crown.

From the *distal,* the apex of the lingual root of the *second* molar is often in line with the tip of the distolingual cusp. The mesiobuccal root, which is wider and longer than the distobuccal root, can be seen behind the distobuccal root.

## D. Occlusal Aspect of First and Second Maxillary Molars

Refer to Figures 7.21 and 7.22, *center,* 7.23**A** and **B,** 7.24**B,** and 7.29 through 7.33 for similarities and differences.

### *LEARNING EXERCISE*

*To follow this description the tooth should be held in such a position that the observer is looking exactly perpendicular to the plane of the occlusal surface, with a line visualized through the tips of the buccal cusps in an exactly horizontal position. Because of the spread of the first molar roots, some of each of the three roots (particularly the lingual root) may be visible (Fig. 7.29) when the tooth is in this position (characteristic of first molars only). In studying these teeth, it must be remembered that the morphology is variable. These variations are discernible in Appendix 8k and Figure 7.29.*

### 1. CONTOUR OF FIRST MOLAR: SQUARE TO PARALLELOGRAM (OR RHOMBOID) AND AS WIDE ON LINGUAL AS BUCCAL

On the maxillary *first* molar, the contour of the occlusal surface is not square, but it gives the general impression of squareness when compared to other teeth.

# Maxillary First Molars (Occlusal)

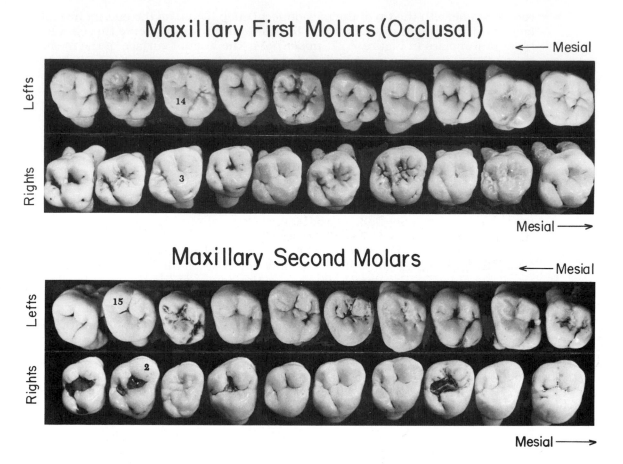

**Figure 7.29.** Maxillary molars (occlusal view). Facial surfaces are *above*, lingual surfaces are *below*. For a simple and quick side determination on maxillary molars oriented as shown (buccal side at *top*): the side (*right* or *left*) of the mesiolingual is the same as the side where the tooth came from. As you can see in the *upper rows* of first and second molars, the larger mesiolingual cusp is to the left side of the distolingual cusp and all of these teeth were extracted from the left side of the arch.

Actually, it is roughly a parallelogram, with two acute and two obtuse angles. The acute angles are the mesiobuccal and distolingual. Can you name the two obtuse angles? The parallelogram is *larger buccolingually than mesiodistally* (arch trait for the maxillary molars) (see Appendix 8k). The oblique ridge transverses between the obtuse angles on the tooth (Fig. 7.30).

On many *first* molars, the lingual side of the crown seen from the occlusal aspect is slightly wider mesiodistally than the buccal side (Figs. 7.23**A** and **B,** *occlusal views*). Try to locate one or two teeth in Figure 7.29 that are not wider on the lingual than on the buccal sides. They are a minority.

## 2. CONTOUR OF SECOND MOLAR: TWISTED PARALLELOGRAM (OR RHOMBOID)

The second molar is also wider buccolingually than mesiodistally, but tapers more from buccal to lingual due to the smaller or absent distolingual cusp.

There is much variation in the morphology of *second* molars, particularly in the size of the distolingual cusp. [Among Dr. Woelfel's hygiene students, 38% of maxillary second molars had no distolingual cusp (808 students' casts with 1396 unrestored second molars).] Five of the 20 second molars in Figure 7.29 have only three cusps.

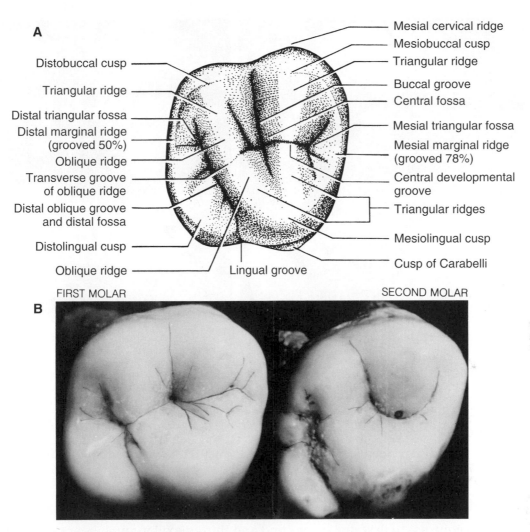

**A.**

Mesial cervical ridge

Mesiobuccal cusp

Triangular ridge

Buccal groove

Central fossa

Mesial triangular fossa

Mesial marginal ridge (grooved 78%)

Central developmental groove

Triangular ridges

Mesiolingual cusp

Cusp of Carabelli

Distobuccal cusp

Triangular ridge

Distal triangular fossa

Distal marginal ridge (grooved 50%)

Oblique ridge

Transverse groove of oblique ridge

Distal oblique groove and distal fossa

Distolingual cusp

Oblique ridge

Lingual groove

FIRST MOLAR

SECOND MOLAR

**B.**

**Figure 7.30. A.** Occlusal surface of a maxillary right first molar with all of the major landmarks named. **B.** *Left:* Maxillary right first molar. *Right:* Maxillary right second molar. Both teeth have all of the morphologic features shown in **A** except for a cusp of Carabelli. Note how the second molar tapers more toward the lingual surface, and has a more rounded mesiolingual angle than the first molar.

The four-cusp type of *second* molars is less square in appearance than the first molar: the obtuse angles at the distobuccal and the mesiolingual cusps are wider, and the acute angles at the mesiobuccal and distolingual cusps are smaller. In other words, the parallelogram is *twisted more* on second molars, with the lingual portion pushed distally. The more acute angle at the mesiobuccal is due in

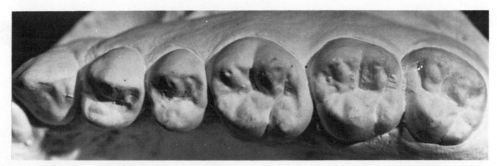

**Figure 7.31.** Comparative size of three maxillary molars in quadrant. This decrease in size from first to third molar is typical in most people.

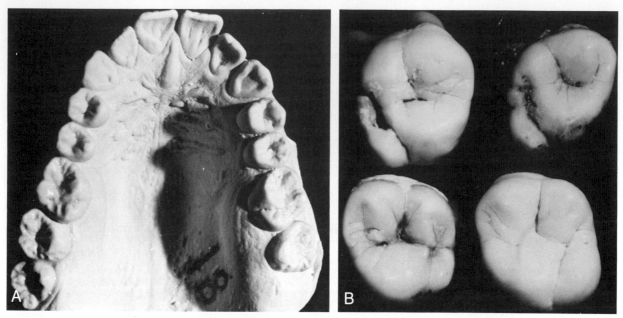

**Figure 7.32. A.** Dental stone cast of maxillary dentition. Notice the decreasing size from first to third molars and the fact that both second molars have only one lingual cusp (tricuspid form). Also note the tubercles on the mesial marginal ridges of the first molars. These were found on 86% of unworn specimens. **B.** *Top:* Two right second molars. *Below:* Two left second molars. Notice the characteristically smaller two distal cusps and the greater twist of the parallelogram outline in these second molars compared to maxillary first molars.

part to a prominent *mesiobuccal cervical ridge* on *second* molars, visible from this view (all 20 second molars in Fig. 7.29). This is helpful in differentiating rights from lefts. The differences in between right and left sides are vividly apparent in Figure 7.32**B.** Also refer to Appendix 8k.

## 3. TAPER TO LINGUAL ON SECOND AND THIRD MOLARS

In contrast to first molars, second and third maxillary molars are noticeably narrower on the lingual side (type trait) (Appendix 8h). The fact that the crown of the second molar tapers from buccal to lingual and from mesial to distal is helpful in differentiating rights from lefts. This taper on second molars may be due in part to the generally smaller distolingual cusp (Fig. 7.32**B**).

When the distolingual cusp is absent, the tooth has only three cusps (six teeth in Fig. 7.29 and both second molars in Fig. 7.32**A** have no distolingual cusps). The three-cusp type (no distolingual cusp) is somewhat triangular or heart-shaped, the blunt apex of the triangle being the lingual cusp.

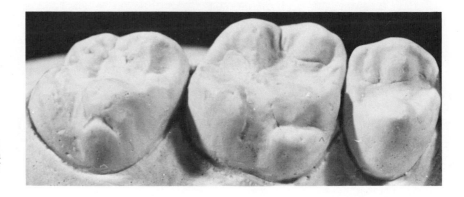

**Figure 7.33.** Maxillary first and second molars, each with a Carabelli cusp. (Courtesy of Dr. Jeff Warner.)

## 4. NUMBER AND SIZE OF CUSPS: NORMALLY FOUR MAJOR CUSPS

The four major cusps of the *first* molar are the mesiobuccal, the distobuccal, the mesiolingual, and the distolingual (Fig. 7.30). The mesiolingual cusp is conspicuously the largest [95% of the 1469 first molars on stone casts]. Most frequently, the distolingual cusp is the smallest [72%]. [The distobuccal cusp was the smallest on 18%, and the mesiobuccal was considered to have the smallest area on 10%.] On *second* molars, there is greater difference in the size of the buccal cusps; the mesiobuccal is noticeably larger (Fig. 7.30**B**). The first molar has a fifth cusp of Carabelli [70% of the time], whereas the second molar does not have this cusp.

## 5. RIDGES: OBLIQUE RIDGE IS UNIQUE TO MAXILLARY MOLARS; EXTENDS FROM MESIOLINGUAL TO DISTOBUCCAL CUSP

On the maxillary *first* molar, each of the four major cusps has a definite *triangular ridge.* The triangular ridges of the mesiolingual cusp and the distobuccal cusp meet and form a diagonal ridge called the *oblique ridge* (characteristic of maxillary molars) (Fig. 7.30**A**). This oblique ridge is smaller on second molars (22). Also on the *first* molar, the mesiolingual cusp usually has a second triangular ridge mesial to the one that meets the triangular ridge of the distobuccal cusp (Fig. 7.30**A**). This second triangular ridge of the mesiolingual cusp meets the triangular ridge of the mesiobuccal cusp, and the two together make up a *transverse ridge.* The groove between the two triangular ridges on the mesiolingual cusp is called the Stuart groove (named after the late Dr. Charles E. Stuart).

## 6. FOSSAE ON FOUR-CUSP MOLARS: FOUR OF THEM

On maxillary molars with four major cusps, there are ordinarily four fossa on the occlusal surface (Fig. 7.30**A**). The *central fossa* is large and near the center of the occlusal surface (major fossa). Its boundaries are the oblique and transverse ridges and the inner buccal cusp ridges. The small *mesial triangular fossa* is just within the mesial marginal ridge (minor fossa). The minute *distal triangular fossa* is just within the distal marginal ridge (minor fossa). The *distal fossa* is an elongated fossa (cigar-shaped) extending between the mesiolingual and the distolingual cusps (major fossa).

## 7. GROOVES ON FOUR-CUSP MOLARS

The *buccal groove in the central fossa* extends buccally from the central fossa and continues onto the buccal surface of the crown as the *buccal groove* (Fig. 7.30). The *central groove* extends mesially from the central fossa over the transverse ridge and ends in the mesial triangular fossa. Occasionally, there will be a continuation of the central groove that runs distally across the oblique ridge to the distal triangular fossa. When present, it is called the *transverse groove of the oblique ridge.* The *distal oblique groove* extends from the distal triangular fossa lingually between the distolingual cusp and the mesiolingual cusp (along the distal fossa) and *continues* onto the lingual surface as the *lingual groove.* These grooves are often fissured and can become the sites of decay. The *fifth cusp groove* separates the fifth cusp (Carabelli) from the mesiolingual cusp. The pit and groove pattern is more variable on *second* molars with more supplemental grooves and pits than on the first molar (22).

## 8. FOSSAE AND GROOVES ON THREE-CUSP MOLARS

On *three-cusp type* second molars, the distal fossae and both the distal oblique and lingual grooves are absent.

## 9. CONTACTS

Mesial and distal contacts are near the center buccolingually. The mesial contact is more buccal on the maxillary first molar.

For a summary of characteristics that differentiate maxillary second molars from first molars, refer to Table 7.6.

# SECTION V. MAXILLARY THIRD MOLAR CHARACTERISTICS

## A. General Information: Smaller, Variable Shape

The size and shape is greatly *variable*. In fact, maxillary third molars have greater morphologic variance than any other tooth (Figs. 7.19 and 7.20, *top rows*).

The maxillary third molar is the *shortest* of the permanent teeth and is *smaller* than the first or second molar (Fig. 7.31). In a study of relative tooth size (23), the second maxillary molar was reported to be larger than the first maxillary molar in 33% of a sample of Ohio Caucasian population, and in 36% of a Pima Indian population. In the mandibular arch, this size sequence was seen in 10% of Ohio Caucasians and in 19% of Pima Indians. [Dr. Woelfel found only two casts of young dental hygienists' mouths, from more than 600 sets of complete dentition casts, in which maxillary second molars were larger than the first molars. On several of these dentitions, the mandibular second molars were slightly larger than the first molars, and there were a few more in which the mandibular third molar crowns were as large as the first molars and larger than the mandibular second molars.]

The distal surface of the third molar is *not* in contact with any tooth. The third maxillary molars occlude only with the mandibular third molars; all other teeth occlude with two teeth EXCEPT mandibular central incisors.

The roots are ordinarily shorter by 2.0 mm [average of 920 teeth] and the root trunk is proportionally longer than the root trunks of the first and second molars.

**Table 7.6.** How to Distinguish Maxillary Second Molars from First Molars

| On second molars | —Both distal cusps are smaller |
|---|---|
| | —Crowns appear to tip distally on roots (buccal view) |
| | —Crowns are smaller, especially mesiodistally |
| | —Crowns are narrower on the lingual side and on the distal side |
| | —Crowns appear more oblong buccolingually because of the reduction of mesiodistal dimension |
| | —Roots seem as long but are less spread apart mesiodistally and faciolingually |
| | —Roots bend more to the distal and have a longer root trunk |
| | —Mesial marginal ridge less often has tubercles (firsts 86%, seconds 38%) |
| | —Cusp of Carabelli is absent (not totally reliable, since 30% of first molars have no fifth cusp) |
| | —Mesial marginal ridge less often has groove (firsts 78%, seconds 67%) |
| | —Buccal groove is shorter and without a pit |
| | —Occlusal parallelogram is twisted more; looks oblong faciolingually (first molar is wider and more square) |
| | —Greater difference in size of buccal cusps (mesiobuccal is widest 92%) |
| | —Smaller oblique ridge and a more varied pit and groove pattern (more wrinkles) |
| | —More prominent mesiobuccal cervical ridge (Fig. 7.30**B**) |

## B. Crown of Maxillary Third Molar

Refer to Figures 7.7, *top*, 7.19 and 7.20, *upper rows*, 7.31, 7.32, 7.34, and 7.35 for similarities and differences.

The great amount of variation in the third molars makes a general description difficult. The crown may have only one cusp or as many as eight (24).

As with the mandibular thirds, the crown of the third molars usually resembles a small first or second molar (Figs. 7.31 and 7.32**A**). The crown, however, *tapers* more from buccal to lingual.

As with the *mandibular* third molars, the *maxillary* third molar can be distinguished from the first or second molar in that arch because it has shorter, less separated roots and more *numerous supplemental grooves* and ridges, particularly on the occlusal surface, which give it a wrinkled appearance. It will also be narrower on the lingual side.

Sometimes the form of the crown is so irregular that it is difficult to identify the mesiobuccal, the distobuccal, and the lingual cusps. The mesiolingual cusp is usually convex, however, and is both larger and longer than the others. The fairly flat buccal side of the buccal cusps and the buccal surface of the crown can be used to properly orient third molars for study and comparison to the other molars (Fig. 7.20, *top row*).

The mesiobuccal cusp is considerably wider and usually longer than the distobuccal cusp. This is very helpful in differentiating rights from lefts when there is only one lingual cusp (Fig. 7.19, *top row*). The oblique ridge is poorly developed and often absent (Fig. 7.20, *top row*).

Occasionally, a small fourth molar (paramolar) will be fused to the maxillary third molar (Fig. 7.34).

## C. Roots of Maxillary Third Molars: Shorter with Longer Root Trunks, Often Curved Considerably to Distal

There are three roots: mesiobuccal, distobuccal, and lingual, which may be separated, as in the first and second molars, but more commonly, they are fused most of their length, with the furcation extending only a short distance cervically from the apices of the roots. This makes a *long* root trunk. Often the roots are entirely fused from the cervix to the apices (10 teeth in Fig. 7.19).

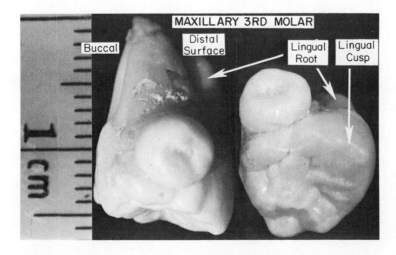

**Figure 7.34.** Unusual maxillary third molar with a paramolar fused to its distal surface. For a separate fourth molar, see Figure 11.8.

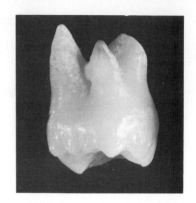

**Figure 7.35.** Maxillary right third molar. Distal surface. Third molars do not always have short roots, and they do not always have fused roots. Occasionally, their morphology is indistinguishable from that of some second molars. Notice the tubercles on the distal marginal ridge.

The roots are noticeably shorter than on the first and second molars [303 teeth averaged 2 mm shorter on their buccal roots and 2.5 mm shorter on their lingual roots]. The roots, fused or not, are often very crooked, and the majority of them curve distally in their apical third (Fig. 7.19, *upper row*).

Some oral surgeons recommend that *all* third molars be removed at an early age (under 25) to facilitate an easier, less traumatic removal and a quicker more comfortable recovery period than that experienced when they are extracted later in life (25). Since many third molars are extracted before the roots are completely formed, you can easily look into the open ends of the root canals.

Many third molars never form or develop. [Among 710 Ohio State University dental hygiene students, there were 185 maxillary third molars and 198 mandibular third molars *congenitally absent*. Many students were missing more than one third molar, so the percentage of the population missing one or more third molars might be close to 20%.]

## LEARNING EXERCISES

*Examine the teeth of your associates and notice the variation in the cusp of Carabelli. Many people have been intrigued by this little cusp.*

*How many second molars do you find with only one lingual cusp (distolingual cusp absent)?*

*Name each of the 17 ridges in Fig. 7.36.*

**Figure 7.36.** Maxillary molar, first or second (*circles* denote cusp tips).

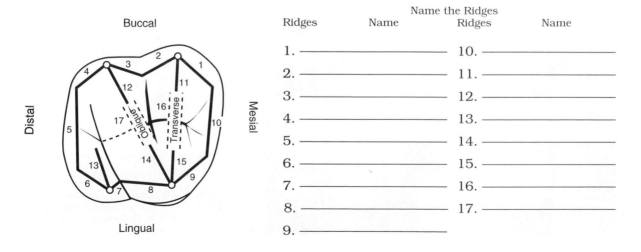

Name the Ridges

| Ridges | Name | Ridges | Name |
|--------|------|--------|------|
| 1. | | 10. | |
| 2. | | 11. | |
| 3. | | 12. | |
| 4. | | 13. | |
| 5. | | 14. | |
| 6. | | 15. | |
| 7. | | 16. | |
| 8. | | 17. | |
| 9. | | | |

*How many molars do you find in your collection of extracted teeth that you are unable to identify as first, second, or third with reasonable assurance? (If you feel no uncertainty about any teeth in a fairly large collection, maybe you need to study more.)*

*Name the three grooves that radiate out from the central fossa in a maxillary first molar.*

*Which cusp has two triangular ridges on the maxillary first molar?*

*Name the two important ridges that these triangular ridges join from the opposite side of the tooth.*

*Which cusp is the largest and longest on a maxillary second molar?*

*Which cusp is most likely to be absent on a maxillary second or third molar (excluding the cusp of Carabelli)?*

*Name the four fossae on a maxillary first molar. Which is the largest? Which one is large and oblong?*

*Which developmental groove connects with the lingual groove running in the same direction?*

*From which two aspect(s) are only two or fewer roots visible on a maxillary first molar?*

*Can you list six ways that maxillary second molars differ from maxillary first molars?*

*List in sequential order the longest to shortest cusps on the maxillary first molar.*

*List in sequential order the largest to smallest cusp area on the maxillary first molar (occlusal view).*

*Which cusp is most likely to be absent on some second molars? When this occurs, which groove and which fossa would not be present?*

*Describe those characteristics of maxillary third molars that would distinguish them from first and second molars.*

*Name the grooves that radiate out of the mesial triangular fossa on the maxillary first molar.*

*Name the grooves that radiate out of the distal triangular fossa on a maxillary first molar.*

*Which are the two largest fossae on a maxillary first molar?*

*Can you list ALL of the ridges that circumscribe or make up the boundary of the occlusal surface of a maxillary first molar? In Figure 7.36, these ridges are numbered 1 through 10.*

*Which two cusps have the triangular ridges that make up or join to form the oblique ridge on a maxillary molar?*

*Which two cusps have the triangular ridges that make up or join to form a transverse ridge on most maxillary molars?*

*If you would like some additional information on how to correctly recognize maxillary and mandibular molars, look at the summary chart Tables 7.3, 7.4, and 7.6.*

# References

1. Tratman EK. A comparison of the teeth of people. Indo-European racial stock with Mongoloid racial stock. Dent Record 1950;70:31–53, 63–88.
2. Masters DH, Hoskins SW. Projection of cervical enamel into molar furcations. J Periodontol 1964;35:49–53.
3. Dahlberg AA. The evolutionary significance of the protostylid. Am J Phys Anthropol 1950;8:NS:15.
4. Dahlberg AA. Geographic distribution and origin of dentitions. In. Dent J 1965;15:348–355.
5. Hellman M. Racial characters of human dentition. Proc Am Philosoph Soc 1928;67:No.2.
6. Everett FG, Jump EG, Holder TD, Williams GC. The intermediate bifurcation ridge: a study of the morphology of the bifurcation of the lower first molar. J Dent Res 1958;37:162.
7. Scott JH, Symons NBB. Introduction to dental anatomy. London: E & S Livingstone, Ltd., 1958.
8. Tratman EK. Three-rooted lower molars in man and their racial distribution. Br Dent J 1938;64:264–274.
9. Turner CG. Three-rooted mandibular first permanent molars and question of American Indian origin. Am J Phys Anthropol 1971;34:239–242.
10. Brand RW, Isselhard DE. Anatomy of orofacial structures. 5th ed. St. Louis: C.V. Mosby, 1994:438.
11. Kraus B, Jordan R, Abrams L. Dental anatomy and occlusion. Baltimore: Williams & Wilkins, 1969:110–114.
12. Jorgensen KD. The Dryopithecus pattern in recent Danes and Dutchmen. J Dent Res 1955;34:195.

13. Garn SM, Lewis AB, Kerewsky RS. Molar size sequence and fossil taxonomy. Science 1963; 142:1060.

14. Dahlberg AA. The dentition of the American Indian. In: Laughlin WS, ed. The physical anthropology of the American Indian. New York: The Viking Fund, 1949.

15. Matsumoto Y. Morphological studies on the roots of the Japanese maxillary second molars. Shikwa Gukuho 1986;86:249–276.

16. Carbonelli VM. The tubercle of Carabelli in the Kish dentition, Mesopotamia, 3000 B.C. J Dent Res 1960;39:124.

17. Garn SM, Lewis AB, Kerewsky RS, Dahlberg AA. Genetic independence of Carabelli's trait from tooth size or crown morphology. Arch Oral Biol 1966;11:745–747.

18. Kraus BS. Carabelli's anomaly of the maxillary molar teeth. Observations on Mexican and Papago Indians and an interpretation of the inheritance. Am J Hum Genet 1951;3:348.

19. Kraus BS. Occurrence of the Carabelli trait in the Southwest ethnic groups. Am J Phys Anthropol 1959;17:117.

20. Meredith HV, Hixon EH. Frequency, size, and bilateralism of Carabelli's tubercle. J Dent Res 1954;33:435.

21. Joshi MR, Godiawala RN, Dutia A. Carabelli trait in Hindu children from Gujurat. J Dent Res 1972;51:706–711.

22. Brand RW, Isselhard DE. Anatomy of the orofacial structures. St. Louis: C.V. Mosby, 1982:159, 163.

23. Garn SM, Lewis AB, Kerewsky RS. Molar size sequence and fossil taxonomy. Science 1963; 142:1060.

24. Kraus B, Jordan R, Abrams L. Dental anatomy and occlusion. Baltimore: Williams & Wilkins, 1969:94.

25. Chiles DG, Cosentino BJ. Third molar question: report of 522 cases. J Am Dent Assoc 1987; 115:575–576.

## General References

Oregon State System of Higher Education. Dental anatomy. A self-instructional program. East Norwalk: Appleton-Century-Crofts, 1982:403–414.

Proskaves C, Witt F. Pictorial history of dentistry. (Cave P, trans.) Koln: Verlag M. Dumont Schauberg, 1962.

Renner RP. An introduction to dental anatomy and esthetics. Chicago: Quintessence Publishing, 1985.

Ring ME. Dentistry: an illustrated history. St. Louis: C.V. Mosby, 1985.

# Clinical Application of Root Morphology

..................
..................
..................
..................
..................
..................
..................

## SECTION I. EXTERNAL ROOT MORPHOLOGY RELATED TO PERIODONTAL THERAPY

(The periodontal portion of this chapter was originally written by Lewis Claman, D.D.S., M.S., Associate Professor, Division of Periodontology, Ohio State University.)

Section I focuses on the disease process (periodontal disease) that can affect the health of periodontium with an emphasis on the relationship of this disease to external root anatomy. The periodontium includes the tissues that surround and support the teeth, including the periodontal ligament (PDL), gingivae, cementum, and alveolar and supporting bone.

### A. Overview of Periodontal Disease

Periodontal disease generally begins with gingival changes. Alterations in the gingiva may occur in a variety of ways and may reflect active early periodontal disease, more advanced disease, or evidence of previous disease that has been arrested. The most common changes in the gingiva are inflammatory and include increased redness and enlargement of interproximal papillae and free gingiva (Fig. 8.1). The surface becomes smooth and glazed, and the gingiva is easily retractable from the tooth when air is directed at it. Bleeding on gentle probing is an important sign that disease is present (Fig. 8.2) (1, 2). It may reflect early and easily treatable periodontal disease, or more severe disease forms. Gingival crevicular

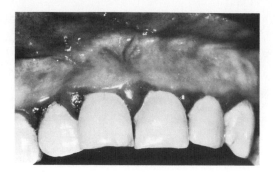

**Figure 8.1.** Inflamed gingiva. Note the contour changes (bulbous papillae, rolled margins), increased size, and glazed surface texture. Clinically, the papillae and margins were red and bled easily when probed (Fig. 8.2). The gingiva separated (retracted) from the teeth easily when air was directed at it.

fluid, not normally found in healthy gingiva, increases with inflammation (3). At times, a purulent exudate (suppuration) may also be expressed from tissues. Another important sign of periodontal disease is an increase in probing depths of the gingival sulcus to greater than 3 mm. Probing depths greater than 5 mm without significant tissue overgrowth frequently accompany more serious forms of periodontal disease. In these disease forms, breakdown has progressed beyond the gingiva and involves destruction occurring in bone and *periodontal ligament* (Fig. 8.3). This is known as *periodontitis.*

When periodontal disease occurs, there may be destruction of the gingival and periodontal ligament fibers, loss of alveolar bone, and apical migration of the junctional epithelium onto the root. This may be clinically observed as *attachment loss* (probing attachment level), which is the distance in millimeters from the cementoenamel junction to the apical aspect of the gingival crevice (sulcus). Although it is difficult to estimate attachment loss if the gingiva covers the cementoenamel junction, once exposure of the root has occurred (gingival recession), attachment loss for each aspect of a tooth is determined by adding gingival recession (Figs. 8.4 and 8.5) to the probing depth (Fig. 2.6). This measurement of periodontal destruction is more accurate than probing (pocket) depths alone, because the level of the gingival margin is considered (4).

Frequently, there is loss of gingival tissue. This is termed *gingival recession* (Fig. 8.4) and may be part of an active, progressive process of periodontal disease, or may reflect previous disease that is now under control. Gingival recession is often seen in older individuals, but severe destruction of the periodontium should not be regarded as a natural consequence of ag-

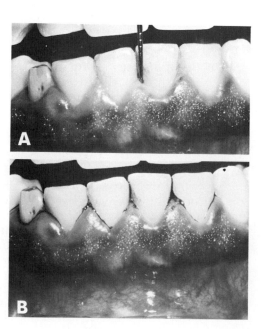

**Figure 8.2.** Bleeding upon probing. **A.** A periodontal probe is inserted and gently swept around the tooth. **B.** The examiner looks for gingival bleeding that occurs within 30 seconds. Bleeding is the most important sign for the presence of active periodontal disease, but does not directly relate to the severity. Note the generalized physiologic melanin pigmentation (*dark regions*) on the attached gingiva.

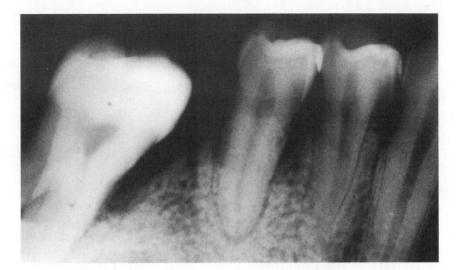

**Figure 8.3.** This radiograph shows advanced periodontal disease as indicated by loss of bone (especially around teeth numbers 29 and 31; note tooth number 30 is missing) which would normally be surrounding all teeth to a level much closer to the cementoenamel junction. Compare this bone destruction to the relatively healthy bone surrounding the teeth in Fig. 8.37.

ing (5). In gingival recession, the papillae may be blunted, rounded, and no longer fill the embrasure. The gingival margin is apical to the cementoenamel junction. A localized area of recession may be related to abnormal tooth prominence, but may also be associated with a lack of attached gingiva, especially if bacterial plaque is present (6) (Fig. 8.5). Abnormal tooth positions do not necessarily indicate disease; they may contribute to other tissue alterations, such as flattened or exaggerated contours and variations in tissue thickness (Fig. 8.6).

## B. Periodontal Considerations of Root Anatomy

### 1. PERIODONTAL SUPPORT

While the anatomy of the crown is significant from an occlusal standpoint, the root anatomy determines the actual support for the teeth. Root attachment area depends on root length, the number of roots, and the cross-sectional diameter of the root from the cementoenamel junction to the apex. It also depends on the presence or absence of concavities and other root curvatures. These features greatly determine the resistance of a tooth to occlusal and other forces, particularly when they are applied in a lateral (buccolingual) direction.

In health, prior to periodontal disease, connective tissue fibers insert into cementum on the entire root surface. This attachment represents insertion of the gingival

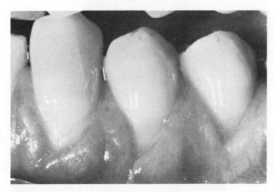

**Figure 8.4.** Area of gingival recession (clefting). The gingiva no longer covers the cementoenamel junction and the root surface is exposed.

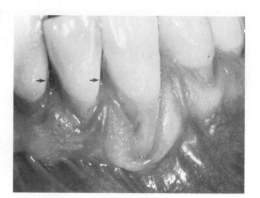

**Figure 8.5.** Severe gingival recession. The prominent canine root and lack of attached gingiva are factors that may have contributed to the recession. Note the blunted papillae (*arrows*). Attachment loss is determined by adding gingival recession to probing depths (mm). (Courtesy of Alan R. Levy, D.D.S.)

fibers (supracrestal) near the cementoenamel junction, and periodontal ligament insertions for the majority of the root (Fig. 1.11). Long roots and wide cross-sectional tooth diameters increase support. Concavities and other root curvatures increase periodontal support in two ways. First, they augment the total surface area. Secondly, the arcuate (bow-shaped) configuration provides multidirectional fiber orientation, which makes the tooth more resistant to occlusal forces. For example, a root with a mesial concavity (Fig. 8.7) is more resistant to buccolingual forces than a tooth that assumes a more conical, convex shape. Likewise, multirooted teeth have increased support and force resistance. For those teeth, the location of the furcation is important; the more coronal it is, the more stability is afforded (Figs. 8.8 and 8.9). Additionally, convergence or divergence of roots influences support. Divergent roots increase stability and allow for more interradicular bone support (Figs. 8.8**A** and 8.9, *left tooth*).

Another important factor for determining tooth stability is the degree of root taper. Teeth with conical roots, such as mandibular first premolars, tend to have the majority of their root area (greater than 60%) in the coronal half of the root, and much less area (only about 40%) in the apical half of the root (Fig. 8.10) (7).

Based on root area alone, one would generally expect to find the maxillary canine to be the most stable single-rooted tooth, and the mandibular central incisors to be the least stable. For posterior teeth, one would expect the maxillary first molar, with its three divergent roots, to be more stable than the third molars, which frequently have fused roots. While these rules generally apply, additional factors, such as the presence or absence of inflammatory periodontal disease and excessive occlusal forces, may greatly influence tooth stability. Also, the density and structure of the supporting bone has an influence on tooth stability.

The periodontal ligament (PDL) is about 0.2 mm wide, decreasing to 0.1 mm in old age. At any age it is wider around both the cervix and the apex than around the middle of the root, depending upon the amount of rotational movements to which the

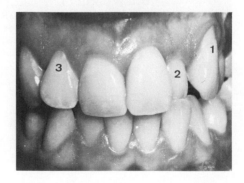

**Figure 8.6.** Examples of contour variations caused by tooth malposition. *1:* Tooth in labial version showing exaggerated escalloping and thin gingiva. *2:* Tooth in lingual version showing flattened gingival contours and thicker tissue. *3:* Rotated tooth showing V-shaped escalloping on the labial gingiva.

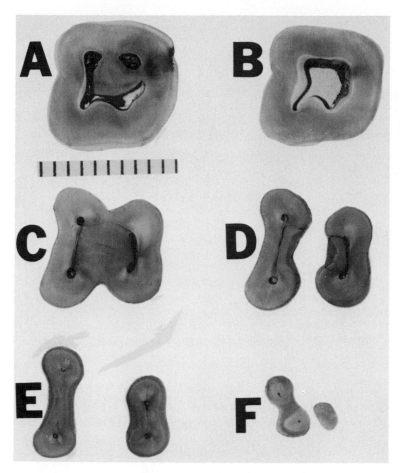

**Figure 8.7.** Series of stained cross-sections of a lower first molar from crown to near apices. For each section, the mesial aspect is *left,* the lingual aspect is *above,* the distal aspect is *right,* and the buccal aspect is *below.* **A.** Cross-section through the crown showing enamel, dentin, and pulp. Caries was present distally. **B.** Cross-section near the cementoenamel junction. Note the shape of the pulp chamber. **C.** Cross-section of the root trunk slightly coronal to the bifurcation (furcation). There is a mesial concavity. Buccal and lingual depressions are coronal to the entrances to the bifurcation. **D.** Cross-section of mesial and distal roots slightly apical to the bifurcation. Note the root canals. Thickened cementum (darkly stained) is apparent on the furcal aspect (between the roots) of both roots. **E.** Cross-section of roots 4 mm apical to the bifurcation. There are concavities on the mesial aspect of the mesial root and the furcal aspects of both roots. **F.** Cross-section of the roots near the apex. The mesial root is longer. The complex shape of molar roots helps provide a greater surface area of attachment and greater tooth stability, but becomes a problem with progressive periodontal disease. There is a 10-mm scale between the top and the middle section on the *left.*

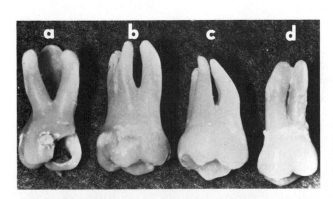

**Figure 8.8.** Variations in root form for maxillary molars. **A.** Divergent roots with the furcation in the coronal one third of the root. **B.** Convergent roots with the furcation in the middle one half of the root. **C.** Very convergent roots. **D.** Fused roots with the furcation in the coronal one-third of the root.

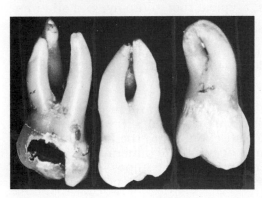

**Figure 8.9.** Additional examples of variations in root convergences and trunk length. The trunk refers to that portion of the root that is coronal to the furcation.

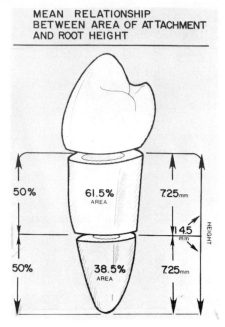

MEAN RELATIONSHIP
BETWEEN AREA OF ATTACHMENT
AND ROOT HEIGHT

50%      61.5%        7.25mm
          AREA

                      4.5
                       mm

50%      38.5%        7.25mm
          AREA

HEIGHT

**Figure 8.10.** Relationship between the area of attachment and root height for lower first premolars. Approximately 60% of the root area is present in the coronal one-half of the root, with only 40% of the area present in the apical one-half of the root. These determinations were made by measuring the areas of many serial cross-sections of tooth roots as shown in Figure 8.7. (Courtesy of Alan R. Levy, D.D.S.)

tooth is subjected. Tipping movements are minimal at the rotational center of the tooth and greater at either the cervical or apical end of the root. Thus, there is a functional difference in the width of the PDL in these three regions. The PDL of a natural tooth in occlusal function is slightly wider than the PDL in a nonfunctional tooth because it does not have an antagonist to stimulate the contents of the periodontal ligament (8).

## 2. PERIODONTAL DISEASE

Some of the factors just described that increase tooth support become potential areas for the development of periodontal diseases, or may perpetuate disease once it has been initiated. Periodontal breakdown resulting in attachment loss and bone loss usually begins in an inaccessible area, one that is neither self-cleansing nor easy for a patient to reach with the oral hygiene aids. It is paramount that both the dentist and the dental hygienist be thoroughly cognizant of root anatomy. A thorough knowledge of root form is important in any periodontal examination. It helps the diagnostician detect periodontal disease at locations which are prone to breakdown but frequently missed. An essential objective in treating periodontal disease involves instrumenting (removing deposits and diseased cementum) on root surfaces that have become affected by periodontal disease. Awareness of furcations and where they are potentially located, concavities, atypical root anatomy, and other aspects of root anatomy help the dentist and the dental hygienist to identify areas at risk for developing periodontal disease. Such knowledge also helps in effective root debridement including planing, instruction for appropriate oral hygiene aids, and in identifying sites that are difficult or impossible to reach or that have not responded to treatment.

*Furcation involvement* in the disease process occurs when there is loss of periodontal ligament to the level of the furcation. It frequently occurs in periodontal disease (Fig. 8.11). Attachment loss and pockets that extend into the furcation create difficult access areas for the patient to reach and accumulate mineralized (calculus) and soft (plaque) deposits. These deposits frequently become impossible to remove and may provide a pathway for periodontal disease to continue to progress apically

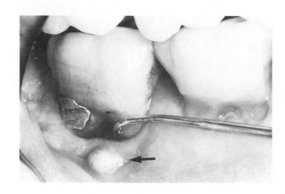

**Figure 8.11.** Clinically severe buccal furcation involvement on a mandibular second molar. The furcation probe is able to engage far into the interradicular area because of periodontal destruction. The clinical periodontal examination should also include probing for furcations that may occur subgingivally and for lingual furcation of mandibular molars and proximal furcations on maxillary molars. Note the abscessed area (*arrow*).

(Fig. 8.12). The location of the furcation is an important consideration (Figs. 8.8 and 8.9). The more coronal the furcation, the more likely it is to become involved with periodontal disease, but the more easily it is treated by traditional periodontal therapy. The more apical the furcation, the more complex the treatment will become. The maxillary first premolar provides a good example of a furcation that is located nearer to the apex (Fig. 6.7**A**). Proximal furcations, once they are involved, with disease are particularly difficult to gain access to because of vertical longitudinal depressions coronal to the furcation and close approximation to adjacent teeth (Figs. 8.7 and 8.13).

Vertical and longitudinal depressions and concave areas occur commonly on the mesial and distal root surfaces of many anterior and most posterior teeth (see Section III of this chapter for a detailed summary of these root depressions). More coronally located root depressions are also found on the mesial surface of maxillary first premolars (both on the root and crown), and on molar root surfaces just coronal to furcations. Recall that mandibular molar furcations are located near the midbuccal and midlingual (between mesial and distal roots); maxilliary molar furcations are located midbuccal (between mesiobuccal and distobuccal roots), mesially (between palatal and mesiobuccal roots), and distally (between palatal and distobuccal roots). Also remember that furcations are closer to the cervix of the tooth on first molars (their root trunks are shorter), and more apical on second and third molars. Exposure of the concave root regions to saliva and subsequent development of periodontal disease make these areas particularly prone to deposit accumulation. Deposit removal becomes quite difficult (Fig. 8.12).

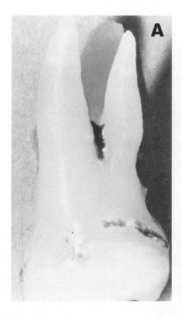
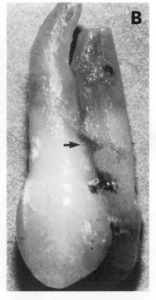

**Figure 8.12. A.** Extracted molar with mineralized deposits (calculus) extending into the furcation. Once disease progresses into the furcation area, instrumentation by the dentist or hygienist becomes exceedingly difficult. **B.** Longitudinal depression on the mesial root of a maxillary first premolar. Notice the calculus deposit (*arrow*) in the depression on the mesial side of the root.

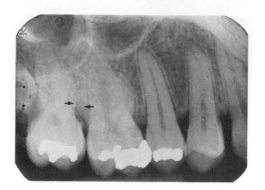

**Figure 8.13.** Radiograph showing close root approximation between the distal root of the maxillary first molar and the mesial root of the second molar (*arrows*). Furcations and concavities are virtually inaccessible when destruction occurs at those locations.

*The degree of root taper* influences the support once periodontal disease has occurred. A CONICAL ROOT MAY HAVE LOST MORE THAN 60% OF THE PERIODONTAL LIGAMENT, EVEN THOUGH IT HAS LOST ONLY 50% OF THE BONE HEIGHT (Figs. 8.7 and 8.10). This is because a small proportion of the root area is present near the apex. For severely conical roots, the apical half of the root may account for even less attachment area than seen in Figure 8.10.

### Influence of Atypical Root Configuration on Periodontal Disease

There are several types of defects in the root structure that weaken periodontal attachment and are potential areas for periodontal disease to develop. Enamel extensions frequently occur on mandibular molars, and enamel pearls often are present on maxillary molars (Fig. 8.14). Both prevent a normal connective tissue attachment and may channel disease into the furcation area. Palatal gingival grooves occur on maxillary incisors and readily collect and retain plaque, which can frequently lead to periodontal destruction (Fig. 8.15). Root fractures also predispose periodontal destruction (loss of attachment of the periodontal ligament) along the fracture line.

## 3. PERIODONTAL THERAPY

Currently there are a wide range of techniques to treat periodontal problems. Nonsurgical periodontal therapy is centered around effective root planing.

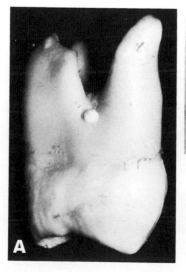

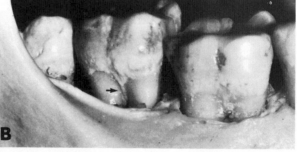

**Figure 8.14.** Enamel oddities on roots. **A.** Enamel pearl in the mesial furcation of a maxillary molar. **B.** Enamel extension (*arrow*) downward into the buccal furcation of a lower second molar. (Courtesy of Charles Solt, D.D.S., and Todd Needham, D.D.S.)

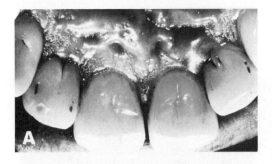

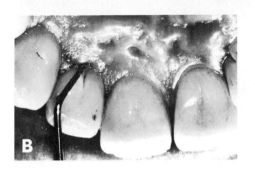

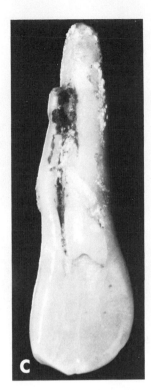

**Figure 8.15.** Palatal gingival groove. **A.** Indentation on the lingual surface of both maxillary lateral incisors. **B.** Periodontal probe in place showing a deep periodontal pocket formed where the groove extends apically on the root. **C.** Groove extending apically on the midpalatal aspect of a maxillary canine. The tooth was extracted because of severe periodontal disease on the palatal aspect. (Courtesy of Leonard K. Ebel, D.D.S.)

Conservative surgical therapy is designed to gain access to the root surface for debridement (9). Resective periodontal surgery is the treatment to correct some of the results of periodontal disease by removal of soft and hard tissue components of the pocket wall. Techniques include gingivectomy (both through the conventional scalpel and the more recent use of the laser) (10), root resections to remove periodontally involved roots on multirooted teeth (11), and periodontal flaps with osseous surgery (12). Regenerative periodontal surgery is intended to attain new cementum, new bone, and a new functional periodontal ligament. Recent advances in the area of periodontal regeneration include guided tissue regeneration through barrier membranes (e.g., GoreTex by W.L. Gore Company, Flagstaff, AZ) (13) and bone grafting materials such as demineralized freeze dried bone (14). Periodontal plastic surgery includes soft tissue reconstructive techniques such as connective tissue grafts designed to cover roots which have been exposed through gingival recession (15).

## 4. ROOT ANATOMY AND PERIODONTAL OCCLUSAL TRAUMA

Injury to the periodontium from occlusal forces is known as *occlusal trauma*. It may result in destructive change in the bone, periodontal ligament, and root. Many of the changes are reversible or ones to which the periodontium can accommodate (16). Occlusal trauma is a disorder that is generally distinct from, but may influence the course of, inflammatory periodontal disease under specific circumstances (17).

Although furcations, concavities, vertical grooves, and other root curvatures tend to increase the area of attachment, making the tooth resistant to occlusal forces, these root anatomy features may also become foci where forces are concentrated. These foci occur because the root curvatures, and the corresponding bone and periodontal ligaments that conform to it, permit the tooth to compress against periodontal ligament and bone in a variety of directions.

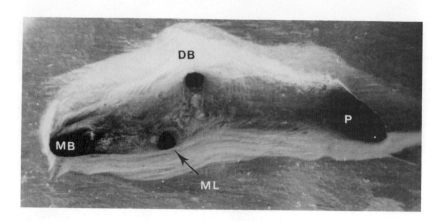

**Figure 8.16.** Scanning electron photomicrograph of the pulp chamber floor of a maxillary molar with four canal orifices. The palatal (*P*), mesiobuccal (*MB*), distobuccal (*DB*), and mesiolingual (*ML-arrow*) orifices are identified for orientation. (Original magnification x20.) (Courtesy of Dr. James Gilles and Dr. Al Reader.)

# SECTION II. INTERNAL PULP CAVITY MORPHOLOGY RELATED TO RESTORATIVE AND ENDODONTIC THERAPY

(This section was modified from material originally written by Al Reader, D.D.S., M.S., Professor, Department of Restorative Dentistry, Prosthodontics & Endodontics, Ohio State University.)

## A. Divisions of Pulp Cavities (for the Purpose of Description)

The *pulp cavity* is the cavity in the central portion of the tooth containing the nerves and blood supply to the tooth. It is divided into the *pulp chamber* (more coronal) and the *root canals* (in the root).

1. *The pulp chamber* of anterior teeth is partly in the crown, but is mostly in the cervical part of the root of posterior teeth. Its wall is the innermost surface of the dentin. There is one pulp chamber in each tooth. Each pulp chamber has a roof at its incisal or occlusal border, and the pulp chambers of multirooted teeth have a floor at the cervical portion with openings for each root canal (Figs. 8.16 and 8.28).

2. *The root canal (pulp canal)* is found in the root of a tooth. The root canal is a continuation of the pulp chamber. The shape and number of root canals in any one tooth have been anatomically divided into four major classifications (Fig. 8.17):

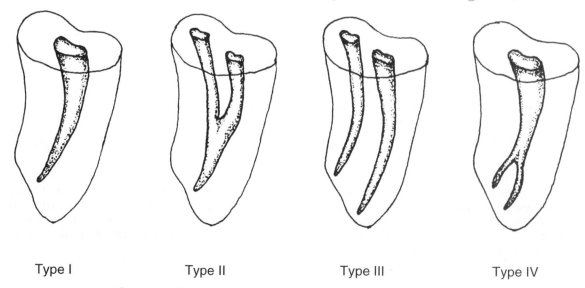

Type I         Type II         Type III         Type IV

**Figure 8.17.** Major configurations of canals occurring in one root.

a. Type I—one canal from the pulp chamber to the apex.

b. Type II—two separate canals leaving the pulp chamber and joining short of the apex to form one canal apically.

c. Type III—two separate canals leaving the pulp chamber and remaining separate to exit the root apically as separate foramina.

d. Type IV—one canal leaving the pulp chamber and dividing in the apical third of the root into two separate canals with separate apical foramina.

*Openings* from the pulp canal to the outside of the tooth include the *apical foramen* at or near the root apex (Figs. 8.18 and 8.20), and the *accessory foramina*, most commonly found near the apex. In maxillary and mandibular molars, the incidence of accessory foramina on the pulpal floor is about 8% (18). On the underneath surface of the furcation (exterior surface), accessory foramina are found 64% of the time (18).

# B. Shape of Pulp Cavities in Sound, Young Teeth by Tooth Type

## *LEARNING EXERCISE*

*Pulp cavities—their size, shape and variations—are best studied by the interesting operation of grinding off one side of an extracted tooth. A dental lathe equipped with a fine-grained abrasive wheel about 3 inches in diameter and $^3/_8$-inch thick can be used to remove any part of the tooth. Simply decide which surface is to be removed, hold the tooth securely in your fingers, and apply this surface firmly to the flat surface of the abrasive wheel. Operating the lathe at a fairly high speed is less apt to flip the specimen from your fingers than operating it at a low speed. If you can devise an arrangement by which a small stream of water is run onto the surface of the wheel as the tooth is ground, you will eliminate flying tooth dust and the bad odor of hot tooth tissue. If such an arrangement is not feasible, keep the tooth moist by frequently dipping the surface being ground in water or by dripping water onto the wheel with a medicine dropper. Look often at the tooth surface you are cutting and adjust your applied pressure to attain the plane in which you wish the tooth to be cut. A high-speed dental handpiece and bur will greatly facilitate your exploration of the insides of teeth.*

*As you frequently examine the cross-section of the tooth, evaluate the anatomy and depth of pits and fissures in the enamel, and watch carefully the configuration of any carious lesion (decay) you see at different levels of grinding. This can be a fascinating pastime, as well as a valuable part of your education. You may want to preserve your ground tooth specimens for future examination when, in your course in oral histology, you study the histology of the hard tooth tissues. Extracted teeth should always be kept moist or wet with buffered neutral formalin as described in the introduction of this text.*

*As you remove different sides of each kind of tooth, carefully examine the pulp cavities. Sketching the cavity outlines as you see them from different planes of cutting is helpful in understanding internal tooth morphology. Notice how the inside shape has irregularities similar to those of the external morphology. On incisors and canines, either the mesial or distal side should be removed from some teeth and the facial or lingual side removed from others. This way, the shape of the pulp cavity can be seen from both the mesiodistal and labiolingual planes. Remember that dental radiographs can picture the pulp chamber and root canal only in the mesiodistal plane (Figs. 8.35).*

*On premolars, the removal of either the mesial or distal side will expose the roof of the pulp chamber, which has pulp horns extending beneath the cusps (Fig. 8.25). On another specimen, removal of the buccal and lingual sides to the level of the buccal and lingual cusp tips will reveal the shape of the pulp cavity in a mesiodistal plane (like a dental radiograph as seen in Fig. 8.34). Compare your direct view with a dental x-ray film of the same tooth.*

*On molars, some specimens should be prepared by removal of the buccal surface (Fig. 8.32) and some by removal of the lingual surface. Some teeth should have the mesial surface removed to the level of the tips of the mesiobuccal and mesiolingual cusps, and others should have the distal surface removed to the level of the distobuccal and distolingual cusps (Figs. 8.29 through 8.31). On other molars, the occlusal surface should be removed so that the openings to the root canals on the floor of the pulp chamber can be seen (Fig. 8.28).*

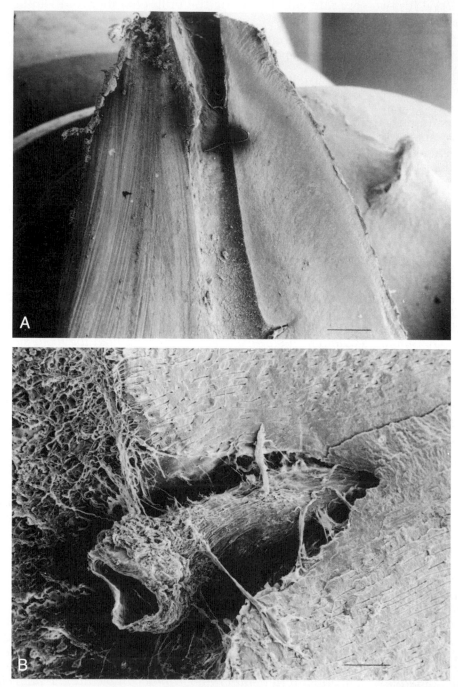

**Figure 8.18. A.** A scanning electron photomicrograph of an instrumented (cleaned) root canal of a maxillary central incisor. After cleaning the root canal, the tooth was split and mounted for viewing with the scanning electron microscope. This view shows the apex of the tooth at the top of the picture and includes the apical third of the root. Near the bottom of the picture (right wall of canal), two accessory canals can be seen. Each canal contains blood vessels. (*Bar* = 1 mm) **B.** A scanning electron photomicrograph at a higher power of one of the accessory canals observed in **A**. The blood vessel can be seen emerging from the dentin. This vessel appears to be a vein due to its thin walls and large size. The adherent "stringy" extensions around the blood vessels are supporting collagen fiber bundles. The dentinal tubules can be observed on the right side of photomicrograph. (*Bar* = 125 μm) (Courtesy of Dr. Dennis Foreman, Department of Oral Biology, College of Dentistry, Ohio State University.)

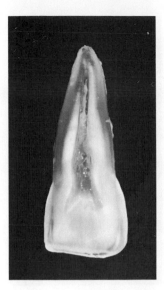

**Figure 8.19.** Maxillary central incisor; facial side removed (young tooth). The high pulp horns and the broad root canal indicate that this is a young tooth. Notice the mesial and distal extensions of the pulp chamber in its incisal border. This outline of the pulp cavity may be seen on a dental radiograph.

## 1. PULP IN ANTERIOR TEETH (INCISORS AND CANINES) (AS SEEN WHEN A TOOTH IS GROUND TO EXPOSE PULP CAVITY)

Refer to Figures 8.19 through 8.24.

### a. Pulp Chamber

#### (1) Cut Labiolingually

The pulp chamber tapers to a point toward the incisal edge (Figs. 8.21 through 8.24 ). In maxillary and mandibular canines, the incisal wall or roof of the pulp chamber is often rounded (Figs. 8.22 and 8.24).

#### (2) Cut Mesiodistally (Similar to View on Many Dental Radiographs)

In maxillary and mandibular central and lateral incisors, the pulp chamber is broad and may have a suggestion of mesial and distal horns (Fig. 8.19). A young tooth may show the configuration of mamelons at the incisal border of the pulp wall (roof of chamber).

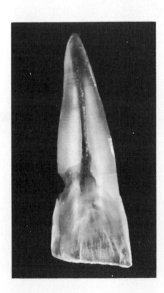

**Figure 8.20.** Maxillary central incisor (old tooth), facial side removed. The pulp chamber is partially filled with secondary dentin and the root canal is narrower than in the tooth shown in Figure 8.19. Also, the incisal edge is worn to a straight line. This is an older tooth than that in Figure 8.19. The damage to the cervical part of the root on the distal side of the tooth has been there for some time because the underlying dentin has been altered by a defense mechanism of the pulp tissues.

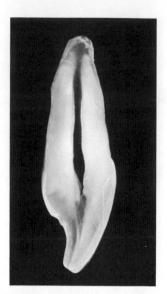

**Figure 8.21.** Maxillary central incisor, mesial side removed. There is attrition on the incisal edge and secondary dentin in the incisal part of the pulp chamber. The root canal is moderately wide. Notice that much of the pulp chamber is located in the cervical third of the root. This is not uncommon. It is not possible to see this view of the pulp cavity on a dental radiograph.

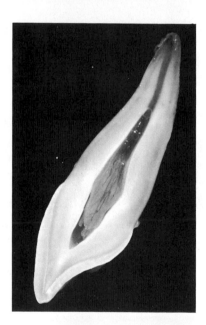

**Figure 8.22.** Maxillary canine, mesial side removed (young tooth). There is no extensive attrition on the incisal edge and the pulp cavity is still large. Observe relative thickness of enamel and dentin in the crown and of the cementum lining the root.

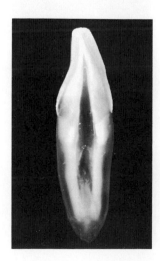

**Figure 8.23.** Mandibular lateral incisor, mesial side removed (young tooth). Curvature of the root prevented cutting the pulp cavity in one plane so that the apical portion was lost. Notice how the pulp cavity extends in a narrow point toward the incisal edge. Even extensive attrition on the incisal edge would not expose the pulp. Should this happen, secondary dentin would form in the incisal part of the pulp chamber and the pulp would be additionally protected.

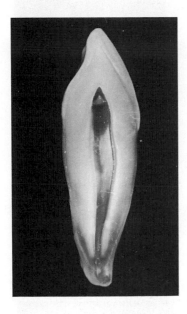

**Figure 8.24.** Mandibular canine, mesial side removed (young tooth). The pulp cavity is large. Only at the incisal tip is there a little evidence of secondary dentin formation. The cementum is extremely thin at the cementoenamel junction, only 50 μm thick (about half as thick as this page). Care must be taken not to remove this thin lining when using scalers or pumice on teeth in this vicinity. The roof of the chamber is slightly more rounded than on incisors.

### b. Root Canal(s)

The number of root canals in each anterior tooth is most frequently one.

Maxillary central incisors, lateral incisors, and canines usually have one canal Type I as seen in Fig. 8.17.

Mandibular central incisors usually have one canal (19–21). Two canals with two separate apical foramina (Type III) (seen in Fig. 8.17) occur 3% of the time (19–20); two canals (usually type II) are present 17–43% of the time (19–21).

Mandibular lateral incisors usually have one canal. However, 20–45% of the time there are two, usually Type II (Fig. 8.17) (19–21). The incidence of two canals with two separate apical foramina (Type III) is about 3% (19–21).

Mandibular canines usually have one canal. However, two canals are found 4–22% of the time (19–21).

## 2. PULP IN PREMOLARS (AS SEEN WHEN THE TOOTH IS GROUND TO EXPOSE THE PULP CAVITY)

Refer to Figures 8.25 through 8.28.

### a. Pulp Chamber

#### (1) Cut Mesiodistally

The occlusal border or roof is curved beneath the cusp similarly to the curvature of the occlusal surface.

#### (2) Cut Buccolingually

The pulp horns in the roof are visible beneath each cusp. The buccal horn is longer than the lingual horn (Fig. 8.25). The pulp chamber

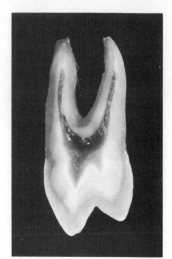

**Figure 8.25.** Maxillary first premolar, mesial side removed (young tooth). The curvature of the tips of the roots prevented cutting the root canals in one plane. The pulp horns are sharp, there is little, if any, secondary dentin, and the floor of the pulp chamber is rounded. The buccal pulp horn is considerably longer than the lingual horn. Notice the floor of the pulp chamber, which has two openings, one for each canal. Also note the constriction of the pulp chamber near the cervix.

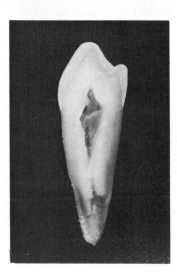

**Figure 8.26.** Mandibular first premolar, distal side removed. Root curvature prevented cutting the root canal in one plane. The pulp horn in the buccal cusp is large; in the lingual cusp it is small. It is unusual to observe much of a pulp horn beneath the nonfunctional lingual cusp on mandibular first premolars.

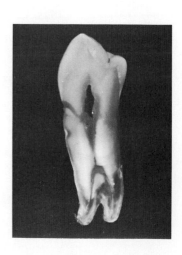

**Figure 8.27.** Mandibular first premolar with root and root canal divided near the apex (Type IV in Fig. 8.17). Mesial side removed. In Figure 6.23**A,** a lower first premolar with two roots and separate canals is seen.

Endodontic access openings

Maxillary teeth | Mandibular teeth

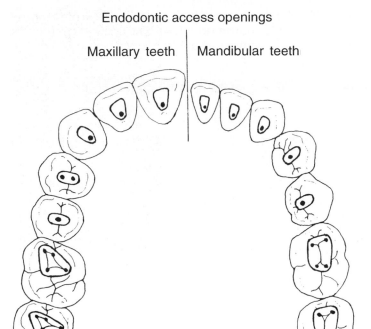

**Figure 8.28.** Ideally shaped access openings for endodontic treatment.

often has the general outline of the tooth surface, sometimes including a constriction near or apical to the cervix.

### b. Root Canal(s)

#### (1) *Maxillary First Premolars*

Maxillary first premolars most often have two roots and two canals.

Approximately 57% of first premolars have two roots and 37% have one root (22). The average incidence of two canals, buccal and lingual, is 90% (both Type I when two roots are present, and either a Type II or Type III with one root) (23). The incidence of three canals is approximately 3% (23). These types of canals are shown in Figure 8.17.

The buccal canal orifice is located just lingual to the buccal cusp tip. The lingual canal is located just lingual to the central fossa (Fig. 8.28).

#### (2) *Maxillary Second Premolars*

Maxillary second premolars most often have one root, but have two canals almost half of the time.

The majority of second premolars have one root. The average incidence of two canals is about 50% (Type II or Type III, as seen in Fig. 8.17) (23). Three canals occur about 1% of the time (23).

When there is one canal, the orifice is located in the exact center of the tooth (Fig. 8.28). If the orifice is located toward the buccal or the lingual, it probably means there are two canals in the root.

#### (3) *Mandibular First and Second Premolars*

Mandibular first and second premolars most frequently have one root and one root canal.

The first premolar has a Type I canal system about 70% of the time and a Type IV canal system 24% of the time (24). The second premolars have one root canal 96% of the time and a Type IV system 2.5% of the time (Fig. 8.17) (24).

The canal orifice is located just buccal to the central fossa (Fig. 8.28).

## 3. PULP IN MAXILLARY MOLARS (FIRST AND SECOND AS SEEN WHEN TEETH ARE CUT IN DIFFERENT PLANES)

Refer to Figures 8.29 through 8.31, and notice how they appear when opened from the occlusal surface for endodontic therapy (Fig. 8.28).

### a. Pulp Chamber

There is a pulp horn well beneath each cusp in the roof of the chamber. Often, the pulp chamber on maxillary molars will not be penetrated by a drill until the dentist reaches the level of the gum line. Thus, the pulp chamber is normally deep to or some distance from the occlusal surface (Figs. 8.29 through 8.31). One exception might be the pulp horn of the mesiolingual cusp.

The pulp chamber of maxillary molars is broader buccolingually than mesiodistally (like the crown) and is often constricted near the floor of the chamber.

The *floor* of the pulp chamber is considerably apical to the cervical line; it is located in the root trunk. It has three or four openings, one for each root canal (Fig. 8.16). When the mesiobuccal root has two canals, there are four openings (Fig. 8.28). The floor is level or flat in young teeth (Fig. 8.29). It may become convex in older teeth with the deposition of additional dentin over time (Figs. 8.32 and 8.33).

### b. Root Canals (Maxillary Molars)

#### (1) Maxillary First Molars

Maxillary first molars most frequently have three roots, but four canals; one each in the distobuccal and palatal root; two in the mesiobuccal root.

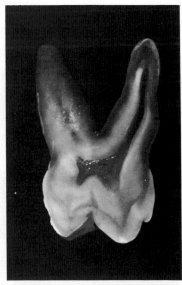

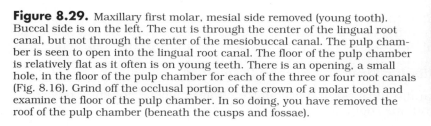

**Figure 8.29.** Maxillary first molar, mesial side removed (young tooth). Buccal side is on the left. The cut is through the center of the lingual root canal, but not through the center of the mesiobuccal canal. The pulp chamber is seen to open into the lingual root canal. The floor of the pulp chamber is relatively flat as it often is on young teeth. There is an opening, a small hole, in the floor of the pulp chamber for each of the three or four root canals (Fig. 8.16). Grind off the occlusal portion of the crown of a molar tooth and examine the floor of the pulp chamber. In so doing, you have removed the roof of the pulp chamber (beneath the cusps and fossae).

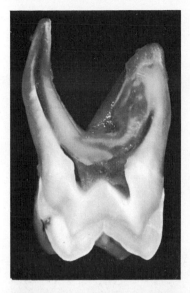

**Figure 8.30.** Maxillary first molar, mesial side removed (young tooth). Buccal side is on the *left*. The cut is through mesiobuccal and lingual root canals. Notice how the lingual canal takes the curvature of the root. The pulp chamber is mostly in the root trunk. Only mesiobuccal and mesiolingual pulp horns extend a little into the part of tooth we define as the anatomic crown. You can determine the extent of the anatomic crown by the location of the cervical border of the enamel. In the groove where the small cusp of Carabelli is attached to the mesiolingual cusp, there is an area of dental caries. Notice the thickness of enamel over the cusps and how very thin it is near the cementoenamel junction.

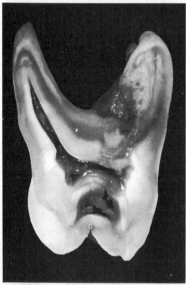

**Figure 8.31.** Maxillary first molar, mesial side removed. Buccal side is on the right. If you grind a number of teeth to expose the pulp cavity, you will easily see why some of them were lost. In this tooth, the carious lesion has spread under the enamel from its point of entry (not seen here) to undermine a large part of the enamel, penetrate through a broad area of dentin, and reach the pulp. Examination of carious lesions by the simple process of judiciously grinding off one side of the tooth makes an extremely interesting study. The occlusal fissure is clearly seen.

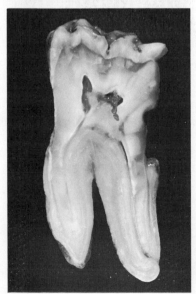

**Figure 8.32.** Mandibular first molar, buccal side removed (old tooth). The apical foramen of the distal root is on the distal side of the root, not at the root tip. Sometimes there are several accessory foramina on a root. The roof of the pulp chamber is about at the same level as the cervical border of the enamel on the mesial side of the tooth. Only the pulp horn extends into the anatomic crown. Most of the pulp chamber is located in the root trunk. The unusual thickening of cementum on the roots is hypercementosis.

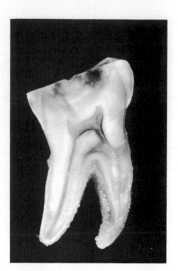

**Figure 8.33.** Mandibular first molar, lingual side removed (old tooth). There appears to be caries in the enamel above the mesiolingual pulp horn, but it has penetrated the dentin only slightly. Again, notice that the roof of the pulp chamber is about at the level of the cervical line. The pulp horns extend occlusal to the cervical line. The rest of the pulp chamber is in the root trunk. The floor of the pulp chamber is convex (a condition founded in older teeth) because of the deposition of secondary dentin.

In the palatal root, the canal is larger and more easily accessible from the floor of the pulp chamber than for the other two roots, but this root and its canal often bend toward the buccal in the apical third, requiring skillful procedures to clean and treat it. The palatal orifice is located beneath the mesiolingual cusp (Fig. 8.28).

The mesiobuccal root has two canals (called mesiobuccal and mesiolingual canals) 56–77% of the time (25). Type III canal systems (Fig. 8.17) have been reported to occur 30–60% of the time (25).

The distobuccal orifice is located on a line between the palatal orifice and the buccal developmental groove at a point just short of the angle formed by the buccal and distal walls of the pulp chamber (Fig. 8.28). The mesiobuccal orifice is located slightly mesial to and beneath the mesiobuccal cusp tip (Fig. 8.28). The mesiolingual orifice is located 2–3 mm distal and slightly to the palatal aspect of the mesiobuccal orifice (Figs. 8.16 and 8.28). Usually, this orifice is difficult to locate because of an overhanging dental shelf. Lightly countersinking the floor of the chamber in this area, with a dental bur, will help in locating the mesiolingual orifice.

### (2) Maxillary Second Molars

Maxillary second molars most frequently have three roots and three canals.

The distobuccal and palatal roots each have one canal. The mesiobuccal root has two canals only 17% of the time (20).

The location of the orifices in the maxillary second molar is similar to the maxillary first molar, except that they are closer together (Fig. 8.28).

## 4. IN MANDIBULAR MOLARS

### a. Mandibular First Molars

Mandibular first molars most frequently have two roots (mesial and distal) and three canals, (one in the distal root and two in the mesial root).

The mesial root usually has two canals: mesiobuccal and mesiolingual. A Type III canal system is present 60% of the time and a Type II (Fig. 8.17) canal system is present 40% of the time (23, 25).

The mesiobuccal orifice is located slightly mesial and close to the mesiobuccal cusp tip (Fig. 8.28). The mesiolingual orifice is just lingual to the mesial developmental groove of the mesial marginal ridge (Fig. 8.28). It is not under the mesiolingual cusp tip, but is in a more central location.

The distal root has two canals approximately 35% of the time (26). If the distal root has one canal, the orifice is large and located just distal to the center of the crown. When two canals are present, the distolingual orifice is small and is located centrally just lingual to the central fossa (Fig. 8.28). Careful inspection of the chamber floor toward the buccal will successfully locate the distobuccal orifice (Fig. 8.28).

Usually the canal configuration is Type II system.

A series of cross-sections of a first molar are shown in Figure 8.7, revealing how the root configuration and canals change at different levels.

### b. Mandibular Second Molars

Mandibular second molars, like first molars, most frequently have two roots and three canals.

The mesial root has two canals 64% of the time. A Type II canal system is present 38% of the time and a Type III canal system is present 26% of the time (24). One canal is present 27% of the time (24). See the types in Figure 8.17. The distal root has one canal 92% of the time (24).

The location of the orifices for mandibular second molars is similar to that of the mandibular first molars (Fig. 8.28).

## C. Pulp Cavities in Third Molars

Maxillary and mandibular third molars vary considerably in form, having from one to seven cusps and as many as seven roots. Third molars will have as many pulp horns as cusps, and as many root canals as roots. Maxillary third molars usually have three root canals and mandibular molars usually have two.

Because third molars complete their development later in life than first and second molars, their pulp chambers and root canals are generally larger than in the other molars. The reason for this is that third molars are 9–11 years younger biologically than first molars. This difference is particularly noticeable on x-ray films made on patients between the ages of 15 and 35 years.

Teeth, other than third molars, exhibiting unusually large pulp chambers on dental x-ray films are immediately suspected to have necrotic pulps, which are a possible source of infection. Without vital pulp tissue, dentin formation ceases, and the pulp chamber size remains constant rather than continuing to decrease in size as is normal for vital teeth.

## D. Pulp Cavities in Deciduous Teeth

Deciduous teeth have thinner amounts of dentin and enamel and since they serve a relatively short time in function, their pulp cavities are proportionally much larger than on secondary teeth (see Figs. 9.8, 9.19, and 9.20). Their pulp horns are closer to the occlusal surface and, on the molars, the mesiobuccal pulp horn is usually longest. Further information is given in Chapter 9.

## E. Why Pulp Cavities Get Smaller in Older Teeth

*Dentin* is a product of specialized cells in the tooth pulp called odontoblasts. *Dentin formation* normally continues as long as the pulp is intact or vital—dentin forms on the wall of the pulp cavity, thickening the dentin and making the pulp chamber and canals smaller. *Dentin formation* over a lifetime may be stimulated to occur more rapidly or in greater quantity by attrition, trauma, caries (i.e., tooth decay), and from calcium hydroxide dental cement.

*The deposition of dentin over time results in reduction in size of the pulp chamber.* In some cases, it may become entirely filled. Reduction in size makes endodontic access openings difficult since there is no chamber to "fall into" as in young teeth.

In a young tooth, the pulp chamber is large and resembles the shape of the crown surface. It has projections called *horns* extending beneath the cusps or mamelons in the roof of the chamber and is usually constricted somewhat at the cervix. In old teeth, it becomes smaller and is more apically located because of deposits of secondary dentin produced by the odontoblasts lining the pulp chamber. The floor of the pulp chamber is nearly flat in young teeth, later becoming convex (compare young specimens in Figs. 8.29 and 8.30, and older specimens in Figs. 8.32 and 8.33).

The diameter of the root canal also decreases in size with age, getting small in older teeth because of the gradual addition of dentin of the internal wall over the years. The canal may be round, flat, or ribbon-shaped. (Figs. 8.20, 8.32, and 8.33).

In a radiographic study of 259 children in England, from their eleventh to fourteenth birthdays, the mesiodistal and roof-to-floor pulp dimensions were recorded with a Lysta-Dent Digitizer. Mesiodistal reduction in size over 3 years was minimal (1–3.5%) compared to a 15% height reduction of the pulp chambers in mandibular first molars. This was mostly the result of secondary dentin deposition on the floor, not the roof, of the chamber (27).

## F. Clinical Application Related to Restorative Dentistry

The dentist, when restoring a tooth, normally avoids exposing any part of the pulp cavity because of the danger of infection. His knowledge of pulp morphology is important to a successful practice because he must prepare the teeth in such a way that the pulpal soft tissues in the teeth are not disturbed. In other words, he always tries to avoid overheating or desiccating the tooth and tries to leave some sound dentin (undecayed) on the floor of the cavity preparation to help support the restoration (composite or amalgam). This is fully explained in Chapter 12.

## G. Clinical Application Related to Endodontics

### 1. ENDODONTICS DEFINED

ENDODONTICS is a specialty branch of dentistry concerned with the morphology, physiology, and pathology of human dental pulp and periapical tissues. Its study and practice encompasses related basic and clinical sciences, including biology of the normal pulp, the etiology, diagnosis, prevention, and treatment of diseases and injuries of the pulp, and resultant pathologic periradicular conditions (28).

An ENDODONTIST is a dentist who specializes in endodontics (root canal therapy). An endodontist is specially trained to treat difficult and complex endodontic cases. This may include difficult root canal anatomy, medically compromised patients, surgical treatments of periapical pathosis and infection, and patients who cannot be successfully treated by the general dentist.

## 2. DIAGNOSIS OF PULPAL AND PERIAPICAL DISEASE

### a. Irreversible Pulpitis

Irreversible pulpitis (inflammation of the pulp that cannot be healed) is a condition of the pulp tissue where root canal treatment is indicated. The tooth is unusually sensitive to cold, hot, or sometimes either stimuli may cause an exaggerated response (prolonged pain). The patient may also experience spontaneous pain in the tooth. The usual cause of this condition is caries (Fig. 8.34), although deep or leaky restorations may also contribute. As the caries approaches the pulp, a normal defense reaction will occur—inflammation and formation of reparative dentin. However, if the caries exposes the pulp, the bacteria will overwhelm the defenses and the tooth usually becomes painful. This prompts the patient to seek emergency treatment from a dentist. The pulp tissue from the crown and root must be removed to gain relief from the pain. The pulp tissue cannot be successfully treated with medications once the pulp is irreversibly damaged.

### b. Periapical Disease

Periapical disease occurs when the pulp has died (becomes necrotic). The pulp has been overwhelmed by the disease process in the crown and the pulp tissue in the root canals gradually dies. The bacteria and pulpal breakdown products contained within the root canals cause the periapical tissue around the tooth to react to this insult. A chronic inflammatory response ensues in the bone with the formation of a granuloma. Since this is less dense than bone, a radiograph will usually reveal a radiolucency (dark area at end of the root; Fig. 8.35). In some cases, the granuloma undergoes degeneration and a cyst is formed. The difference between a granuloma and cyst cannot be determined in a radiograph.

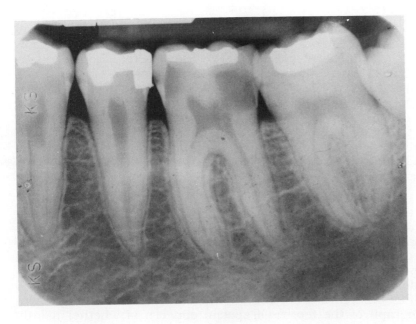

**Figure 8.34.** Radiograph of a lower right first molar. The distal carious lesion has exposed the pulp. There is also mesial caries on this tooth and on the second molar. The third molar is partially impacted.

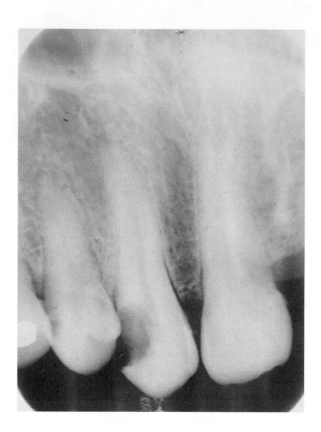

**Figure 8.35.** Radiograph of a maxillary left canine. The dark area on the distal aspect of the root apex means the pulp has become necrotic and a granuloma or cyst has developed in the bone.

When the bacteria from the root canal overwhelm the defenses of the periapical tissues, or the patient's immune system is compromised, the bacteria invade the surrounding bone and soft tissue, resulting in severe pain and facial swelling. This prompts the patient to seek emergency treatment. Cleaning the root canals, draining the area of infection, and antibiotic treatment will usually provide relief.

## 3. ENDODONTIC THERAPY

### a. Goal of Endodontic Therapy

The GOAL of endodontic therapy is to relieve pain, control infection, and preserve the tooth so it may function normally during mastication. Endodontic treatment is preferred to extraction because if the tooth was extracted, there would be a delay for healing before a replacement tooth (prosthesis) could be made. Endodontic therapy is less expensive than having a tooth extracted and subsequently replaced. Once a tooth has had endodontic therapy, it is not a "dead tooth." Although it cannot respond to stimuli like hot or cold, and cannot form reparative dentin, the periodontal support is the same as if it never had endodontic treatment. Therefore, if the periodontium remains healthy, the treated tooth generally will last for the lifetime of the patient.

### b. Access Openings

To gain access to the pulp chamber and the root canals of teeth, the dentist makes an opening in the crown of the tooth. On anterior teeth, the opening is made on the lingual surface and on posterior teeth through the occlusal surface. These access openings vary considerably from cavity preparations used in operative dentistry. The shape (outline form), size, position, and depth of the access opening is determined by studying ideal openings of maxillary and mandibular teeth (Fig. 8.28) and modifying them to conform to what is present on the initial radiograph of the tooth. Of special concern is whether a pulp chamber is present. In older teeth, or teeth that have large or deep restorations, the formation of secondary or reparative dentin may obliterate the pulp chamber making endodontic access difficult. In many cases, the tooth may be crowned and this masks the pulp chamber on the radiograph. Care must be exercised in locating the pulp chamber in these teeth. Once the access opening is complete, the dentist locates the root canal orifices on the floor of the pulp chamber. The knowledge of the number of root canals present in teeth is CRITICALLY IMPORTANT to successful endodontic treatment. Not locating and cleaning all the canals may result in continued discomfort for the patient or unsuccessful endodontic treatment with ensuing periapical disease.

### c. Endodontic Treatment

Once the canal orifices have been located, endodontic files are carefully inserted into the root canals. The file length is approximated by measuring the length of the corresponding root and crown on the preoperative radiograph. A radiograph is made with the files in the root (Fig. 8.36). The positions and length of the files are adjusted to be approximately 1 mm from the radiographic apex of the root. This apical position corresponds to the cementodentinal junction and is a natural constriction of the canal apically (Fig. 3.2, *right side*). The canals are then cleaned and shaped, at this length, with incrementally larger diameter files until the root canal system is clean. Following this cleaning procedure, the root canals are filled with gutta percha (a rubber-type material) and a zinc oxide sealer (Fig. 8.37). The access opening in the crown is filled with a permanent restoration (composite material in anterior teeth) or in posterior teeth, a crown is usually placed to protect the tooth from fracture.

## LEARNING EXERCISES (OPTIONAL)

*It is interesting to keep a record of peculiarities you see in teeth you have ground to expose the pulp cavities.*

*Watch carefully for accessory foramina (foramina in places other than the root tip). Look particularly on the sides of the root in the apical third and in the furcation of multirooted teeth. You will probably need to use a magnifying glass to find the small apical foramen in most teeth.*

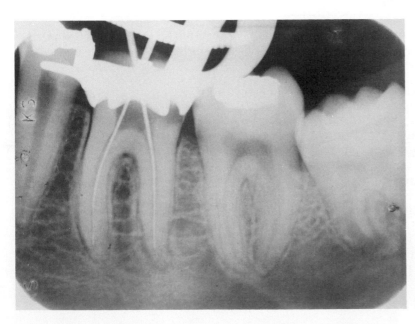

**Figure 8.36.** Radiograph of a lower right first molar. Endodontic files have been placed within the root canals to the cementodentinal junction apically (same tooth as Fig. 8.34).

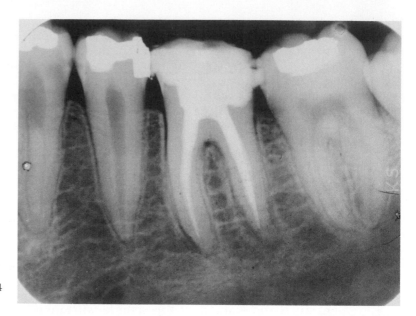

**Figure 8.37.** Radiograph of a lower right first molar. The root canals have been filled with gutta percha and sealer (same tooth shown in Figs. 8.34 and 8.36).

# SECTION III. LOCATION OF ROOT AND CERVICAL CROWN CONCAVITIES, FURCATIONS, DEPRESSIONS, AND CANALS

The following tooth drawings identified by the Universal numbering system, include cross-sections of the roots at the cervix and in the apical half. Tooth surfaces are labeled:

M = mesial; D = distal; F = facial; and L = lingual

## A. Maxillary Central Incisors

Cross-section of the root at the cervix is triangular with the mesial side longer than the distal side, consistent with the slight distal placement of the cingulum.

There are no prominent root grooves on this incisor, though the *mesial* surface may be flattened or have a slight longitudinal depression.

The distal root surface is convex.

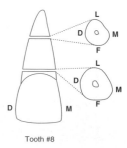

Tooth #8

## B. Maxillary Lateral Incisors

Cross-section of the root at the cervix is "egg-shaped" or ovoid, with the widest portion on the labial.

A shallow longitudinal depression is often found on the middle of the mesial surface extending about half of the root length.

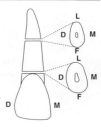

Tooth #7

## C. Mandibular Incisors

In cross-section, the cervical portion of the root is ovoid, considerably broader (about 2 mm) labiolingually than mesiodistally.

Longitudinal depressions are present on both proximal sides with the *distal* depression more distinct than the mesial.

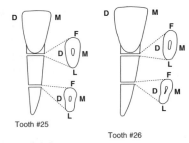

Tooth #25

Tooth #26

## D. Maxillary Canines

Cervical cross-section is broad labiolingually and appears ovoid.

Developmental grooves are present on both the mesial and *distal* sides providing better anchorage. The groove may be more distinct on the distal.

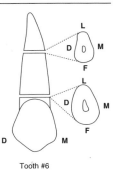

Tooth #6

## E. Mandibular Canines

Roots are wide labiolingually in the cervical half.

Longitudinal depressions are present on both sides, often more deep on the distal.

Variations in double-root depressions include clearly separated roots labiolingually to deep proximal grooves.

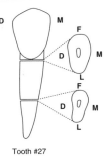

Tooth #27

## F. Maxillary First Premolars

*Most have two roots and two canals,* or when one root is present, two pulp canals are usually found. The mesial and distal depressions occur on both one- and two-rooted first premolars.

The bifurcation occurs in the apical third to half of the root.

The *mesial developmental depression of the crown* continues across the cervical line to join the deep depressions between the roots, or between the buccal and lingual segments of the single root.

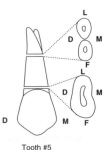

Tooth #5

## G. Maxillary Second Premolars

Often there is a shallow developmental groove on the *mesial* side of the root, but it does *not* extend onto the crown, as on the first premolar.

A root depression can also be found on the distal side, usually deeper than on the mesial.

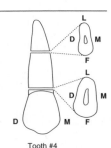

Tooth #4

## H. Mandibular First Premolars

In cross-section, the cervical portion of the root is ovoid, and is widest buccolingually.

Longitudinal depressions are often present on *both* sides, deeper on the distal. Sometimes these depressions may be quite deep and end in a bucco-lingual apical bifurcation.

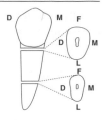

Tooth #28

## I. Mandibular Second Premolars

The root is rarely bifurcated.

Longitudinal depressions are not common on the mesial root surface, but are frequent on the *distal* surface in the middle third.

The cervical cross-section of the root of the three-cusp premolars is particularly wide on the lingual, more so than on two-cusp types.

Cross-section of the cervical portion of the root is ovoid buccolingually.

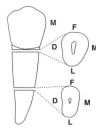

Tooth #29

## J. Mandibular First and Second Molars

Mandibular molars normally have two roots: mesial (broader and longer with two root canals) and distal. Both roots are broad buccolingually.

Prominent root depressions are common on the mesial and distal surfaces of the mesial root of both molars (where there are usually two root canals, and this root may be divided into buccal and lingual part).

Root bifurcations are found near midbuccal and midlingual.

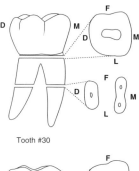

Tooth #30

Enamel of buccal and lingual cervical lines may extend into the bifurcation.

Buccal and lingual depressions on a relatively short root trunk extend from cervical lines to buccal and lingual furcations.

The root trunk is shorter on *first* molars than on second molars; the furcation is nearest to the cervical line on the buccal of first molars; the cervical line is more occlusal on the lingual of first molars.

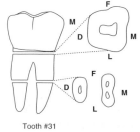

Tooth #31

Roots of *second* molar are narrower and less widely separated with a distal inclination.

*First* molar roots have more separation than second molar roots.

*Distal* root surface contours are more variable, but may be convex.

# K. Maxillary First and Second Molars

Normally three roots: mesiobuccal, distobuccal (shortest) and lingual (longest).

Trifurcations found near mid-buccal, mid-mesial and mid-distal.

Separation between roots is more pronounced on *first* molars; on *second* molars, the buccal roots are more nearly parallel and inclined distally in their apical third.

The root trunk is broader (longer) than on mandibular molars, so the furcation between mesiobuccal and distobuccal root may be at the junction of the cervical and middle thirds of the mesiobuccal root, especially on second molars.

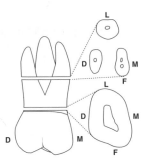

Tooth #3

Often a depression extends from the trifurcation to the cervical line and sometimes into the enamel of the crown on first molars.

The *mesiobuccal root* has mesial and distal side root depressions (and on first molars usually has two root canals while on second molars has one canal).

Distal of *distobuccal* root contour is more variable, and is normally convex.

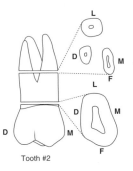

There is usually a slight longitudinal depression on the lingual side on the *lingual* root which has one canal.

Tooth #2

## LEARNING EXERCISE

*Draw a horizontal cervical cross-section of the following teeth:*

   a. Maxillary central incisor

   b. Maxillary lateral incisor

   c. Mandibular central incisor

   d. Mandibular lateral incisor

# References

1. Van Der Velden U, Winkel E, Abbas F. Bleeding/plaque ratio—a possible prognostic indicator for periodontal breakdown. J Clin Periodontol 1985;12:861.
2. Lang NP, Joss A, Orsamic T., Gusbert, FA and Siegrist BE: Bleeding on probing—a predictor for the progression of periodontal disease. J Clin Periodontol 1986;13:590.
3. Fine D, Mandel I. Indicators of periodontal disease activity: an evaluation. J Clin Periodontol 1986;13:533.
4. Haffajee A, Socransky S. Attachment level changes in destructive periodontal diseases. J Clin Periodontol 1986;13:461.
5. Burt BA. Periodontitis and aging: reviewing recent evidence. JADA 1994;125(Mar):273–279.
6. Kennedy J, Bird W, Palcanis K, Dorfman H. A longitudinal evaluation of varying widths of attached gingiva. J Clin Periodontol 1985;12:667.
7. Levy A, Wright W. The relationship between attachment height and attachment area of teeth using a digitizer and digital computer. J Periodontol 1978;49:483.

8. Renner RP. An introduction to dental anatomy and esthetics. Chicago: Quintessence Publishing, 1985:162.

9. Ramfjord SP, Nissie R. The modified widman flap. J Periodontol 1974;45:601.

10. Zakariasen KL. New and emerging techniques: promise, achievement and deception. JADA 1995; 126(Feb):163.

11. Basaraba N. Root amputation and tooth hemisection. Dent Clin North Am 1969;13:121.

12. Oschenbein C. Current status of osseous surgery. J Periodontol 1977;48:577.

13. Pontoriero R, Lindhe J, Nyman S. Guided tissue regeneration in degree II furcation involved mandibular molars. A clinical study. J Clin Periodontol 1988;15:247.

14. Mellonig JL. Freeze-dried bone allografts in periodontal reconstructive surgery. Dent Clin North Am 1991;35:505.

15. Langer B, Langer L. Subepithelial connective tissue flap for root coverage. J Periodontol 1985;56:15.

16. Zander H, Polson A. Present status of occlusion and occlusal therapy in periodontics. J Periodontol 1977;48:540.

17. Ericsson I, Lindhe J. Effect of long-standing jiggling on experimental marginal periodontitis in the beagle dog. J Clin Periodontol 1982;9:497.

18. Perlich MA, Reader A, Foreman DW. A scanning electron microscopic investigation of accessory foramens on the pulpal floor of human molars. J Endodontics 1981;7:402–406.

19. Benjamin KA, Dowson J. Incidence of two root canals in human mandibular incisor teeth. Oral Surg 1974;38:123–126.

20. Rankine-Wilson RW, Henry P. The bifurcated root canal in lower anterior teeth. JADA 1965;70:1162–1165.

21. Bellizzi R, Hartwell G. Clinical investigation of in vivo endodontically treated mandibular anterior teeth. J Endodontics 1983;9:246–248.

22. Vertucci FJ, Gegauff A. Root canal morphology of the maxillary first premolar. JADA 1979;99:194–198.

23. Bellizzi R, Hartwell G. Radiographic evaluation of root canal anatomy of in vivo endodontically treated maxillary premolars. J Endodontics 1985;11:37–39.

24. Vertucci FJ. Root canal anatomy of the human permanent teeth. Oral Surg 1984;58:589–599.

25. Neaverth EJ, Kotler LM, Kaltenbach RF. Clinical investigation (in vivo) of endodontically treated maxillary first molars. J Endodontics 1987;13:506–512.

26. Skidmore AE, Bjorndal AM. Root canal morphology of the human mandibular first molar. Oral Surg 1971;32:778–784.

27. Shaw L, Jones AD. Morphological considerations of the dental pulp chamber from radiographs of molar and premolar teeth. J Dent 1984;12:139–145.

28. The American Association of Endodontists. An annotated glossary of terms used in endodontics. 4th ed. Chicago: American Association of Endodontists, 1984.

## General References

Estrela C, Pereira HL, Pecora JD. Radicular grooves in maxillary lateral incisor: case report. Braz Dent J 1995;6(2):143–146.

Pecora JD, Saquy PC, Sousa Neto MD, Woelfel JB. Root form and canal anatomy of maxillary first premolars. Braz Dent J 1991;2(2):87–94.

Pecora JD, Sousa Neto MD, Saquy PC, Woelfel JB. In vitro study of root canal anatomy of maxillary second premolars. Braz Dent J 1992;3(2):81–85.

Pecora JD, Woelfel JB, Sousa Neto MD. Morphologic study of the maxillary molars. Part I: External anatomy. Braz Dent J 1991;2(1):45–50.

Pecora JD, Woelfel JB, Sousa Neto MD, Issa EP. Morphologic study of the maxillary molars. Part II: Internal anatomy. Braz Dent J 1992;3(1):53–57.

# Primary Dentition (Deciduous Teeth)

Your best specimens for the study of crown morphology can be found in the mouth of a 2–6-year-old who is willing to open his or her mouth wide, long, and often enough to permit your examination. Extracted primary teeth, even those with roots resorbed (gradual physiologic root destruction by the underlying erupting permanent tooth) and attrition (occlusal wear), are difficult to find. Plastic tooth models, if available, are very helpful and have the added advantage of complete roots.

Primary teeth emerge in children between the ages of 6 months and 2 years (Table 9.1). Beginning at age 6, these teeth are gradually replaced by the teeth of the permanent dentition (Figs. 9.5 and 9.6). Primary teeth are often called deciduous teeth. Deciduous comes from the Latin word meaning to fall off. Deciduous teeth fall off or are shed like leaves from a deciduous tree. Common nicknames for them are "milk teeth," or "temporary teeth," which, unfortunately, denote a lack of importance.

The primary teeth are actually in the mouth functioning for from 5.9 years ( for mandibular central incisors) to 9.8 years (for maxillary canines), the average being 8 years for maxillary teeth and 7.6 years for mandibular teeth (1). When people live to be 70 years of age, they will have spent 6% of their life masticating solely with primary teeth. This small proportion of time should not infer a lack of importance of primary teeth, however, because they play a very important role in "reserving" space for the permanent teeth, which assures proper alignment, spacing, and occlusion of the permanent teeth. When primary molars are lost prematurely, the results can be devastating (Figs. 9.3 and 9.4).

**Table 9.1.** Sequence of Tooth Eruption*

Of course, many variations occur, but the usual order of appearance of the teeth in the oral cavity is as follows:

| Primary Teeth | Months | Permanent Teeth | Years |
|---|---|---|---|
| Mandibular central incisor | 6 | Mandibular and then maxillary first molars | 5¾–6 |
| Mandibular lateral incisor | 7 | Mandibular central incisor | 6 |
| Maxillary central incisor | 7½ | Maxillary central and mandibular lateral incisors | 7–8 |
| Maxillary lateral incisor | 9 | Maxillary lateral incisor | 8–9 |
| Mandibular first molar | 12 | Mandibular canine | 9–10 |
| Maxillary first molar | 14 | Maxillary first premolar | 10–11 |
| Mandibular canine | 16 | Maxillary second premolar and mandibular first premolar | 10–12 |
| Maxillary canine | 18 | | |
| Mandibular second molar | 20 | Mandibular second premolar and maxillary canine | 11–12 |
| Maxillary second molar | 24 | Mandibular second molar | 11–13 |
| No more teeth for 3¾ years | | Maxillary second molar | 12–13 |
| (See top of next column) | | Third molars | 17–21 |

*Dates modified from Ash MM. Dental anatomy, physiology and occlusion. 6th ed. Philadelphia: W.B. Saunders, 1984. For complete development dates, see Table 9.3.

## DENTAL FORMULA OF THE HUMAN PRIMARY DENTITION

As stated in Chapter 1, the number and type of primary teeth in each half of the mouth is represented by this formula (Figs. 9.1 and 9.2):

$$\text{Incisors } \frac{2}{2} \text{ Canines } \frac{1}{1} \text{ Molars } \frac{2}{2} = \frac{5 \text{ maxillary teeth per side}}{5 \text{ mandibular teeth per side}}$$

THERE ARE NO PRIMARY PREMOLARS. When primary teeth are replaced by teeth of the permanent dentition, the primary molars are replaced by permanent premolars. The permanent molars have no predecessors in the primary dentition and erupt distal to the primary molars. Therefore, the permanent molars are not succedaneous teeth.

To review, the permanent dentition or secondary dentition formula is:

$$\text{Incisors } \frac{2}{2} \text{ Canines } \frac{1}{1} \text{ Premolars } \frac{2}{2} \text{ Molars } \frac{3}{3} = \frac{8 \text{ maxillary teeth per side}}{8 \text{ mandibular teeth per side}}$$

## IMPORTANT FUNCTIONS OF SOUND PRIMARY TEETH

1. Efficient mastication of food.

2. Maintenance of a normal facial appearance.

3. Formulation of clear speech.

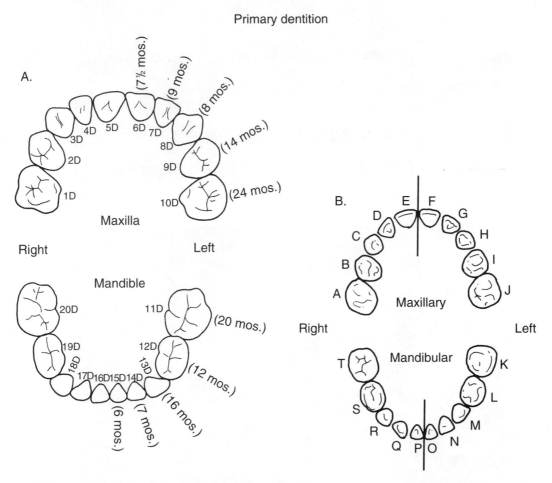

**Figure 9.1. A.** Diagram of maxillary and mandibular primary dental arches. The numbers in parentheses indicate the ages at which each tooth may be expected to emerge into the oral cavity. The numbers *1D* through *20D* inside the arches indicate one of several ways in which the teeth may be coded (rather than named) for purposes of record keeping. Starting at *1D*, the teeth are right second molar, first molar, canine, lateral incisor, and central incisor (which is *5D*). The remaining teeth are similarly coded. **B.** The universal numbering system described in Chapter 2. Two other methods for numbering the deciduous dentition are given in Table 2.1.

4. Maintenance of a proper diet. Missing or badly decayed primary teeth may be one reason that your children reject foods that are difficult to chew. (These are the only teeth that children have until approximately their 6th birthday.)

5. Avoidance of infection and concomitant pain. An abscess from a primary tooth can cause dark spots (Turner's spots) on the permanent tooth developing beneath it (Fig. 11.25**B**).

6. Maintenance of space and arch continuity for the emergence of permanent teeth. Soon after the first permanent molars emerge, their mesial drift and eruptive forces start to push the primary teeth together. If this were to continue, there would be insufficient space for the premolars to come in (erupt) (Figs. 9.3 and 9.4). The flared roots of the primary molars (Fig. 9.9) however, resist the mesial displacement. This, coupled with the fact that the primary molars are wider mesiodistally than their premolar successors (see Table 9.2), helps preserve sufficient space for the premolars and permanent canines (2).

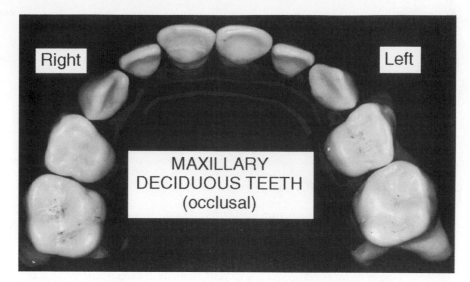

**Figure 9.2. A.** Maxillary deciduous teeth (occlusal view). Notice the striking resemblance of the second deciduous molar to a first permanent molar. The anterior teeth are much wider mesiodistally than faciolingually.

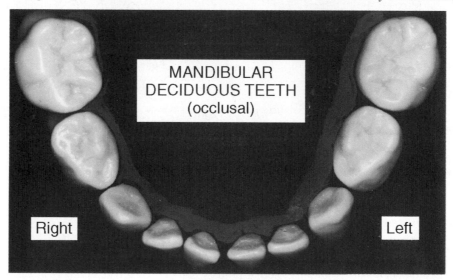

**Figure 9.2. B**. Mandibular deciduous teeth (occlusal view). Notice the resemblance of the second deciduous molar to a first permanent molar.

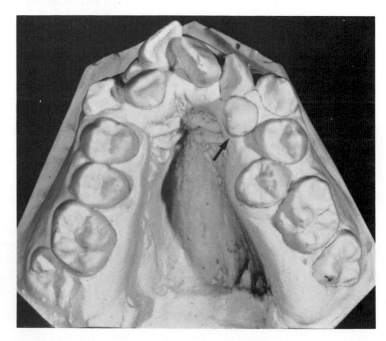

**Figure 9.3.** Extreme crowding of a maxillary permanent dentition in a 12-year-old child. The left deciduous canine (*arrow*) was not shed because its successor emerged labially to it. Both 12-year molars (three-cusp type) are in the process of emerging. Correction of the tooth alignment deformities in Figures 9.3 and 9.4 would require extensive and prolonged orthodontic therapy.

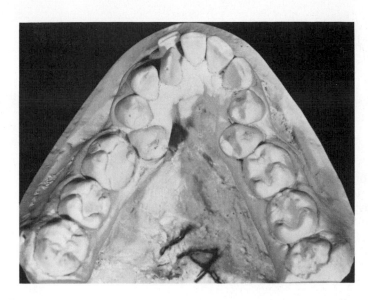

**Figure 9.4.** A crowded mandibular secondary dentition caused by the premature loss of deciduous molars. Notice that the left lateral incisor almost contacts the right central incisor and that the left first premolar is only 2.5 mm from contacting the first molar.

**Table 9.2.** Deciduous Tooth Size Compared to Their Successors

| | Crown Length | | Root Length | | Overall Length | | Mesio distal Crown | | Facio lingual Crown | | Mesio distal Cervix | | Facio lingual Cervix | | Average of all Measurements |
|---|---|---|---|---|---|---|---|---|---|---|---|---|---|---|---|
| | mm | %* | mm | %* | mm | %* | mm | %* | mm | %* | mm | %* | mm | %* | %* |
| **Maxillary Teeth** | | | | | | | | | | | | | | | |
| Central Incisor | 6.4 | 57 | 11.3 | 82 | 17.2 | 73 | 7.4 | 86 | 5.0 | 70 | 5.7 | 89 | 4.4 | 70 | 75.3 |
| Lateral Incisor | 7.4 | 76 | 10.9 | 81 | 16.8 | 75 | 5.8 | 88 | 4.9 | 79 | 4.0 | 85 | 4.5 | 78 | 80.3 |
| Canine | 7.6 | 72 | 13.5 | 78 | 20.2 | 80 | 7.4 | 97 | 5.4 | 67 | 5.3 | 95 | 5.0 | 66 | 78.8 |
| First Molar | 6.0 | 70 | 12.5 | 93 | 17.1 | 80 | 8.1 | 114 | 9.5 | 103 | 5.9 | 123 | 8.9 | 108 | 98.7 |
| Second Molar | 6.4 | 83 | 10.4 | 74 | 15.9 | 75 | 9.7 | 147 | 10.3 | 114 | 7.1 | 151 | 9.6 | 118 | 108.8 |
| **Mandibular Teeth** | | | | | | | | | | | | | | | |
| Central Incisor | 6.1 | 69 | 10.5 | 83 | 16.0 | 77 | 4.5 | 85 | 4.5 | 79 | 3.5 | 100 | 4.2 | 78 | 81.6 |
| Lateral Incisor | 7.3 | 78 | 10.6 | 78 | 16.5 | 75 | 4.9 | 86 | 4.8 | 79 | 3.7 | 94 | 4.5 | 78 | 81.4 |
| Canine | 8.2 | 74 | 11.7 | 74 | 18.7 | 72 | 6.1 | 90 | 5.7 | 74 | 4.2 | 81 | 5.0 | 67 | 76.0 |
| First Molar | 7.1 | 81 | 9.7 | 67 | 15.9 | 71 | 8.7 | 124 | 7.4 | 96 | 7.2 | 150 | 5.3 | 78 | 95.3 |
| Second Molar | 6.6 | 80 | 10.0 | 68 | 15.5 | 70 | 10.3 | 145 | 9.2 | 112 | 7.6 | 152 | 7.1 | 97 | 103.4 |

Measurements are derived from 2392 maxillary and 2180 mandibular permanent tooth specimens compared to plastic model replicas of deciduous teeth made by the Shofu Dental Manufacturing Company reflecting the size of Japanese primary teeth. In most instances, these measurements on the plastic model teeth were 0.5–1 mm larger than measurements made by G.V. Black at the turn of the century (deciduous teeth).

*Percentage is based on the average size for the permanent successor as equaling 100%. In instances in which the deciduous tooth dimension is greater than its successor, the percentage is over 100, even as high as 152% on the mandibular second molar mesiodistal cervix dimension, indicating that this part of the deciduous molar is 1.5 times larger than the corresponding region on its successor the mandibular second premolar.

# ERUPTION TIME OF PRIMARY DENTITION

The first primary teeth to erupt are usually the mandibular central incisors, at about 6 months of age. The last teeth to emerge, thus completing the primary dentition, are the maxillary second molars, at about 24 months of age (complete data in Table 9.3).

The complete primary dentition is in the mouth from 2 years to $5^3/_4$ or 6 years of age, when no permanent teeth are present. Shortly after the 4th birthday, as the maxilla and the mandible grow larger, spaces develop between the primary teeth. This frequently concerns parents, but is perfectly natural in providing space for the permanent incisors and canines, which are considerably wider than their predecessors (Figs. 9.5 and 9.6).

# MIXED DENTITION: PRESENCE OF PRIMARY AND PERMANENT TEETH

The first permanent teeth to erupt are usually the mandibular first molars and then maxillary first molars. They appear distal to the second primary molars when a child is between $5^3/_4$ and 6 years of age. They are commonly called 6-year molars. It is important to recognize that these are permanent teeth and to care for them accordingly. With their eruption commences the mixed dentition period.

**Table 9.3.** Deciduous Tooth Formation and Eruption Times

| | Tooth | Hard Tissue Formation Begins | Crown Completed | Eruption | Root Completed |
|---|---|---|---|---|---|
| **Deciduous Dentition — Maxillary Teeth** | Central incisor | 4 mos. in utero | 4 mos. | $7^1/_2$ mos. | $1^1/_2$ yrs. |
| | Lateral incisor | $4^1/_2$ mos. in utero | 5 mos. | 9 mos. | 2 yrs. |
| | Canine | 5 mos. in utero | 9 mos. | 18 mos. | $3^1/_4$ yrs. |
| | First molar | 5 mos. in utero | 6 mos. | 14 mos. | $2^1/_2$ yrs. |
| | Second molar | 6 mos. in utero | 11 mos. | 24 mos. | 3 yrs. |
| **Deciduous Dentition — Mandibular Teeth** | Central incisor | $4^1/_2$ mos. in utero | $3^1/_2$ mos. | 6 mos. | $1^1/_2$ yrs. |
| | Lateral incisor | $4^1/_2$ mos. in utero | 4 mos. | 7 mos. | $1^1/_2$ yrs. |
| | Canine | 5 mos. in utero | 9 mos. | 16 mos. | 3 yrs. |
| | First molar | 5 mos. in utero | $5^1/_2$ mos. | 12 mos. | $2^1/_4$ yrs. |
| | Second molar | 6 mos. in utero | 10 mos. | 20 mos. | 3 yrs. |
| **Permanent Dentition — Maxillary Teeth** | Central incisor | 3–4 mos. | 4–5 yrs. | 7–8 yrs. | 10 yrs. |
| | Lateral incisor | 10–12 mos. | 4–5 yrs. | 8–9 yrs. | 11 yrs. |
| | Canine | 4–5 mos. | 6–7 yrs. | 11–12 yrs. | 13–15 yrs. |
| | First premolar | $1^1/_2$–$1^3/_4$ yrs. | 5–6 yrs. | 10–11 yrs. | 12–13 yrs. |
| | Second premolar | 2–$2^1/_4$ yrs. | 6–7 yrs. | 10–12 yrs. | 12–14 yrs. |
| | First molar | birth | $2^1/_2$–3 yrs. | 6–7 yrs. | 9–10 yrs |
| | Second molar | $2^1/_2$–3 yrs. | 7–8 yrs. | 12–15 yrs. | 14–16 yrs. |
| | Third molar | 7–9 yrs. | 12–16 yrs. | 17–21 yrs. | 18–25 yrs. |
| **Permanent Dentition — Mandibular Teeth** | Central incisor | 3–4 mos. | 4–5 yrs. | 6–7 yrs. | 9 yrs. |
| | Lateral incisor | 3–4 mos. | 4–5 yrs. | 7–8 yrs. | 10 yrs. |
| | Canine | 4–5 mos. | 6–7 yrs. | 9–10 yrs. | 12–14 yrs. |
| | First premolar | $1^3/_4$–2 yrs. | 5–6 yrs. | 10–12 yrs. | 12–13 yrs. |
| | Second premolar | $2^1/_4$–$2^1/_2$ yrs. | 6–7 yrs. | 11–12 yrs. | 13–14 yrs. |
| | First molar | birth | $2^1/_2$–3 yrs. | 6–7 yrs. | 9–10 yrs. |
| | Second molar | $2^1/_2$–3 yrs. | 7–8 yrs. | 11–13 yrs. | 14–15 yrs. |
| | Third molar | 8–10 yrs. | 12–16 yrs. | 17–21 yrs. | 18–25 yrs. |

*Logan and Kronfeld (slightly modified by McCall and Schour)

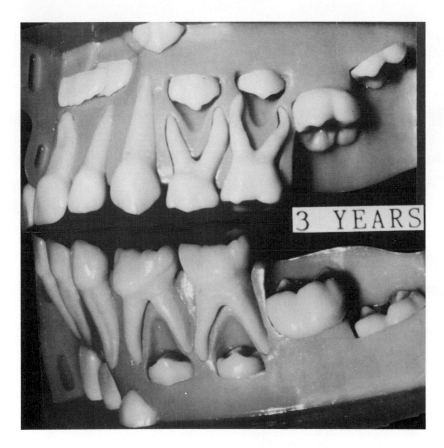

**Figure 9.5.** Models depicting the stage of development of the dentitions of a 3-year-old child. All primary teeth have emerged into the oral cavity, and they have full roots, prior to resorption. Notice the various amounts of crown development and positions of the partially formed crowns of the permanent dentition. (Models courtesy of 3M Unitek, Monrovia, CA.)

Permanent incisors begin to replace primary incisors at about 6–7 years of age (mandibular preceding maxillary). Next, permanent mandibular canines replace primary mandibular canines at about 9–10 years of age, followed at age 10–12 by the permanent premolars which replace primary molars. Finally, the maxillary canines are the last primary teeth to be lost at $11\frac{1}{2}$ to $12\frac{1}{2}$ years of age. The mixed dentition is therefore present from $5\frac{3}{4}$ or 6 years until 12 years of age. Usually 24 teeth are present in the mixed dentition (including the four permanent 6-year molars).

The roots of primary teeth are completely formed in just 1 year after emergence of the crown into the mouth. The intact roots as seen in Figure 9.5 are short-lived—in just 3 years they start to resorb, usually at the apex, or on one side near the apex. Resorption of the root occurs as the crown of the permanent tooth that is to replace it begins to move occlusally to infringe upon the primary root. Increasing loss of root attachment from root resorption results in the eventual loosening of the primary teeth, so they "fall off" the jaw. Usually, the crowns of the permanent successors are close to the surface, ready to emerge within a few months (Figs. 9.6 and 9.8).

## GENERAL CHARACTERISTICS OF PRIMARY TEETH

1. Primary teeth are smaller in size than the analogous permanent teeth (Table 9.2).

2. They are whiter in color than the analogous permanent teeth.

3. They are less mineralized than the analogous permanent teeth, and become very worn (3, 4). There is considerable attrition because of the expanding growth of the jaws and the various positions of occlusion of the teeth before they are shed. Attrition, therefore, is not a dentition trait, but a fact of life or normal occurrence (4).

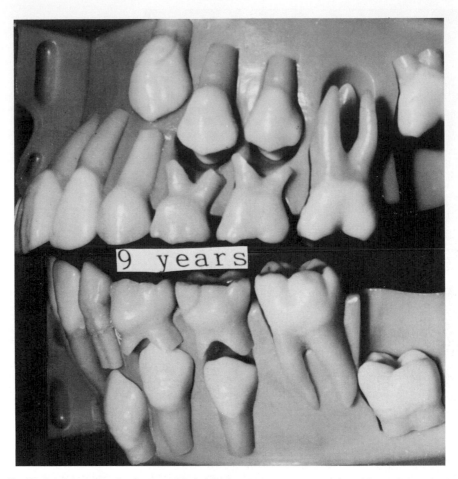

**Figure 9.6.** Tooth development of a 9-year-old child. The permanent central and lateral incisors and first molars have emerged into a functional level. The deciduous canines and molars are still functioning (*mixed dentition*) although much of their roots have resorbed. You can see at this time why the maxillary canine is often the last permanent tooth to erupt except for the third molars (not shown). (Models courtesy of 3M Unitek, Monrovia, CA.)

**Figure 9.7.** Dentition of a teenager with partial anodontia (congenitally missing lateral incisors and second premolars). Observe the similarity in occlusal morphology between the deciduous second and permanent first molars, as well as their different size. These deciduous second molars may continue to function for many years without the succedaneous teeth to replace them.

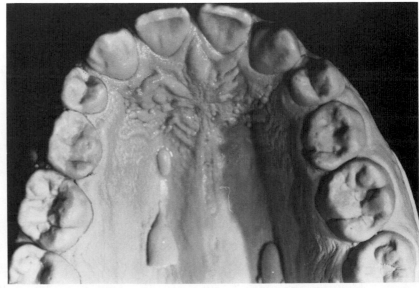

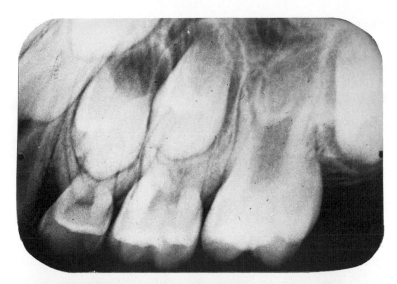

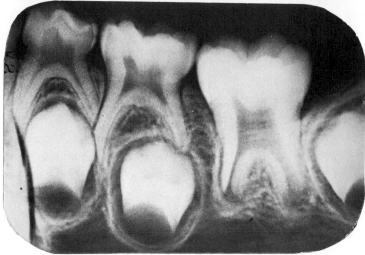

**Figure 9.8.** Radiographs made of an 8-year-old child showing the first and second deciduous molars and first permanent molars in the mouth. Notice the premolar crowns between the partially resorbed roots of the deciduous molars. Part of the permanent second molar crowns is seen on the far *right*. The lesser enamel thickness and larger pulp cavities are evident in the deciduous molars. (Courtesy of Professor Donald Bowers, Ohio State University.)

4. They have shorter crowns with respect to their roots.

5. The crowns have a marked constriction at the cervix, appearing as if they are being squeezed with a rubber band.

6. The enamel seems to bulge close to the cervical line, rather than gradually tapering (3).

7. The layers of enamel and dentin are thinner than on permanent teeth.

8. The pulp cavities are proportionally larger.

9. Primary teeth have more consistent shapes than the permanent dentition (fewer anomalies) (3).

10. The crowns on primary teeth appear bulbous, often having labial or buccal cingula (3).

## A. On the Anterior Teeth

11. Usually there are no depressions or perikymata on the labial surface of the crowns of the incisors. These surfaces are smooth.

12. There are no mamelons on the incisal edges.

13. The cervical ridges on facial surfaces are prominent (running mesiodistally in the cervical third) (Appendix 9a).

14. The cingula are prominent or seem to bulge and occupy about one-third of the cervicoincisal length (Appendix 9a).

15. The roots are long in proportion to crown length, and are narrow mesiodistally (Appendix 9b and 9f).

16. The roots bend labially in their apical one-third to one-half by as much as 10° (Appendix 9c; Fig 9.12).

## B. On the Posterior Teeth

17. The molar crowns are wide mesiodistally, yet very short cervico-occlusally (Appendix 10a).

18. The second molars are decidedly larger than the first molars (Appendix page 10, compare firsts to seconds; Figs. 9.2 and 9.9).

19. The molar crowns have a narrow chewing surface (occlusal table) buccolingually (Appendix 10c).

20. The molar occlusal anatomy is shallow. In other words, the cusps are short, the ridges are not pronounced, and the fossae are correspondingly not as deep (Appendix 10, all molars).

21. The buccal cusps on molars are not pointed or sharp, and their cusp slopes meet at a very wide obtuse angle (sometimes almost a straight line when viewed from the buccal) (Appendix 10d).

22. There are few grooves or depressions in the crowns.

23. The mesial cervical ridge is prominent (it is easy to distinguish rights from lefts) (Appendix 10e).

24. Microscopically, the enamel rods at the cervix slope occlusally, unlike in permanent teeth where these rods slope cervically.

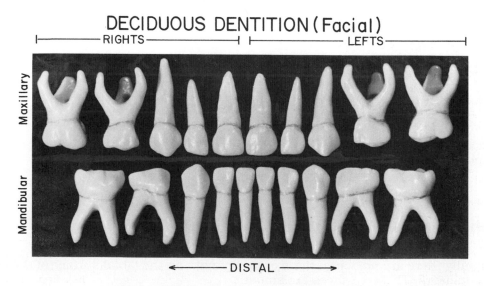

**Figure 9.9.** Deciduous dentition (facial view).

25. The root furcations are near the crown, with little or no root trunk (Appendix 10f).

26. The roots are widely spread beyond the outlines of the crown (Appendix 10g).

27. The roots are thin and slender (Appendix 10g).

28. The second molar roots are spread more widely than the first deciduous molar (the opposite of the permanent molars) (5).

## PRIMARY INCISORS: UNIQUE PROPERTIES

### A. Labial Aspect of Primary Incisors

Refer to Figure 9.9 and Appendix page 9.

#### 1. Crown Proportion

In contrast to permanent maxillary central incisors, primary maxillary central incisors are the only incisors (primary or permanent) that are wider mesiodistally than they are long incisocervically (Appendix 9e). The crowns narrow near the cervix, and are more symmetrical than primary lateral incisor crowns which are longer than they are wide.

#### 2. Root to Crown Proportion

The roots of primary incisors are much longer relative to the crown length than on permanent teeth (Appendix 9f)—primary incisor roots are about twice the length of the crown. The roots of maxillary lateral incisors appear proportionally even longer. On primary extracted or shed teeth, there is usually some root resorption (Fig. 9.10). Often the entire root is gone.

#### 3. Outline Shape of Crowns (Fig 9.10)

Incisal edges of primary maxillary central incisors are flat except for some rounding at the distoincisal angle. Distoincisal angles of lateral incisors are even more rounded. Mesial sides of maxillary central incisor crowns are fairly flat, whereas the distal sides are more convex. The lateral incisor crowns are similar in shape, but less symmetrical and smaller than central incisors in the same dentition.

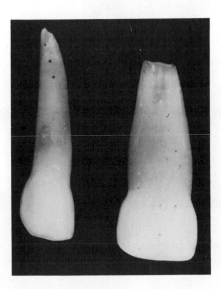

**Figure 9.10.** Primary maxillary right lateral incisor (at *left*) and right central incisor. Compare the labial surfaces. The central incisor crown is short and wide. There has been some resorption of the root tips on both teeth, but even so, they are twice as long as the crown. The lateral incisor is less symmetrical and is longer than it is wide.

The crowns of the mandibular incisors resemble permanent mandibular incisor crowns, but are much smaller. As with permanent mandibular incisors, primary lateral incisor crowns are a little larger than the crowns of central incisors and less symmetrical (with more rounded distoincisal angles) than the central incisors of the same dentition (Fig. 9.9).

### 4. Contact Areas

The locations of proximal contact areas on primary incisors (Fig. 9.9) are comparable to those of their permanent successors.

### 5. Labial Surfaces

Labial surfaces of maxillary central incisors are smooth; usually there are no depressions. Mandibular incisors are also relatively smooth, but may have shallow depressions on their labial surfaces in the incisal third.

## B. Lingual Aspect of Primary Incisors

Refer to Figure 9.11.

### 1. CINGULUM

The cingula of primary maxillary central incisors are often proportionally large, so that lingual fossae are in only the incisal and middle thirds of the lingual surface. The lingual surface of mandibular incisors also has a cingulum and a slight lingual fossa.

### 2. MARGINAL RIDGES

On maxillary central incisors, marginal ridges are often distinct and prominent (like shovel shaped incisors). In mandibular incisors, marginal ridges are more faint (Fig 9.11).

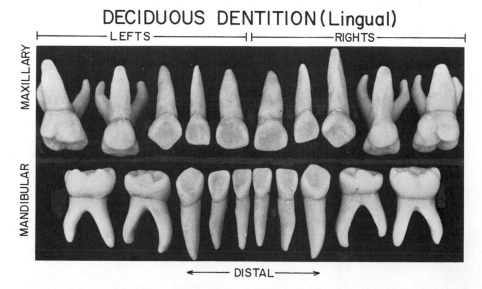

**Figure 9.11.** Deciduous dentition (lingual view). Notice that the lingual cusps are not as long as the mesiobuccal cusps on the molars.

### 3. TAPER TO LINGUAL

As with permanent incisors, the roots and crowns of primary incisors are somewhat narrower on the lingual side than on the labial side.

## C. Proximal (Mesial and Distal) Aspect of Primary Incisors

Refer to Figure 9.12.

### 1. PROPORTION OF CROWNS

Although the faciolingual dimension of these crowns appears small from these aspects, crowns are wide labiolingually in their cervical one third because of large cingula.

### 2. CERVICAL RIDGES

Convex labial cervical ridges are prominent on all primary incisors.

### 3. INCISAL EDGE LOCATION

Similar to permanent maxillary anterior teeth, incisal ridges of maxillary central incisors are located labial to the root-axis line, whereas incisal ridges of mandibular incisors are located on the root axis line (Fig. 9.12).

### 4. CERVICAL LINE (CEMENTOENAMEL JUNCTION)

As on permanent teeth, the convexity of the cervical line toward the incisal is greater on the mesial than on the distal. The cervical line is positioned more apically on the lingual than on the labial side.

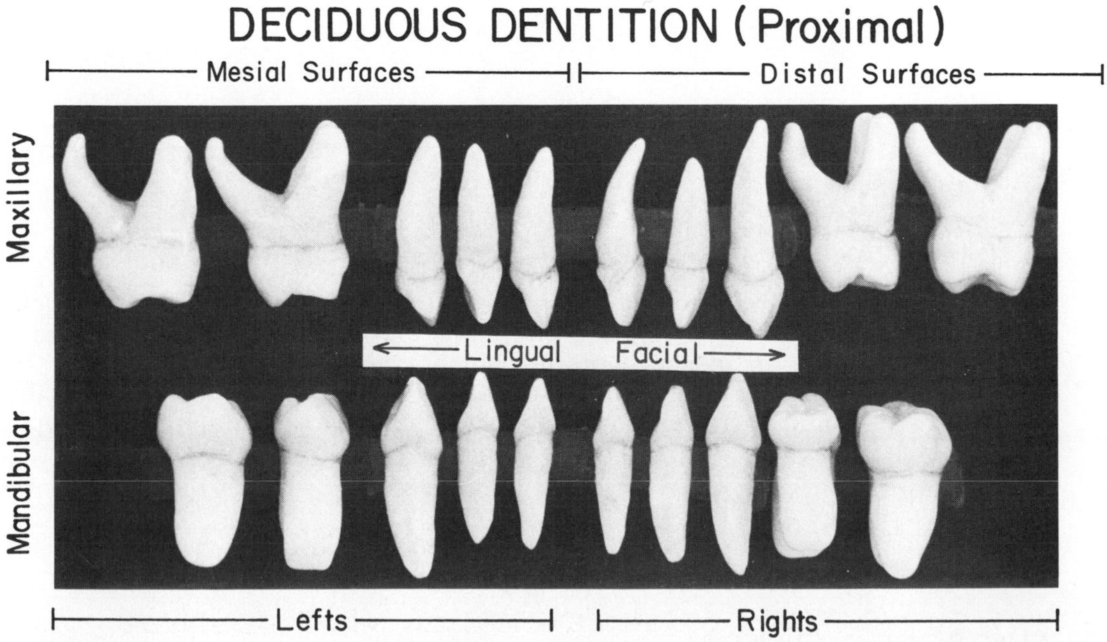

**DECIDUOUS DENTITION ( Proximal )**

Mesial Surfaces — Distal Surfaces

Maxillary

Lingual   Facial

Mandibular

Lefts   Rights

**Figure 9.12.** Deciduous dentition (proximal view). Notice on the molars that more of the occlusal surfaces are visible from the distal view than from the mesial view. Also notice that the roots of anterior teeth bend labially, especially in the maxillary dentition.

## 5. ROOT SHAPE

The roots of *maxillary* incisors are S-shaped, bending lingually in the cervical third to half, and labially by as much as 10° in the apical half (5). Roots of the *mandibular* incisors, in contrast, are straight in their cervical half, but then bend labially about 10° in their apical half (5). This bend helps make space for the developing secondary incisors, which should be in a lingual and apical position (Appendix 9c and d).

## D. Incisal Aspect of Primary Incisors

Refer to Figure 9.2.

### 1. CROWN OUTLINE

Incisor crowns have a smoothly convex labial outline. The one mm thick incisal ridge is slightly curved.

### 2. TAPER TO LINGUAL

The crowns have lingual surfaces that become narrower toward the lingual, at the cingulum.

### 3. PROPORTION

Crowns of primary maxillary *central* incisors are much wider mesiodistally than faciolingually (by 2.4 mm) compared to maxillary lateral incisors which are only 0.9 mm wider mesiodistally (see Table 9.2). Both mandibular incisor crowns have mesiodistal and faciolingual dimensions that are essentially equal.

# PRIMARY CANINES: UNIQUE PROPERTIES

## A. Labial Aspect of Primary Canines

Refer to Figures 9.13 and 9.14 and Appendix page 9.

### 1. OUTLINE SHAPE

Maxillary canine crowns may be as wide as they are long. They are constricted at the cervix. They have convex mesial and distal outlines, with distal contours more broadly rounded than mesial contours which are somewhat angular (Fig. 9.13). Mandibular canine crowns are longer incisocervically than wide mesiodistally (by 2.1 mm) and are 1.3mm narrower mesiodistally than maxillary canine crowns (Appendix 9g; Fig. 9.14).

### 2. CERVICAL LINES

Cervical lines on maxillary canines are nearly flat on the labial surface.

### 3. CUSP RIDGE OUTLINES

*Maxillary* canine cusps are often very sharp (pointed) with two cusp ridges meeting at an acute angle. The mesial cusp slopes of these maxillary canines are longer than

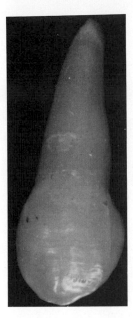

**Figure 9.13.** Primary maxillary right canine. Labial surface. Notice the longer mesial cusp ridge and the more cervically positioned contact area, and the rounded distal contours compared to the more angular mesial contours.

the distal cusp slopes (*which is the opposite of permanent canines*). These mesial cusp slopes are flat to concave and less steeply inclined (6) than the shorter distal slopes, which are more convex. *Mandibular* canines also have sharp cusp tips pointed like an arrow (Fig. 9.14). As on the permanent mandibular canines, the mesial cusp slope is shorter than the distal cusp slope. See Appendix 9h.

## 4. CONTACT AREAS (APPENDIX 9I)

Distal contact areas of primary canines rest against the mesial surfaces of primary molars since there are no primary premolars. Mesial and distal contact areas of primary maxillary canines are near the center of the crown cervicoincisally, with the mesial contact more cervically located (*a condition unique to this tooth and the permanent mandibular first premolar*). See Appendix 9i.

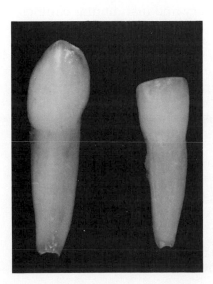

**Figure 9.14.** Primary mandibular right canine (at *left*) and right lateral incisor (labial surfaces). The root tips have resorbed. Some primary mandibular canines bear a closer resemblance than this one to their permanent successor.

## 5. ROOTS

Maxillary canine roots prior to resorption are the longest of the primary teeth (13.5 mm) tapering to a blunt apex. The roots of mandibular canines are more tapered and pointed, and 1.8 mm shorter than maxillary canine roots (Fig. 9.9; Table 9.2).

## B. Lingual Aspect of Primary Canines

### 1. CINGULUM

The cingulum on a maxillary canine crown is bulky with well-developed mesial and distal marginal ridges which are less prominent than on permanent canines.

### 2. LINGUAL RIDGE

A lingual ridge, with adjacent mesial and distal fossae, is located on *maxillary* canine crowns somewhat distal to the middle of the crown. Distal fossae on these teeth are narrower and deeper than mesial fossae which are broader and shallower (5, 6). In contrast, lingual ridges are barely discernible on *mandibular* canines, with faint marginal ridges and usually a single concavity or fossa (Fig. 9.11) (7).

## C. Proximal (Mesial and Distal) Aspect of Primary Canines

Refer to Figure 9.12.

### 1. PROPORTION

The cervical third of primary canines is much thicker than on incisors.

### 2. CUSP TIP POSITION

On maxillary canines, cusp tips are positioned considerably labial to the root axis line, whereas the cusp tip of mandibular canines is most often located slightly lingual to the root axis line.

### 3. LABIAL CERVICAL RIDGE

Labial cervical ridges are prominent on both maxillary and mandibular canines, bulging similar to lingual cingula.

### 4. OUTLINE

The S-shaped lingual crown outline of maxillary canines is more concave than on permanent canines.

### 5. CERVICAL LINES

Cervical lines of both maxillary and mandibular canines curve incisally more on the mesial side than on the distal side, and are more apical on the lingual than on the labial (Fig. 9.12).

### 6. ROOTS

The roots of maxillary and mandibular canines are bulky in the cervical and middle thirds, tapering mostly in the apical third where they are bent labially, similar to primary central and lateral incisors. (Fig. 9.12).

## D. Incisal Aspect of Primary Canines

Refer to Figure 9.2.

### 1. CROWN OUTLINE

Crown contours of maxillary canines are somewhat angular and taper noticeably toward the cingulum. The mesial half of these crowns are thicker faciolingually than the distal half (similar to permanent maxillary canines). Cingula are centered mesiodistally.

From the incisal aspect, mandibular canine crowns have a diamond shape and are nearly symmetrical, except for the mesial position of the cusp tips and they appear to have slightly more bulk in the distal half (Fig. 9.2). Cingula are centered or just distal to the center.

### 2. CROWN PROPORTIONS AND SIZE

Primary maxillary canine crowns are broader faciolingually than incisor crowns, but are still 2 mm wider mesiodistally than faciolingually (Fig. 9.2; Table 9.2). The 1.5-mm thick mesial and distal cusp ridges curve toward the lingual at both ends. Mandibular canine crowns are only 0.4mm wider mesiodistally than faciolingually. The smallness of these teeth, compared to their permanent counterparts, is quite noticeable.

## PRIMARY MOLARS

Refer to Figures 9.15 through 9.19.

Recall that first and second primary molars erupt just distal to primary canines. It could be said that these primary molars are saving a place in the arch for the teeth that will succeed them, namely the permanent first and second premolars respectively.

Primary first molars are smaller than primary second molars which is different than in the permanent dentition (Appendix 10b). Primary first molars are more unique in their shape. One author feels that primary maxillary first molars are the most atypical of human molars (8), while another author feels they resemble somewhat the permanent premolars (9). It is agreed that primary mandibular first molars resemble no other tooth in either dentition.

Primary second molars have considerable similarities to permanent first molars in their respective arches, and since they are both present in the mouth during the time of mixed dentition (or longer in the case of retained primary teeth), it is important to distinguish between the primary second molars and the teeth that erupt just distal to them—the permanent first molars. One obvious difference between primary and permanent molar crowns is the presence of a prominent mesial cervical ridge on the buccal surface of primary molars. This bulge is sometimes called a buccal cingulum (4). Also, primary second molars are smaller than permanent first molars in the same dentition, and are normally positioned as the fifth tooth from the midline (whereas first permanent molars are sixth from the midline). Other more subtle differences are presented later.

When considering arch traits, primary *maxillary* molars generally have three roots (as in the permanent dentition), whereas *mandibular* molars have only two roots. As stated earlier, primary molar roots are thinner and more widely spread than permanent molar roots to make room for the developing premolars crowns which are forming beneath them (Appendix 10g). Extraction of a deciduous molar when roots are complete and before they have started to resorb may cause the germ of the permanent premolar to be removed along with the deciduous molar (7). Also, root furcations of primary molars are nearer to the cervix with little root trunk (Appendix 10f).

Each type of primary molar will be discussed in detail at this time, emphasizing the traits that further differentiate each type.

## A. Primary Maxillary Second Molar

Refer to Figure 9.15 and Appendix page 10.

Primary maxillary second molars are located over the crown of the developing second premolars, just distal to primary first molars and, after age 6, just mesial to permanent first molars. Primary second maxillary molars resemble permanent maxillary first molars (Fig. 9.7), but are smaller [by 13.2% when all dimensions are averaged]. They are similar in most respects, with the cusp ridges and fossae corresponding to those of permanent first molars. There are even cusps of Carabelli on maxillary primary second molars (Fig. 9.15**C** and **D**).

Primary maxillary second molars differ from permanent first molars as follows:

### 1. ACCENTUATED CROWN TAPER

Due to the prominent mesiobuccal cervical ridge and small occlusal table, these primary molars, when viewed from the proximal aspect, appear to taper narrower much more toward the occlusal (Appendix 10c and e; Fig. 9.12) (5). From the occlusal aspect, the crown also tapers more from mesial to distal, accentuated by the mesial bulge of the strongly prominent mesiobuccal portion of the mesial marginal ridge (Fig 9.7) (5).

Further, the mesiolingual corner of the occlusal surface is flattened as though it were compressed toward the distal (5) (Appendix 10h; Figs. 9.2**A** and 9.7), displacing the mesiolingual cusp more distally than on the permanent first molars. As a result, the oblique ridge is straighter in its course buccolingually (5), and the oblong distal fossa is smaller buccolingually. This also results in more taper from buccal to lingual.

### 2. RELATIVE CUSP SIZE

The mesiobuccal cusp is almost equal in size or slightly larger than the mesiolingual cusp (Appendix 10i). (Recall that the mesiolingual cusp is largest on permanent maxillary first molars.)

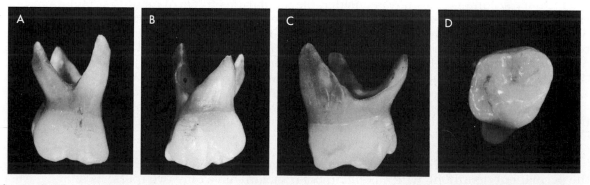

**Figure 9.15. A.** Primary *maxillary* right *second* molar. Buccal surface. **B.** Lingual surface. **C.** Mesial surface. Notice the spread of the roots. The crown of the permanent maxillary second premolar develops in the space bounded by these roots. Some root resorption has occurred (especially on the lingual root). **D.** Occlusal surface. From this aspect the primary maxillary second molar resembles a miniature permanent first molar (even with a Carabelli cusp).

## B. Primary Mandibular Second Molar

Refer to Figure 9.16 and Appendix page 10.

Primary mandibular second molars are located over the crowns of developing second premolars, just distal to primary first molars and, after age 6, just mesial to permanent first molars. These primary molars resemble permanent mandibular first molars, but are smaller [by 17.3% when all dimensions are averaged]. They are similar in most respects, with the cusp ridges and fossae corresponding to those of permanent first molars.

Primary mandibular second molars differ from permanent first molars as follows: There is a more prominent mesial cervical ridge, the roots are more slender and more widely spread, and the three buccal cusps (mesiobuccal, distobuccal, and distal) are of nearly equal size (Appendix 10j). The middle buccal cusp (called the distobuccal) is the widest (largest). As in the permanent mandibular molars, these cusps are separated by mesiobuccal and distobuccal grooves. The mesiolingual and distolingual cusps are about the same size and height, slightly shorter than the buccal cusps (5). A lingual groove separates these cusps.

### 1. MESIAL AND DISTAL ANATOMY

The mesial marginal ridge is high and is crossed by a groove that may extend about one-third of the way down the mesial surface (9). The contact area with the first primary molar is in the shape of an inverted crescent just below the notch of the marginal ridge (9). This mesial surface is generally convex but flattens cervically (9).

Since the crown is shorter on the distal side, and the distal marginal ridge is lower (more cervical) than the mesial marginal ridge, all five cusps can be seen from the distal aspect. The distal contact with the first permanent molar is round in shape and is located just buccal and cervical to the distal marginal groove (furrow) (9).

The cervical line is almost flat on both the mesial and distal sides of the crown but slopes occlusally toward the lingual.

### 2. ROOTS

The roots are about twice as long as the crowns and are thin mesiodistally. The mesial root is broad and flat with a blunt apex and has a shallow longitudinal depression. The distal root is broad and flat, and is narrower and less blunt at the apex than the mesial root. The root furcation is very close to the cervical line with very little root trunk.

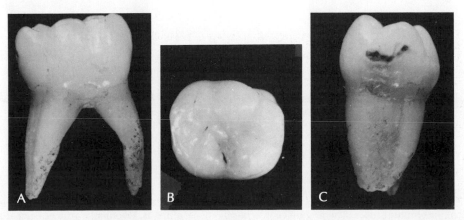

**Figure 9.16.** Primary *mandibular* right *second* molar. **A.** Buccal surface. The short root trunk and the widespread roots, as well as the small size, distinguish this tooth from the permanent mandibular first molar. The mesiobuccal, distobuccal, and distal cusps are often about the same size. **B.** Occlusal surface. Buccal side at *top;* mesial side at *left.* **C.** Distal surface. Buccal side at *right.*

## C. Primary Maxillary First Molar

Refer to Figure 9.17 and Appendix page 10.

Primary maxillary first molars are located over the crowns of developing first premolars, just distal to primary canines and mesial to primary second molars. They are quite unique in appearance. According to one author, they do not resemble any other molars (8). According to another author, they resemble maxillary first premolars which will replace them (9). The crowns are slightly larger than the premolars that will replace them (mesiodistally by 14%).

### 1. CROWN PROPORTION AND TAPER

From the buccal aspect, these crowns appear very wide relative to their height, and are noticeably shorter occlusocervically toward the distal. They are widest buccolingually toward the mesial (due in part to the wide mesial cervical bulge).

The mesiobuccal cusp has a buccal ridge (running occlusocervically) that extends to the cervical line. There is also a prominent cervical ridge (running mesiodistally) on the wider portion of the buccal surface. Due to this prominent bulge at the cervical, when viewed from the proximal, these crowns taper considerably from the wide cervical third to the narrow occlusal third (Appendix 10c and e). The crown outline is flat from the buccal ridge to the occlusal margin. The lingual outline is more gradually convex in the cervical and middle thirds and flat in the occlusal third (Fig. 9.17**C**).

The crown also tapers to become narrower mesiodistally toward the lingual. The lingual surfaces of these crowns are very convex mesiodistally and slightly convex cervico-occlusally.

### 2. CUSP SIZE AND SHAPE

The two main cusps are a wide mesiobuccal cusp and a narrow, slightly more distinct, mesiolingual cusp, and two more indistinct cusps, the distobuccal and distolingual (frequently absent). (A three-cusp type of primary maxillary first molar has no distolingual cusp.) The mesiobuccal cusp is always the longest (but second

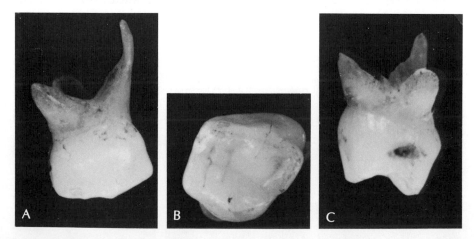

**Figure 9.17.** Primary *maxillary* right *first* molar. **A.** Buccal surface. The mesiobuccal root is less resorbed than the distobuccal and lingual roots. The lingual root is barely discernible. **B.** Occlusal surface. Buccal side at *top;* mesial side at *right.* The prominent cervical ridge below the mesiobuccal cups gives the tooth an angular appearance. **C.** Distal surface. Buccal side at *right.* The roots are partly resorbed. Within the space enclosed by these three widespread roots, the crown of the permanent maxillary first premolar developed.

sharpest) (Fig. 9.17**C**) (5). The mesiolingual cusp is the second longest, but sharpest, cusp. (See depiction of cusps described on back of Appendix 10k.) There is no buccal groove on the buccal surface, but a scallop or notch which divides the large mesiobuccal cusp from the indistinct distobuccal cusp (Appendix 10-L). This notch is distal to center. The distolingual cusp, when present, is inconspicuous, and is often only a small nodule on the distal marginal ridge. A groove between the two lingual cusps is present only when the distolingual cusp is definite.

The mesial marginal ridge is nearly as wide buccolingually as the distance between cusp tips. It may be crossed by a marginal groove. The mesial contact is flat where it contacts the canine in the occlusal third. The distal crown outline is decidedly more convex than the mesial, and contacts the second molar in the middle third.

## 3. OCCLUSAL OUTLINE

See Figures 9.2**A** and 9.17**B.**

The crown is oblong and wider faciolingually by 1.4mm than mesiodistally (Appendix 10m); therefore, the occlusal surface is basically rectangular except for the rounded mesiolingual corner (Appendix 10n) (similar to the tapered mesiolingual corner in the primary maxillary second molar). This rounding is reflected in the mesial marginal ridge, which does not run straight toward the lingual, but rather obliquely in a distolingual direction. In contrast, the distal marginal ridge runs in a straight direction buccolingually, joining both the buccal and lingual borders at right angles (7).

## 4. OCCLUSAL ANATOMY

See Figures 9.2**A** and 9.17**B.**

The triangular ridge of the narrow distobuccal cusp becomes the distal marginal ridge on three-cusp molars. When a distolingual cusp is present (four-cusp type), the triangular ridges of the distobuccal cusp joins the more distal of the two triangular ridges from the mesiolingual cusp as a barely discernible transverse ridge (9). The lingual half of the distal marginal ridge becomes the distolingual cusp. In these teeth, a distolingual groove separates the large and minute lingual cusps.

There are three fossae on these first molars: a medium size central fossa, a large and deep mesial triangular fossa, and a minute distal triangular fossa, each with a pit: central, mesial, and distal, respectively (Appendix 10o).

The grooves of these teeth usually form an "H" pattern. The crossbar of the "H" is the central groove which connects the central and mesial triangular fossae. [Some textbooks say there is no central groove and that the crossbar is made up of a mesial and distal groove instead (9).] Supplemental grooves running buccolingually just inside of the mesial marginal ridge form the mesial side of the "H," and the buccal groove (dividing the buccal cusps) combined with the distolingual groove (between the mesiolingual and distolingual cusps on four-cusp type molars only) form the distal side of the "H."

## D. Primary Mandibular First Molars

Refer to Figure 9.18 and Appendix 10.

Primary mandibular first molars are located over the crown of the developing permanent first premolars, and are just distal to primary canines and mesial to primary second molars. These first molars do not resemble any other primary or permanent tooth. According to one

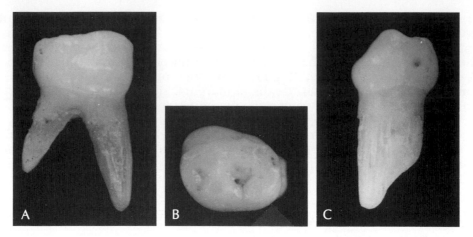

**Figure 9.18.** Primary *mandibular* right *first* molar. **A.** Buccal surface. The distal root has been considerably shortened by resorption. Notice that the crown is longer mesially (*right side*) than distally. **B.** Occlusal surface. Buccal side at *top;* mesial side at *left*. The buccal cervical ridge (*top left side*) on the mesiobuccal cusp is conspicuous. **C.** Mesial surface. Again the cervical ridge is outstanding. Notice how the crown appears to tilt lingually. If the root apex was not partially resorbed, the root would appear to taper to a more blunt end.

author, their chief differentiating characteristic may be their overdeveloped mesial marginal ridge (Appendix 10q) (9).

## 1. CROWN PROPORTION AND TAPER

The crowns of these first molars are wider mesiodistally than high cervico-occlusally [by 1.6 mm] (Appendix 10a). They taper to become shorter on the distal, due in part to the slope of the cervical line gingivally from distal to mesial (accentuated by the very prominent horizontal mesiobuccal cervical ridge), and also due to the cervical slope of the occlusal border from mesial to distal.

As with the primary maxillary molars, these teeth have a taper or rounding of the mesial surface, tapering to become narrower on the lingual (Appendix 10s); this convergence is not evident on the distal side (2). The lingual surface is convex mesiodistally and cervico-occlusally. The cervical line on the lingual is nearly straight from mesial to distal.

## 2. CUSP SHAPE AND SIZE

The mesiobuccal cusp of these first molars is always the largest and longest cusp, occupying nearly two-thirds of the buccal surface (Appendix 10t; Fig. 9.18**A**). It is characteristically compressed buccolingually, and its two long cusp ridges extend mesially and distally serving as a blade when occluding with the maxillary canine (5). The smaller distobuccal cusp is separated from the mesiobuccal cusp by a depression rather than a distinct groove. The mesiolingual cusp is larger, longer and sharper than the distolingual cusp, and there is a slight groove between these two lingual cusps which ends in a depression near the cervical border. The distobuccal and distolingual cusps are nearly the same height (much shorter than the mesiobuccal and mesiolingual cusps).

## 3. PROXIMAL CONTOURS AND CONTACTS

The *mesial* marginal ridge is so well developed that it resembles a cusp (2) (Appendix 10q). This ridge is concave and more occlusally positioned than the distal marginal ridge. (Compare mesial and distal views in Figure 9.12 for marginal ridge heights and lengths.) The *distal* marginal ridge is short buccolingually, is less prominent than the longer mesial marginal ridge, and is located more cervically, so more of the occlusal is seen.

The mesial contour is nearly flat buccolingually and cervico-occlusally, whereas the distal side is convex. The mesial contact area with the canine is located more cervically than the distal contact area (Fig. 9.18**A**), which is in the middle of the crown.

The cervical line on the mesial is convex toward the occlusal and slants occlusally toward the lingual. On the distal, the cervical line is practically flat or horizontal from buccal to lingual, where it is also slightly more occlusal in position.

## 4. ACCENTUATED LINGUAL CUSP TIP

The crown appears to lean decidedly toward the lingual (accentuated by the prominent mesiobuccal cervical ridge), placing the buccal cusp tips well over the root base (6). Recall that all mandibular posterior teeth—primary and permanent—appear to lean lingually, even more so with primary teeth. The lingual cusp tip may be even outside the lingual margin of the root (Fig. 9.18**C**). The buccal crown contour is nearly (but not quite) flat from the buccal crest of curvature to the occlusal surface.

## 5. OCCLUSAL ANATOMY

Refer to Figures 9.2**B** and 9.18**B.**

The general shape of the occlusal surface is oval (wider mesiodistally than buccolingually) (Appendix 10r). From the occlusal view, the mesiobuccal angle is acute and prominent because of the mesial cervical ridge on the buccal surface. The distobuccal angle is obtuse. The occlusal table (chewing surface inside cusp ridges and marginal ridges) is small buccolingually. It is considerably smaller than the crown outline. The shape of the occlusal table is that of a rhomboid (9).

The cusps are often difficult to distinguish, but careful examination of an unworn tooth will reveal (in order of diminishing size) mesiobuccal , mesiolingual, distobuccal, and the smallest (also shortest) distolingual cusp. There is one transverse ridge between the mesiobuccal and mesiolingual cusps (Appendix 10u). The occlusal table distal to the transverse ridge is larger than that portion mesial to the transverse ridge (Appendix 10v). The distal spur of the distolingual cusp forms the lingual third of the distal marginal ridge ending in a furrow (5). The lingual groove invariably marks the widest portion of this tooth (5).

## 6. GROOVES, FOSSAE, AND PITS

Refer to Figure 9.18**B.**

Primary mandibular first molars have a small mesial triangular fossa and pit, and a larger distal fossa that extends almost into the center of the occlusal surfaces (Appendix 10v). In the distal fossa, there is a central pit and a small distal pit near the distal marginal ridge. There is no central fossa.

A central groove separates the mesiobuccal and mesiolingual cusps and connects with a mesial marginal groove (furrow). There is a short buccal groove and a short lingual groove on the occlusal surface. The buccal groove does not extend onto the buccal surface, and the lingual groove becomes a shallow depression on the lingual surface.

Both marginal ridges have furrows or grooves between them and cusp ridges of lingual cusps (6) similar to the supplemental grooves in the triangular fossae of other posterior teeth. These grooves serve as escapeways during mastication.

## 7. ROOTS

There are two roots—mesial and distal—with the mesial root wider (square and flat) and longer than the distal root. The distal root is more rounded, less broad, thinner, and shorter than the mesial root.

## PULP CAVITIES OF PRIMARY TEETH

Refer to Figures 9.8, 9.19, and 9.20.

Primary anterior teeth have pulp cavities that are similar in shape to the pulp cavities of the permanent teeth, but are much larger in proportion because of the thinner, more uniform enamel covering, and the thinner portion of dentin in the deciduous teeth. There are slight projections on the incisal border corresponding to the lobes, and there is usually no demarcation or constriction between the single canal and pulp chamber except on the mandibular central incisor (9).

Primary molar teeth, when compared with permanent molars, have pulp chambers much less elongated vertically relative to the size of the tooth. In *permanent* molars, much of the pulp chamber is located in the root trunk; in *primary* molars there is little or almost no root trunk. In these teeth, the pulp chambers are mostly in the tooth crown.

The pulp chambers of primary molars have long and often very narrow pulp horns extending beneath the cusps (Fig. 9.19). Great care must be taken when preparing these teeth for restorations to avoid exposing the pulp horn to the oral cavity.

### LEARNING EXERCISE

*Compare the relative size and shape of the pulp chambers of primary molars (Figs. 9.8, 9.19, and 9.20) with the size and shape of the permanent molar chambers (Figs. 8.29 through 8.34).*

*If you are fortunate to have a collection of primary teeth, study the morphology for variations. In addition to the root resorption, examine the occlusal surface for wear facets from attrition and the interior pulp chamber (after sectioning) for size, pulp horns, and thickness of enamel and dentin.*

*Compare the distinguishing characteristics in Table 9.4 with your collection of deciduous teeth. If you don't have any teeth to study, try to recognize these traits as seen in Figures 9.2, 9.9, 9.11, and 9.12.*

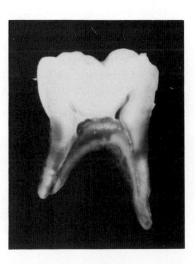

**Figure 9.19.** Primary *mandibular* right *second* molar. Buccal side ground off to expose pulp cavity. An interesting feature is the long narrow shape of the pulp horns, which often extend even higher or closer to the occlusal surface than seen in this cross-section.

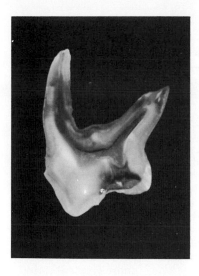

**Figure 9.20.** Primary *maxillary first* molar; mesial side removed. The root canals of the mesiobuccal root and of the lingual root (*right side* of picture) are exposed. An extensive carious lesion beneath the enamel of the lingual cusp (initial point of entry not seen here) has reached the pulp horn.

**Table 9.4.** How to Identify Deciduous Teeth

| Teeth | Maxillary Arch | Mandibular Arch | How to Tell Rights from Lefts | |
|---|---|---|---|---|
| | | | **Maxillary Teeth** | **Mandibular Teeth** |
| Central Incisor | Short, wide, symmetrical crown<br>Large cingulum, long bulky root<br>Root bends facially in apical one-third | Long, narrow, symmetrical, very small crown<br>Long, thin, straight root<br>Labial root bend in apical third | 90° mesioincisal angle<br>More cervical distal than mesial contact<br>More rounded distoincisal angle<br>Crown outline flat on mesial side, convex on distal side<br>More mesial cervical curvature | Difficult to discern |
| Lateral Incisor | Narrow and oblong asymmetrical crown<br>Root bends facially in apical one-third | Same shape as uppers except smaller cingulum<br>More acute mesioincisal angle<br>Labial root bend in apical third | Flat mesial and rounded distal crown outline<br>Distal contact more cervical than mesial<br>Acute mesioincisal angle<br>More mesial cervical curvature<br>Cingulum slightly to distal | More rounded distoincisal angle<br>Distal contact more cervical than mesial<br>Distal crown bulge<br>Cingulum slightly distal |
| Canine | Wide crown, sharp centered cusp<br>Rounded contacts in middle of tooth<br>*Longer, steeper mesial cusp arm*<br>Flat labial cervical line<br>Cingulum centered<br>Mesial contact is more cervical<br>Root bends facially in apical one-third | Longer, narrower, less symmetrical crown<br>Cusp tip toward mesial<br>Short mesial cusp arm<br>Distally located cingulum<br>Contacts in incisal one-third<br>Distal contact is more cervical<br>Less labial root bend (apical third) | Longer mesial cusp slope<br>Mesial contact more cervical than distal<br>More mesial cervical curvature<br>Deeper and narrower distal than mesial fossa | Shorter mesial cusp slope<br>Flat mesial crown outline<br>Distal contact more cervical than mesial<br>Cingulum toward distal |

**Table 9.4.** How to Identify Deciduous Teeth—*Continued*

| Teeth | Maxillary Arch | Mandibular Arch | How to Tell Rights from Lefts | |
|---|---|---|---|---|
| | | | **Maxillary Teeth** | **Mandibular Teeth** |
| First Molar | 3 roots—MB, DB, L Unique crown shape 3 cusps—MB (very large), DB, ML Crown oblong faciolingually, tapering toward lingual Crown wider (F-L) mesially than distally H-shape occlusal grooves | 2 roots—mesial and distal Unique crown shape 4 cusps—MB, DB, ML, DL Crown very wide mesiodistally and narrow faciolingually Crown wider (F-L) distally than mesially Well-developed high mesial marginal ridge | Crown longer on mesial than distal (facial) Crown wider (F-L) mesially than distally Mesial cervical crown bulge Distal marginal ridge more cervical than mesial Distobuccal root is smallest and shortest | Crown longer on mesial than distal (facial) Crown wider (F-L) distally than mesially Mesial cervical crown bulge Larger distal than mesial fossa Pointed mesiolingual cusp Distal marginal ridge more cervical than mesial Longer, wider (F-L) mesial root |
| Second Molar | 3-roots—MB, DB, L Crown resembles small, short permanent maxillary first molar | 2 roots—mesial and distal Crown closely resembles permanent mandibular first molar | Large mesiolingual cusp Crown longer on mesial than distal (facial view) Mesial cervical crown bulge Distal marginal ridge more cervical than mesial Distobuccal root is smallest and shortest | Crown longer on mesial than distal (facial view) Mesial cervical crown bulge Identify and position distal cusp (fifth cusp) Distal marginal ridge more cervical than mesial Longer, wider (F-L) mesial root |

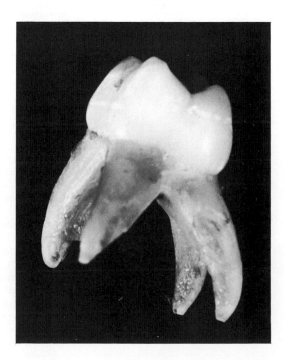

**Figure 9.21.** Primary *mandibular* left *second* molar. This is the mesial side of the tooth; the buccal surface is at the *right*. The four roots are widely spread with little resorption. No history is known about this specimen. Only when you hold this tooth in your hand and turn it around can you identify it as a mandibular molar.

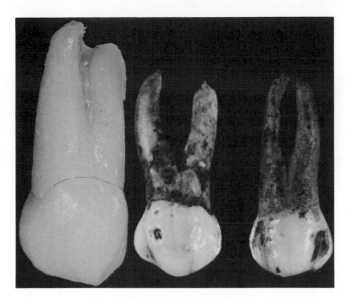

**Figure 9.22.** Facial view of three double-rooted primary maxillary canines (10). The left one was extracted from a 9´-year-old black child at Children's Hospital in Columbus, Ohio. It is a right side tooth with mesial surface facing the other two teeth. The matched pair on the right are 2580 years old and came from a 5-year-old American Indian child found in Wood County, Ohio. Their mesial sides face each other in the photograph. (Courtesy of Dr. Ruth B. Paulson.)

*Prepare a tooth of each type to study the shape of the pulp cavities. In the primary molar teeth, which, as you see, have little to no root trunk, how is the location of the pulp chamber different from the location of the pulp chamber in permanent teeth? Look carefully at both (see Figs. 9.8, 9.19, and 9.20).*

*What might happen if a primary molar is extracted before its roots have begun to resorb?*

*What parts of the roots of primary teeth seem to undergo resorption first? What causes them to resorb?*

*What may happen if a primary tooth has a severe abscess?*

*Figure 9.21 shows the mesial side of a mandibular left second molar. There are two mesial roots and two distal roots. In the extracted primary teeth that you have had an opportunity to examine, have you found any other anomalies? Other anomalies are seen in Figure 9.22.*

## References

1. Hellman M. Nutrition, growth and dentition. Dental Cosmos Dec. 1923.
2. Brand RW, Isselhard DE. Anatomy of orofacial structures. St. Louis: C.V. Mosby, 1982:180–204.
3. Osborn JW, ed. Dental anatomy and embryology. Oxford: Blackwell Scientific Publications, 1981:144–151.
4. Huang L, Machida Y. A longitudinal study of clinical crowns on deciduous anterior teeth. Bull Tokyo Med Dent Univ 1987;28:75–81.
5. Jorgensen KD. The deciduous dentition—a descriptive and comparative anatomical study. Acta Odontologica Scandinavia 1956;14(Suppl 20):1–192.
6. Pagano JL. Anatomia dentaria. Buenos Aires: Editorial Mundi S.A., 1965:471–540.
7. DuBrul EL. Sicher's oral anatomy. 7th ed. St. Louis: C.V. Mosby, 1980:238–244.
8. Kraus B, Jordan R, Abrams L. Dental anatomy and occlusion. Baltimore: Williams & Wilkins, 1969:115–131.
9. Finn S. Clinical pedodontics. Philadelphia: W.B. Saunders, 1957:54–80.
10. Paulson RB, Gottlieb LJ, Sciulli PW, et al. Double-rooted maxillary primary canines. ASDC J Dent Child 1985; 52:195–198.

# Functional Occlusion and Malocclusion

Occlusion between teeth in an ideal Class I relationship was discussed earlier in Chapter 3, Section VII. In this chapter, the more advanced aspects of tooth and jaw relationships during function are discussed, as well as the terminology and concepts associated with malocclusion (which literally means "bad" occlusion).

## A. Jaw Relationships—The Relationship of the Mandible to the Maxillae

The maxillae are firmly and immovably attached at suture lines to each other and to the other bones of the facial skeleton. The maxillae move only as the head moves, not independently as for the mandible. The mandible articulates with the skull at the craniomandibular joints; it moves and changes its position in relation to the maxillae and cranium.

Jaw relation refers to the position of the mandible relative to the maxillae and should be thought of as a bone-to-bone relationship, as well as a tooth-to-tooth relationship.

### 1. VERTICAL RELATION OR VERTICAL DIMENSION

Vertical relation or vertical dimension refers to the amount of separation or opening between the mandible and maxillae.

#### a. Vertical Relation of Occlusion

*Vertical relation* (or vertical dimension) *of occlusion* is the amount of separation between the mandible and maxillae when the teeth are in natural maximum contact (centric occlusion).

### b. Vertical Relation of Rest Position

*Vertical relation* (or vertical dimension) *of rest position* (mandibular physiologic rest position) (1) is the amount of separation between the mandible and maxillae when the mandible and all of its supporting muscles (eight muscles of mastication plus the supra- and infrahyoids) are in their resting posture.

In a normal, erect posture, when no conscious effort is made to close or to open the jaw (Fig. 10.1**A**), there is a 2–6 mm (average) space between the occlusal surfaces of the maxillary and mandibular teeth. Of course, when the teeth are gone (in an edentulous person) there would be a 1 cm or more distance between the residual toothless ridges with the mandible resting (2). Unless we are nervous, eating, talking, yawning, or using our muscles to perform other less natural functions (i.e., parafunctional movements) such as playing a clarinet, the mandible is in this comfortable resting position most of the time (over 23 hours each day). A simple change, such as looking up at the sky, will change the resting position of the jaw, in this instance separating the teeth farther (Fig. 10.1**B**) due to stretching the skin and underlying fascia on the neck below the mandible.

### c. Interocclusal Distance

*Interocclusal distance* or freeway space is the normal 2–6 mm space between the incisal and the occlusal surfaces of the maxillary and mandibular teeth with the mandible in physiologic rest position.

## 2. HORIZONTAL RELATIONS

Horizontal relations refer to both the anteroposterior and lateral positions of the mandible relative to the maxillae (also called eccentric relations, i.e., "out of centric").

### a. Centric Relation

*Centric relation* is the most posterior position of the mandible relative to the maxillae at a given vertical dimension. It is really any position with the jaw retruded maximally and rotated open without moving bodily forward (or translating) (Figs. 10.2, *top,* and 10.8**B**). This is a relationship of the bones of the *upper and lower*

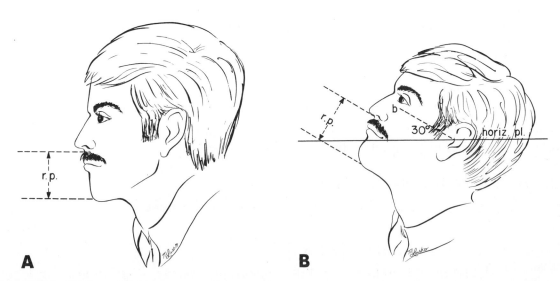

**Figure 10.1.** **A.** The man assumes a normal posture with his mandible in physiologic rest position and the posterior teeth separated (interocclusal distance). **B.** This man is looking up at an airplane and his mandible is again in physiologic rest position with his posterior teeth separated, more so than in **A,** because of the stretch of fascia, skin, and the supra and infrahyoid muscles. The resting position of the mandible varies with such factors as body posture, fatigue, and stress.

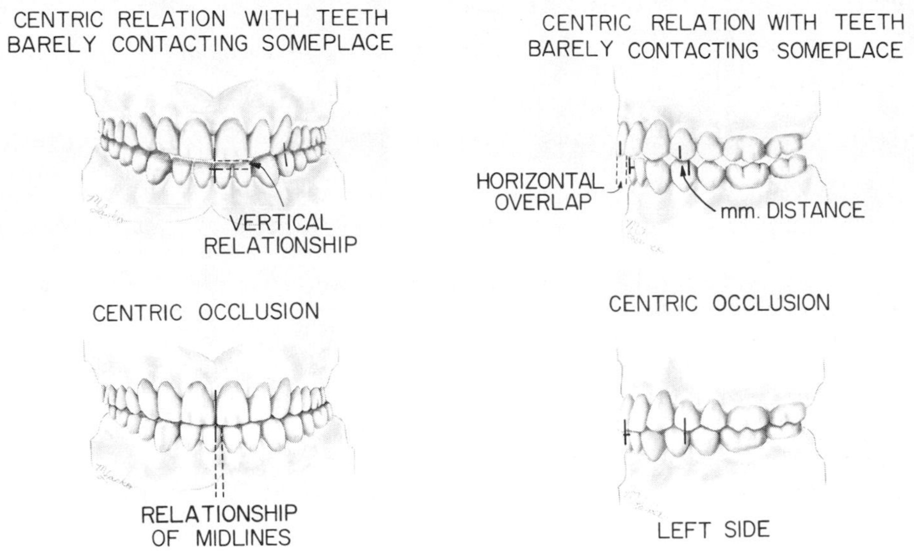

CENTRIC RELATION WITH TEETH
BARELY CONTACTING SOMEPLACE

VERTICAL
RELATIONSHIP

CENTRIC RELATION WITH TEETH
BARELY CONTACTING SOMEPLACE

HORIZONTAL
OVERLAP

mm. DISTANCE

CENTRIC OCCLUSION

RELATIONSHIP
OF MIDLINES

CENTRIC OCCLUSION

LEFT SIDE

**Figure 10.2.** *Upper left* and *upper right:* Mandible has closed in the most retruded position until the first tooth contact between any upper and lower teeth (centric relation, prematurity, or deflective contact). *Lower left* and *lower right:* The mandible has continued to close from the first tooth contact into maximum intercuspation (centric occlusion) and, as a result, the mandible has deviated forward and to the left. The deviation of the mandible was caused by deflective tooth interferences, which guided the terminal (most upward) portion of jaw closure. Two or more opposing teeth first contact and then they all slide into centric occlusion. In the centric occlusion figures, observe the normal anterior and posterior maxillary to mandibular tooth relationships as described in the text.

*jaws without tooth contact* or with teeth only barely contacting before closing teeth into maximum intercuspation (4, 6, 7). The presence or absence of teeth, or the type of occlusion or malocclusion, are not factors. This relationship can be obtained by using a gauge of variable thickness inserted between overlapping incisors to help retract the mandible (Figs. 10.3**B** and **C,** 10.4, *below,* and 10.14**B** and **C**).

## LEARNING EXPERIENCE

*Tip your head way back, retrude your mandible forcibly, and close very slowly until the first teeth touch gently with the jaw in centric relation. This first gentle tooth contact or contacts (jaw retruded) may differ from your normal maximum biting contacts or occlusion (see an extreme example in Fig. 10.4, below).*

### b. Centric Occlusion

As stated in Chapter 3, *centric occlusion* is the maximum intercuspation or contact attained between maxillary and mandibular posterior teeth. The posterior teeth fit together most tightly (Figs. 10.2, *below,* and 10.4, *above*). (Other names for this are: most occlusal position, intercuspal position, acquired or habitual occlusion, and natural bite.)

This is the position in which your teeth fit together best. Your mandible is usually forward from the centric relation position by 1–2 mm (3–5). Usually one can fit two casts of a person's upper and lower teeth together in the centric occlusion (maximum contact) without looking into the mouth (Fig. 10.4, *above*).

### c. Centric Relation Occlusion

Centric relation occlusion (when centric relation and and centric occlusion coincide) is the simultaneous even contact between maxillary and mandibular teeth into maximum interdigitation with the mandible in centric relation (most retruded position) (4, 6–9).

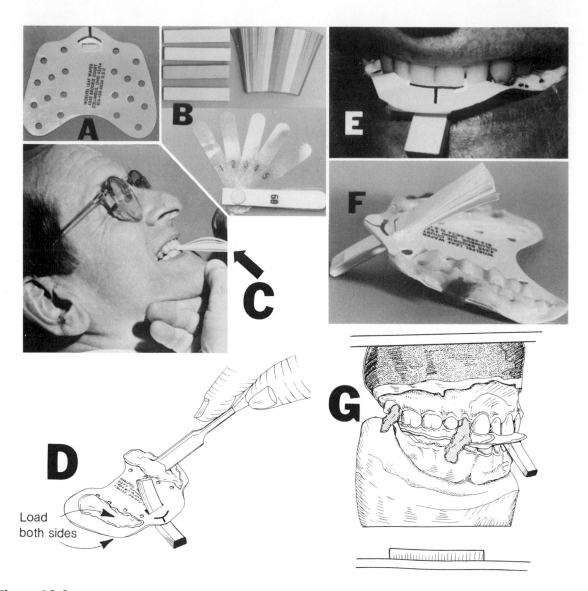

**Figure 10.3.** Procedure for making a centric relation jaw registration (checkbite) for mounting casts on an articulator for analysis and possible tooth alteration or movement. **A.** A Woelfel Leaf Wafer used to carry a leaf gauge (**B**) of predetermined thickness and the registration medium into the mouth. **B.** Paper leaf gauges *above* (color coded for thickness) and *below* is a numbered plastic leaf gauge. **C.** Patient, with head tipped back, is arcing his mandible in the hinge position and closing on the leaf gauge of minimal but sufficient thickness to separate all teeth to negate any engram (learned habit) closure. **D.** The recording media is applied to tooth indentations on the wafer. **E.** The patient closes firmly onto the leaf gauge as the recording material sets. **F.** The centric relation checkbite (recording material is a polyether rubber). **G.** The leaf wafer checkbite is used to orient the lower to upper cast for assembly on an articulator. The *shaded* regions are a brittle, strong, sticky wax used until the plaster sets between the lower cast and the articulator. The results of a similar mounting on another patient are seen in Figure 10.4.

Most people do not have this type of ideal occlusal relationship or balance between the jaw muscles, condyle position, and fitting together of their teeth unless they have just had a well-executed equilibration (8), or a complete dental arch rehabilitation replacing or reorienting all occlusal surfaces (Fig. 10.5), so that maximum contact will occur with the jaw in centric relation. Edentulous people who wear complete dentures (false teeth) are provided with centric relation occlusion so that they can learn to pull the mandible back and close into a repeatable position enabling the dentures to remain tightly secured.

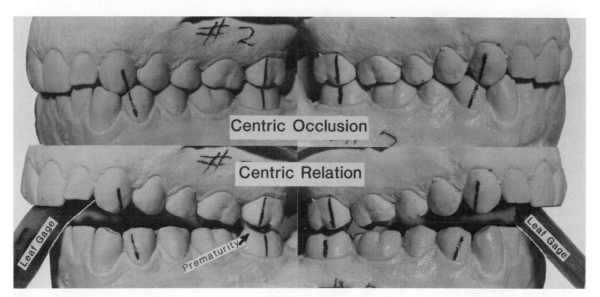

**Figure 10.4.** This patient had trismus and limited jaw opening over a 4-year period. Casts of his dentition are hand held in the centric occlusion position *above*. After wearing a maxillary occlusal splint for 18 months, his mandible stabilized into a comfortable centric relation position and he was able to open at the incisors 55 mm (an increase of 20 mm). A centric relation registration with a 5.7-mm leaf gauge, and subsequent articulator mounting of his casts, revealed the severe deflective left second molar contact (*below*), which is impossible to correct by an equilibration. His mandible would deflect forward 2 mm and to the right 1 mm as the teeth came into centric occlusion (*above*).

When teeth are not present, vertical and horizontal jaw relations still exist. Dentists who make dentures attempt to duplicate the patient's jaw relationships when teeth were present. An articulator is a mechanical device that holds casts of the two arches, permitting duplication of the patient's jaw relations. It is easier to study these relationships with the patient's mouth in your hands (the dental stone casts), than with your hands in the patient's mouth. How else could you determine whether or not the maxillary and mandibular *lingual* cusps fit together tightly or properly in the centric occlusion relationship?

### d. Other Horizontal Relations

#### (1) Protrusive Relation

Protrusive relation is that position with the mandible moved anteriorly and downward (as when incising food) so that both mandibular condyles and discs are forward in their glenoid or articular fossae, functioning against and beneath the articular eminences. Movement in both joint compartments occurs when the mandible is protruded, with most of the movement (translation) occurring in the upper joint space. As the mandible moves forward, the incisal edges of the mandibular anterior teeth glide against the lingual fossae of the maxillary anterior teeth (Fig. 4.4). When the mandible is fully protruded, the incisal edges of the mandibular incisors are in front of the maxillary anterior teeth. (Fig. 10.6).

The average maximum forward protrusion for 1114 young men and women was 8.3 mm with a range from 2.5 to 16.0 mm (Table 10.1). These extremes represent a very tight joint compartment (smallest protrusion) and a very large jaw with loose ligamentous attachments (16-mm protrusion).

*Incisal guidance* is a measure of the amount of movement and angle at which the lower incisor and mandible must move from the

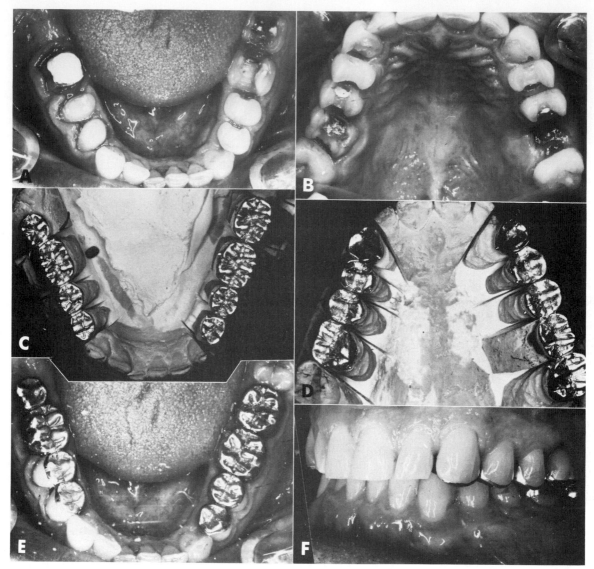

**Figure 10.5.** Several stages of a full mouth rehabilitation involving tooth preparations on 15 teeth with the finished product having 17 units. **A** and **B.** Preparations on 15 teeth ready for the reversible hydrocolloid impressions. **C** and **D.** Completed castings with gnathologic morphology including two replacement teeth (pontics) for teeth 14 and 31. The preparations and gold castings were as follows: one DO inlay-onlay (*21*), three ³/₄ crowns (*6, 11, 15*), three full cast crowns (*28, 29, 30*), eight MOD inlay-onlays (*3, 4, 5, 12, 13, 18, 19, 20*), and two pontics (*14, 31*). The pontic for tooth 31 is very small for a molar pontic because it has no posterior support, only the three splinted or soldered units anterior to it (*28, 29, 30*). Notice the ideal embrasure design and the multiple small ridges (cutting blades) and grooves or escapeways (gnathologic design) that provide for the highest possible masticatory efficiency while directing all forces parallel to the long axes of the teeth. **E.** Mandibular gold castings in place including the pontic replacing tooth 31. **F.** All 17 units cemented in place with the teeth in centric relation occlusion. When the mandible moves either to the right or left, all of the teeth come apart or separate (disclude) with the exception of the canines, which have been lengthened and thickened lingually to provide this canine protection. Prior to having this extensive treatment, the patient wore a maxillary bite plane (Fig. 10.10) for 4 months to assure comfort, stability, and compatibility between his craniomandibular joints and the new occluding surfaces. (Courtesy of Dr. John Regenos, Cincinnati, Ohio.)

overlapping position in centric occlusion to an edge-to-edge relationship with the maxillary incisors. [The average incisal guidance angle for 1114 dental hygiene and dental students was 50° as shown in Figure 10.7, *right.* Many of these people did not have Class I occlusion.] The average canine guidance angle was a little steeper at 56° and 57°. To have a so-called canine protected occlusion, it is usually necessary to have a canine angle of over 60°.

# MAXIMUM PROTRUSION

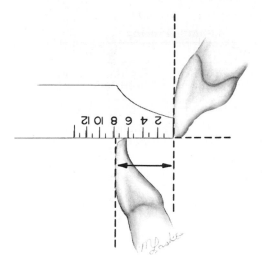

**Figure 10.6.** Relationship of mandibular to maxillary central incisor when the mandible is maximally protruded. The mandible has protuded 11mm because the mandibular central incisor was 3mm lingual to the maxillary incisor in centric occlusion (see Fig. 10.7).

### (2) *Lateral Relation*

In *lateral relation*, the mandible is moved to the right or left side and slightly downward (as when masticating food). If the mandible moves to the right side, the right condyle remains relatively stationary (while rotating), and the left condyle and disc move forward, downward, and inward within the articular fossa (orbiting or balancing side condyle). Table 10.1 on maximum jaw movement reminds us that the *mandible can move almost twice as far sideways as it can directly forward.* On 945 subjects, the maximum movement to either side was 8.1 mm (both sides laterally 16.2 mm) compared to an average forward protrusion of 8.3 mm.

#### (a) *Working Side*

The *working side* is the side toward which the mandible moves (side where chewing or work occurs). Usually the posterior upper and lower teeth are aligned with the upper buccal cusps directly over the lower buccal cusps and with the lower lingual cusps directly beneath the upper lingual cusps during working side tooth contacts (group function). The condyle on the working side does not move much; it rotates on its vertical axis and moves laterally (Bennett movement) 1–2 mm or less.

#### (b) *Balancing Side*

The *balancing side* is the side away from which the mandible moves. On the balancing side, the upper lingual cusps are aligned over the lower buccal cusps, but usually will not contact during the opposite side working tooth relation. Any balancing side tooth contacts are thought to be destructive to both the involved teeth and damaging to the craniomandibular joint on the opposite side. The balancing side mandibular condyle moves medially, downward, and forward perhaps 5–12 mm.

#### (c) *Eccentric Relations*

*Eccentric relations* refers to any deviation of the mandible from the centric occlusion position. This would include lateral and protrusive movements and any combination thereof.

**Table 10.1.** Capability of Mandibular Movement of 1114 Students

| No. and Type of Students | Incisor Overlap | | Canine Overlap | | | |
|---|---|---|---|---|---|---|
| | | | Horizontal | | Vertical | |
| | Horiz. (mm) | Vert. (mm) | Right (mm) | Left (mm) | Right (mm) | Left mm) |
| 796 Dental Hygiene Students | | | | | | |
| Average | 2.78 | 3.27 | 2.01 | 2.02 | 3.23 | 3.19 |
| Low | minus 2.5 | minus 1.0 | minus 1.0 | minus 1.0 | minus 1.0 | minus 1.0 |
| High | 9.0 | 13.0 | 6.2 | 6.2 | 11.0 | 9.0 |
| 318 Dental Students | | | | | | |
| Average | 2.88 | 3.60 | 4.05 | 4.25 | — | — |
| Low | minus 6.5 (prognathic) | minus 2.0 (open-bite) | 0.0 | 0.0 | — | — |
| High | 10.0 | 8.0 | 8.5 | 9.0 | — | — |

Average of 1114 Students:

## B. Normal Movement Within the Craniomandibular Joint

The articular disc divides the articular space into upper and lower compartments (44). The result of this division is the formation of two joint spaces (Fig. 1.13). In a healthy joint, with no clinical manifestations of joint disorder, the actual space between the top of the mandibular condyles and the top of the temporal fossae (determined from radiographs) was 2.5 mm, 1.5 mm to the anterior inferior surface of the eminence and 7.5 mm to the center of the external auditory meatus [teeth in centric occlusion, averages from 50 subjects, 100 joints] (45).

The craniomandibular joint is a ginglymoarthrodial joint, permitting both hinge-like rotation and sliding movements. Ginglymus means rotation, and arthrodial means freely moving. The rotational movements occur in the lower joint space, whereas the sliding movements occur in the upper joint space.

### 1. MOVEMENT WITHIN THE LOWER JOINT SPACE

In the lower compartment, *only a hinge-type* or *rotary motion* can occur. This *rotational* or terminal hinge-axis opening of the mandible is possible only when the mandible is retruded in centric relation with a conscious effort or by the dentist's control. This rotational movement of the mandible, around an axis connecting the two condyles, is like a swing rotating back and forth around a supporting pole (the swing's axis) that passes through both condyles. The maximum separation of the incisors for this pure-hinge opening averaged only 22.4 mm which was 44% of maximum opening on 352 subjects (Fig. 10.8**B**; Table 10.2). With practice, a person who has crepitus on one or both sides can repeatedly open the jaw during hinge movement without any clicking noise because the discs remain in position as the retruded condyles rotate beneath them. However, this pure hinge type of movement normally does not occur.

| Maximum Jaw Opening (mm) | Maximum Lateral Jaw Movement | | Maximum Jaw Protrusion (mm) | Entire Lateral Jaw Movement (mm) | Ratio of Lateral to Protrusive Movement |
| | Right Side (mm) | Left Side (mm) | | | |
| --- | --- | --- | --- | --- | --- |
| 51.01 | 7.68 | 7.71 | 8.44 | 15.39 | 1.89:1 |
| 27.0 | 2.5 | 2.0 | 3.0 | 7.0 | 0.9 |
| 68.5 | 14.0 | 15.2 | 16.0 | 28.4 | 4.89 |
| 50.99 | 9.12 | 9.32 | 7.95 | 18.44 | 2.32:1 |
| 35.5 | 2.0 | 3.0 | 2.5 | 6.0 | |
| 71.0 | 14.0 | 15.4 | 13.5 | 32.0 | |
| 50.29 | 8.09 | 8.17 | 8.30 | 16.26 | 2.01:1 |

## 2. MOVEMENT WITHIN THE UPPER JOINT SPACE

The discs and mandibular condyles, when pulled simultaneously by the lateral pterygoid muscles, can slide forward (*translatory motion*) down over the articular eminences (protrusion), or can move backwards together (retraction) during opening

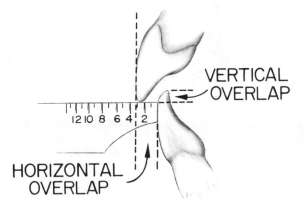

CENTRIC OCCLUSION

VERTICAL OVERLAP

12 10 8 6 4 2

HORIZONTAL OVERLAP

| INCISAL AND CANINE GUIDANCE ANGLE ON 1114 STUDENTS | | |
| --- | --- | --- |
| *Incisal Angle (Central Incisors)* | *Canine Rise Angle* | |
| | *Right Side* | *Left Side* |
| Average | 50° | 56° | 57° |
| Low | minus 26° (open bite) | 0° | 0° |
| High | 86° | 84.2° | 83° |

**Figure 10.7.** *Left side:* Side view of maxillary and mandibular incisors with the posterior teeth in centric occlusion. *Right side:* Incisal guidance angle is the angle formed between the occlusal plane (*numbered line on left*) and a line from the upper incisal edge to the lower incisal edge. It is only 37° on the left, which is less steep than in many dentitions. Usually a canine guidance angle of 60° or more is necessary to provide canine protection which causes disclusion (separation) of the premolars and molars.

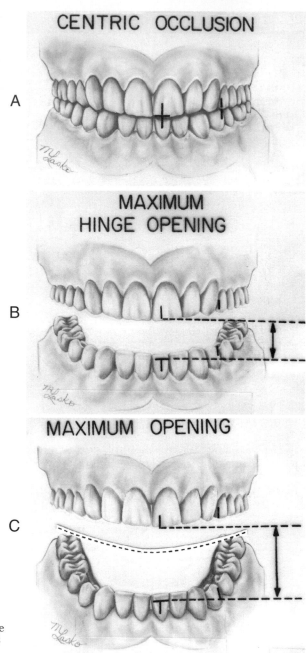

**Figure 10.8. A.** Centric occlusion. **B.** Maximum hinge opening. **C.** Maximum normal opening. *Curved line* in **C** denotes the curve of Wilson.

and closing of the mouth respectively. A sliding motion, when it occurs unilaterally, results in a lateral movement and a *grinding motion* of the teeth. Both translatory *and* hinge opening movement occur when the patient opens beyond maximum hinge opening (Fig. 10.8**B**) and continues to the maximum normal opening (Fig. 10.8**C**).

## LEARNING EXERCISE

*Place your fingers in front of your ears and open and close your jaw and slide to each side. When you open widely as in yawning, you may feel the bump as the condyles move forward (translate) and slide down under the articular eminences.*

*This combined hinge and translatory motion follows a curved path primarily dictated by the shape of the condyle against the posterior inferior slope of the articular eminence (i.e.,*

**Table 10.2.** Terminal Hinge (Rotary) Opening Capability on 352 Dental Hygiene Students

| Type of Jaw Opening | Average | Range | Condylar Rotation Degrees Average | Range |
|---|---|---|---|---|
| Maximum Opening at Incisors | 51.0±6.3 mm | 27.0–68.5 mm | NA[†] | NA[†] |
| Hinge Opening at Incisors | 22.4±5.7 mm | 9.5–40.5 mm | 12.7* | 4.4–24.2* |
| Percentage of Maximum Incisor Opening | 44.0% | 18.9–50.6% | — | — |

*Results obtained by Dr. Woelfel (1980–1986).
[†]Unknown because translation has taken place in upper joint compartment.

*on the anterior portion of the glenoid ([articular] fossa). Most functional movements of the mandible involve translatory motions with curved components because of the shape of the articular fossae and eminences and because no conscious effort is made to open in a retruded manner (12, 13).*

## 3. TOTAL JOINT MOVEMENT

Refer to Figures 10.8 and 10.9.

All functional motion occurs simultaneously in both the upper and lower portions of the craniomandibular joints (combined translatory and rotary movement). This includes, eating, swallowing, yawning, relaxing the jaw, and talking.

A specific characteristic of human jaw opening is this combination of both hinge and sliding movement. Even in the highest order of apes (chimpanzee), the mandible drops open in a simple hinge movement. In the human, this type of pure hinge opening *is possible only* by voluntary control or by dentist guidance. Pure hinge opening is usually limited to about half of the maximum incisor opening (Table 10.2). Any point beyond this involves both translation and rotation (Fig. 10.8**B** and **C,** and 10.9**A,** *right, sagittal view*).

Perhaps the most exhaustive study to date on the craniomandibular joint is the study by Turell (29), which includes color pictures of many human craniomandibular joints—some healthy, some with displaced discs, and others diseased with osteoarthritis. This project involved joints from 100 people who had been dead for less than 12 hours at the time of dissection and analysis. Joint conditions were compared with existing occlusal relationships and were found to be directly related. Older people with their teeth and natural organic occlusion had normal joints. Internal derangement was determined to be more common in the elderly only because of occlusal interferences, loss of teeth, heavy attrition, and noncorrected malpositions of teeth. It was concluded that impact loading of the craniomandibular joints from poor occlusion caused many of the alterations seen in osteoarthrosis (29).

## C. What Is Involved in the Act of Chewing?

### 1. INCISING

The mandible drops downward. Food is placed between the opposing anterior teeth. The jaw is protruded (by the lateral pterygoid muscles) and then closed in a protrusive position until the incisal edges of the anterior teeth meet the morsel. The mandible is then moved up and posteriorly, thus cutting a portion of the food free.

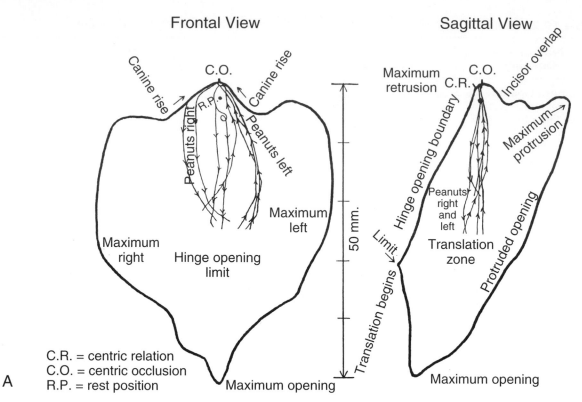

**Figure 10.9. A.** Frontal and sagittal envelopes of motion are the outer boundaries for movement of the mandible usually made by following the pathway of a mandibular central incisor. In the frontal envelope (*left*), beginning in the *C.O.* position (centric occlusion) at the top and following clockwise: The mandible with the teeth in contact slides to the left as far as possible, as the jaw begins to open from the left side down to maximum opening of 51 mm. From this point, the jaw moves to the right as far as possible as it begins to close (lateral and open from tooth contact). Then, from the closed right side position, the teeth slide together as the jaw slowly moves back and upward (canine rise) into the starting point (C.O.). The sagittal envelope of motion (*right*), begins from the most posterior position (centric relation), moves forward and upward slightly into centric occlusion. The teeth are held together as the mandible slowly protrudes maximally, then opens in the protruded position down to the maximum opening of 51 mm. From this point, the jaw is slowly closed and retruded firmly which develops the curved translation portion of closure followed by the straight hinge opening boundary (rotary motion only), back to the starting point (C.R.). Four chewing strokes are shown as the patient chewed on 3 gram portions of peanuts, first on the left and then on the right sides (*arrows* denote direction of chewing strokes).

## 2. MASTICATING (CHEWING)

Food is transferred by the tongue to the posterior teeth; it is held in position on one side by the cheek (buccinator muscle) and the tongue.

The teeth are brought together, engaging the food in a lateral position (Fig. 10.9**A,** *left, frontal view*). This is the working side. The upper buccal cusps are directly over the lower buccal cusps in this lateral position.

The closing motion slows (32) as the mandible is forcibly closed (by the masseter and medial pterygoid muscles) and the canine overlap and posterior tooth cusp inclines guide the slide into centric occlusion (maximum interdigitation of the posterior teeth; *C.O.* in Fig. 10.9**A** and **B**). As this happens, the crushed food squirts out into the buccal and lingual embrasures and down over the tooth curvatures into the cheek and onto the tongue where it can be tasted, mixed with saliva, placed back over the teeth, and chewed some more.

The various incline planes, cusp ridges, triangular ridges, and grooves of opposing teeth reduce the food to bits. Ridges act as cutting blades, whereas the grooves

Frontal envelopes of motion for three young men

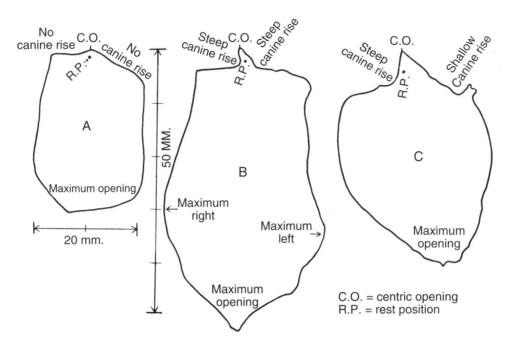

B

**Figure 10.9. B.** These frontal envelopes of motion demonstrate the wide range of variability between the movement capabilities of three men's mandibles. Subject *A* has the smallest and narrowest range of movement for his mandible (32 mm vertically, 21 mm sideways). No rise in the upper central part indicates he had a group function occlusion (no canine protection nor deeply overlapping canines). Subject *B* could open his mandible 53 mm and move it laterally 31 mm and he would have a canine protected occlusion (steep portion on either side of the *C.O.*). Patient *C* had a medium-sized envelope of motion with canine protection on the right side and group function occlusion with shallow canine rise on the left. He preferred to chew mostly on the left side where his envelope is lopsided.

(major and supplemental) serve as escape pathways (places for crushed food to squirt out buccally and lingually), thus significantly lessening lateral forces that are potentially damaging to the teeth and to their supporting bone.

Once the posterior teeth contact in centric occlusion (*C.O.* in Fig. 10.9**A** and **B**), there is a pause of about 1/6 second (silent period). Next, the mandible opens and moves laterally to commence the next chewing stroke. The duration of each chewing stroke varies from 0.7 to 1.2 seconds in most people (32). Usually we masticate for a while on one side and then switch the food over to the opposite side and chew there for several strokes.

When you face someone and observe the chewing pattern, the mandible generally travels in the shape of a lopsided teardrop somewhat pointed at the top (teeth together after crushing the food bolus). This teardrop tends to be somewhat straight upon the opening stroke with considerable convexity or bulge toward the side on which the patient is chewing. This is seen in Figure 10.9**A,** which shows actual motion of the mandible as the patient chewed peanuts on the right and left sides. The *heavy outlines* give the maximum range the mandible can move in any chosen direction, called an *envelope of motion*. In the frontal view (Fig. 10.9**A,** *left*), the chewing cycles occupy only 25 of the maximum 51-mm opening range for this man. Laterally, the chewing strokes on peanuts utilize only 12 mm of the total side-to-side range of his mandible.

In the sagittal view (*right envelope* in Fig. 10.9**A**), the hinge opening boundary indicates this man could rotate his mandible open (without translation) 30 mm, as this line marks the movement of the lower incisor. Observe that in chewing, the patient's opening stroke is 7 mm anterior and the closing stroke is 10 mm anterior to the hinge opening boundary. However, as the jaws are closed to crush the food bolus, the mandible is slightly posterior to the centric occlusion position. Crushing of the food bolus occurs in the centric occlusion position (*C.O.* in Fig. 10.9**A**).

## LEARNING EXERCISE

*Look in a mirror and see if you are able to move your mandible in a circle similar to the envelope of motion seen on the left in Figure 10.9**A.** Your side or sagittal view would, of course, have to be viewed by a friend.*

## 3. SWALLOWING

Swallowing (deglutition) begins as a voluntary muscular act (when we decide to) and is completed involuntarily (by reflex action). The mechanics are as follows:

1. The anterior part of the mouth is sealed (lips closed).

2. The teeth are closed into their maximum intercuspal position (centric occlusion).

3. The soft palate is raised.

4. The hyoid bone is raised to close off the trachea (windpipe).

5. The posterior part of the tongue is engaged in a piston-like thrust causing the bolus to be pushed into the oral pharynx.

6. The act of swallowing takes place.

7. Once the bolus is in the pharynx, the superior portion of the posterior wall presses forward to seal the pharynx, and then the esophageal phase of swallowing commences. This is accomplished by involuntary peristalsis that moves the food bolus through the entire length of the digestive tract.

8. The mandible usually drops open assuming its physiological resting posture. Several swallows are necessary to empty the mouth of a given food mass. However, we swallow a number of times every hour without eating or drinking anything.

## LEARNING EXERCISE

*Bite off a piece of firm food and analyze your jaw movements by looking in a mirror as you prepare the food for swallowing. This process is called mastication, to be followed by deglutition (swallowing). Feel the hyoid bone move as you swallow.*

## D. Parafunctional Movement and Contacts

The opening movements of the mandible are quite complex, but are subconsciously controlled by our neuromuscular system. Branches of the fifth cranial nerve in the periodental ligaments provide proprioception (i.e., a sense of position) which signal directive movements to the muscles of mastication. Subsequently, traumatic or deflective contacts (evident in Fig. 10.4) are consistently avoided during normal function (chewing, talking, and swallowing) (4, 6–9). Unfortunately, when a person develops a bruxing habit, these potentially damaging tooth contacts are exercised almost constantly and are called parafunctional contacts, i.e., occurring outside of the normal function of chewing, talking, etc. In a healthy person without occlusal problems, functional tooth contacts over a 24-hour period, including eating three meals, will total only 7–8 minutes. Parafunctional tooth contacts, in contrast, may amount to several hours per day and are potentially damaging to both teeth and to the craniomandibular joints. Symptoms from problems of this nature can be tired muscles, trismus (limited opening), sore tooth or teeth, joint pain, loose tooth (fremitus), heavy facets, facial, head, and even neck pain. The pain can sometimes be severe (10, 11, 14–17).

*Parafunctional contacts* are undesirable and should be avoided. The human jaw muscles are very powerful. The largest maximum bite strength ever recorded was that of a 37-year-old man who maintained a force of 975 pounds for 2 seconds (12). The average biting force for 20 subjects was 192 pounds (range: 55–280 lbs). Biting strength in bruxer-clenchers can be as much as six times higher than the nonbruxer, so it takes little imagination to understand why bruxing can be a dangerous and damaging habit (12). Natural dentition chewing forces are well below maximum bite force on average foods, ranging from $^1/_2$ to 33 pounds, seldom exceeding 100 pounds (13).

## E. Treatment Modalities

Treatment for bruxing, myofacial, and craniomandibular joint problems may involve or include (a) conscious effort by the patient to avoid clenching, (b) biofeedback, (c) tranquilizers, (d) muscle relaxants, (e) occlusal corrections (including orthodontics), tooth equilibration (selective recontouring of enamel), (f) jaw muscle exercise, (g) patient education, (h) nutritional guidance, (i) psychological counseling, and (j) occlusal bite-plane therapy (Fig. 10.10) (15, 16, 18). To succeed and to correct a patient's unfortunate parafunctional bruxing habit is not an easy task and takes time, skill, and patience at best. Often, wearing a properly constructed occlusal bite plane for a few days will offer tremendous relief from severe headaches or even some backaches.

A *maxillary bite plane (orthopedic splint)* is a thin, horseshoe-shaped, transparent plastic device that fits over the upper teeth and provides a smooth flat surface for the mandibular teeth to contact (Fig. 10.10). This negates input to proprioceptive sensors in the teeth (4, 6–9, 17, 19), permitting the mandible to seek its most neuromuscularly comfortable and stable position (centric relation). Once this has been accomplished, diagnosis of the etiology is made and corrective measures instituted. The basic principle is to get the teeth to come together evenly with the jaw in the most comfortable position. This temporary splint procedure is noninvasive, is relatively easy to accomplish, and is entirely reversible.

## F. Dislocation of the Mandible (Luxation or Subluxation)

During an extreme opening of the mandible, the disc and head of the condyle may slip out of the articular fossa and forward beyond the articular eminence. Thus, the mandible will be *dislocated* or *subluxed* (luxation). Unless the closing muscles contract with the jaw in this extreme forward position, no problem will exist. If they do suddenly contract, however, the mandible would become painfully locked in this subluxed position and could be released only by another person who would depress the mandible with heavy force by pushing downward with the thumbs on the buccal shelf next to the first molars. This dislocation occurs in the upper joint compartment. Recall that the disc is loosely attached to the condyle and normally travels with it.

The loose capsular tissue surrounding the joint does not usually tear when dislocation occurs, but there would be a lot of pain until the contracted muscles relax after the mandible is depressed and repositioned by the thumbs of the rescuer. The patient's jaw opening muscles are not nearly as powerful as the closing muscles and, therefore, are unable to unlock a mandibular dislocation. Perhaps you have seen an alligator trainer hold the alligator's jaws closed with one hand (comparatively weak lateral pterygoid muscles).

### LEARNING EXERCISE

*Feel the function of the craniomandibular joint by placing a finger on either side of your face just in front of your ears and opening and closing your mouth and moving the mandible*

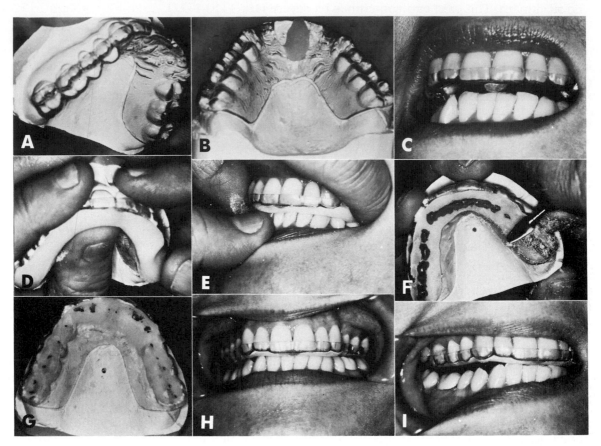

**Figure 10.10.** Stages of construction design and adjustment of a maxillary bite plane for a patient experiencing craniomandibular joint problems (crepitus, trismus or limited mandibular opening, joint pain, and/or certain types of headaches). **A.** Thin plastic sheet (1.5–2.0 mm thick) has been heated and vacuum-molded (sucked down) onto a clean dry accurate cast of the maxillary teeth. The center palatal portion and excess on the sides and posteriorly has been removed leaving only a 3-mm overlap on the facial surfaces of the teeth. The occlusal surfaces are roughened with a carbide bur so that the occlusal portion to be added to it will adhere securely (see **D** and **E**). **B.** A triangular-shaped anterior ramp of cold-curing acrylic resin has been added lingually between the central incisors to maintain vertical dimension and to guide the mandible posteriorly like a leaf gauge or sliding guide. **C.** Contact with the anterior ramp shows an excessive increase of the vertical dimension. This is adjusted leaving only a point of contact with the mandibular incisors so they will contact at an incline of about 45° upward and posteriorly. **D.** The softened dough roll of orthodontic cold-curing clear acrylic resin is adapted over the roughened occlusal and incisal portion of the template with the anterior portion slightly longer and thinner than the posterior part. **E.** The template with the molded softened acrylic resin dough is placed in the mouth and the patient closes gently two or three times into centric relation and just far enough upward so that the mandibular incisors are stopped and the mandible is guided posteriorly by the previously adjusted narrow anterior ramp. The resin dough is permitted to harden. **F.** With the acrylic resin hardened, the bite plane is returned to the cast, the cusp indentations are marked with a bright red felt marker, and all excess acrylic except the imprints of the tips of the cusps is ground off making a flat plane. **G.** The anterior portion must also be relieved of all tooth imprints and sloped sharply upward toward the lingual to provide a ramp for disclusion during lateral jaw movement (**I**). The posterior imprints are correct for initial placement of the bite plane. While on the cast, the roughened acrylic resin is lightly buffed with a rag wheel and polishing compound. **H.** Initial placement of the maxillary bite plane with the patient closing in centric relation. The mandibular posterior teeth contact uniformly on a flat smooth plane. The mandibular anterior teeth are just barely out of contact until the jaw moves forward or to either side. **I.** The patient slides the mandible to the left and all teeth on the right side disclude (separate) as the lower left canine slides up the lingual ramp. A bite plane such as this is worn by the patient 24 hours each day except when eating. Usually painful craniomandibular symptoms subside within a few days. The bite plane is periodically adjusted and definitive dental work (restorations, bridges, equilibration, orthodontics, etc.) is postponed until the patient has remained comfortable for several weeks and upon return visits shows little if any adjustment of the maxillary bite plane to be necessary. (Courtesy of Dr. Richard W. Huffman, Professor Emeritus, Ohio State University.)

*from side-to-side. Then put your fingers in your ears and move the mandible sideways. Do you feel more movement when the jaw moves toward that side or when it moves away from that side? How do you account for this difference?*

*Now try to reproduce this action with the skull. (Of course, the skull has lost the disc, which is not bone.) If you are moving the mandible correctly, the condyle will move down onto the articular eminence. (See reference 30 for interesting information on this subject.)*

*Notice how important the teeth are in determining certain movements that occur in the joints. Measure how far you can open maximally in the incisor region. Then practice opening with a pure hinge motion holding your mandible forcibly retracted. This pure hinge opening is a most important one to record (Fig. 10.14) when making extensive dental restorations for a patient. It is called centric relation.*

*How far are you able to open in the incisor region before you feel the condyles slide or slip forward (translation in the upper part of the joints)? Compare this limited amount of opening with your maximum opening in the incisor region and compare with Dr. Woelfel's measurements shown in Table 10.2.*

*Try to find a copy of reference 31 in your library. It has a Glossary, a review of most significant research on the temporomandibular joint, 488 references, and contains original research on the joints of 318 oral rehabilitation patients compared to those of 61 other patients. It is a fascinating treatise.*

## G. Types of Malocclusion

Refer to Figure 10.11.

Malocclusion (incorrect alignment or tooth interferences) results from abnormalities in the size or arrangement of teeth, in the relative sizes of the dental arches and their alignments, or in the types of occlusal relationships acquired naturally or from incorrect orthodontic treatment. Malocclusion is often detrimental to oral health and adversely affects appearance, comfort, and function. It could even cause ringing in the ears, sinus pain, dizziness, and migraine-type headaches. Myofacial pain dysfunction syndrome (MPD) is a common disorder and it originates in the jaw muscles (10, 11). The pain is usually alleviated simply when the patient wears a maxillary biteplane (orthopedic splint), as discussed earlier under E and shown in Fig. 10.10.

Three types of malocclusion are recognized. They were first classified by Dr. Edward H. Angle in 1887. It may seem confusing in that a normal occlusal relationship is called a *Class I Occlusion* (normal or ideal tooth and jaw relationships), but one of the three classifications of malocclusion is Class I Malocclusion (dental type) (9).

### 1. CLASS I MALOCCLUSION (also called Dental Malocclusion)

As stated in Chapter 3, normal Class I occlusion (ideal relationships) is when the maxillary and mandibular *first* molars are in normal alignment anteroposteriorly with the tip of the upper mesiobuccal cusp directly over the mesiobuccal grove on the lower molar and with the distal surface of the upper first molar posterior to the corresponding surface on the lower molar (Fig. 10.11, *left*). The patient's profile would be straight or *orthognathic*.

Class I malocclusion *(dental malocclusion)* would exhibit this same first molar relationship, but would have malalignments of teeth within the Class I relationship such as (a) crowded arch (Fig. 10.12), (b) a loss of arch continuity, (c) poor alignment of the anterior teeth (aesthetic malocclusion, Fig. 10.12), (d) abnormal buccolingual tooth relationships such as crossbite or buccal version (Fig. 10.13) and/or (e) premature occlusal contacts (either centric or eccentric) (*below* in Fig. 10.4).

In contrast to Class I ordental malocclusion, Class II and Class III malocclusions are considered to be *skeletal malocclusions* because of the considerable difference in size, or the abnormal positional relationship, of the maxillae and the mandible (Fig. 10.11).

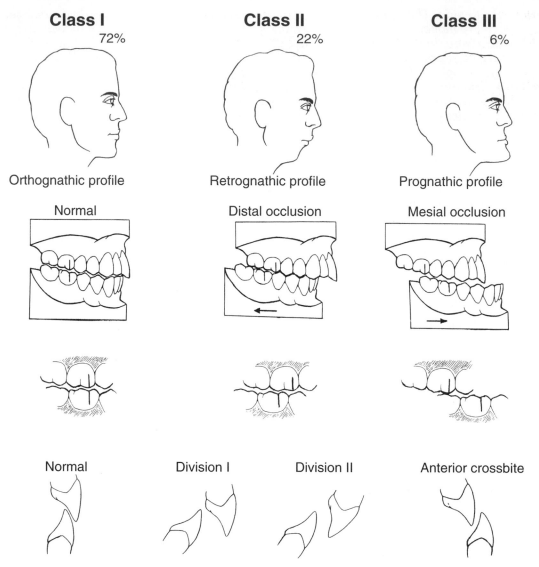

**Figure 10.11.** Angle's classification of occlusion and malocclusion. **Top row:** expected facial profile. **Second row:** occlusal relationships of casts in centric occlusion. **Third row,** below each cast: a close-up of the first molar relationships. **Fourth row,** *on the left:* Class I malocclusion has this expected normal incisor relationship; *in the center:* the two divisions of Class II malocclusion; and, *on the right:* the anterior crossbite that is frequently found in Class III malocclusions.

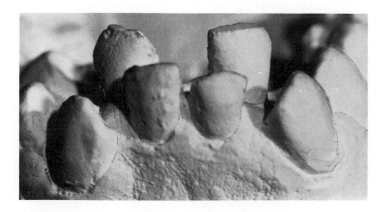

**Figure 10.12.** A type of Class I malocclusion. Extreme anterior crowding in a mandibular dentition. The mandibular lateral incisors emerged lingual to rather than beneath their deciduous predecessors, which were subsequently extracted and had nearly half of their roots intact.

Normal

Buccal version

Crossbite

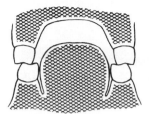
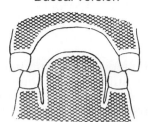
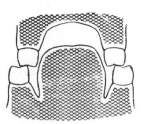

**Figure 10.13.** Cross-section views of the normal occlusion with the buccal surfaces of maxillary molars buccal to mandibular molars (*left*); maxillary molars in buccal version or more buccal than normal (*middle*) common with Class II malocclusion; and posterior crossbite with mandibular molars positioned buccally to maxillary molars (*right*), common with Class III malocclusion.

## 2. CLASS II MALOCCLUSION (also called Distal Occlusion or Mandibular Retrognathism)

Refer to Figure 10.11, *middle column.*

This is a skeletal type of malocclusion with a relatively small mandible as compared to the maxillae. The mandibular teeth are in a distal and sometimes lingual (Fig. 10.13, center) relationship to their normal maxillary opponents. The patient's curved retrognathic profile appears to have a receded chin. Often there is an abnormally large horizontal overlap of the maxillary to mandibular incisors (5–10 mm). Some evidence indicates that people with this type of malocclusion have more crepitus because of the frequent necessity to protrude the jaw more in order to properly enunciate and to incise. There are two subdivisions of this type of malocclusion:

**a. Class II, Division I**

Refer to Figure 10.11, *lowest row.*

The maxillary incisors have a labial inclination. Also people with this subdivision of malocclusion have a long face, tapered arch with high palate, a large horizontal overlap, super eruption of mandibular incisors, a hypotonic upper lip, and an overactive lower lip (20).

**b. Class II, Division II**

Refer to Figure 10.11, *lowest row.*

The incisors have a lingual inclination. Also these people have a short, wide face, square arch, somewhat less horizontal overlap than in Division I, a deep vertical overlap, severe curve of Spee, anterior crowding, and well-developed chin musculature (20).

## 3. CLASS III MALOCCLUSION (also called Mesial Occlusion or Mandibular Prognathism)

Refer to Figure 10.11, *right column.*

In addition to a massive mandible, people with this class of malocclusion have a long narrow face, a tapered upper arch with a high vault, increased activity of their upper lip, and decreased activity of their lower lip.

This is a skeletal type of malocclusion with the mandible relatively large compared to the maxillae and with the *mandibular teeth in a mesial, and often facial, relationship to their upper counterparts.* The anterior teeth may be in an edge-to-edge or crossbite relationship (facial to uppers) (Figs. 10.11, *right in lowest row,* and

10.13, *right*). The patient's profile will be concave with a very prominent chin. Other terms for this anterior relationship are underbite, crossbite, or edge-to-edge bite. Crepitus with Class II malocclusion is not common since little, if any, protrusion is required to clearly enunciate or to incise.

Class II and Class III malocclusions usually require much longer term orthodontic correction or surgical intervention than Class I malocclusions, owing to the greater disparity from an ideal relationship of the corresponding teeth in the maxillae and mandible. Corrections made surgically (e.g., using a surgical technique called a sliding osteotomy) for Class II and III malocclusions will dramatically and suddenly improve appearance, provide better tooth relationships and, eventually, better function as well.

From eight unrelated surveys of the prevalence of malocclusion done by orthodontists on 21,328 children ages 6 to 18 in the United States between 1951 and 1971, Dr. Woelfel averaged the results and derived the following information:

71.7% had malocclusion (range: 31–95%)

28.3% had acceptable occlusion

72.3% had Angle's Class I malocclusion (range: 62–88%)

22.0% had Angle's Class II malocclusion (range: 8–32%)

5.7% had Angle's Class III malocclusion (range: 2–12%)

## H. Terms Commonly Used in Discussions about Occlusion and Malocclusion

**Normal occlusion** (Figs. 10.2, *bottom*, 10.8**A,** and 10.11, *left*) is a Class I relationship of the maxillary and mandibular first molars in centric occlusion. Ideally, one should also include canine protection or canine rise when the mandible moves forward or to either side so that there are no molar or premolar contacts (see Fig. 10.10**I**). Normal occlusion is an absence of large or many facets, bone loss, closed vertical dimension, crooked teeth, bruxing habits, loose teeth, and freedom from joint pain (17).

**Intercuspal position** or habit bite (Fig. 10.4, *above*) is the same as *centric occlusion* or position of *maximum intercuspation* of the posterior teeth, which is approximately 1 mm anterior to the centric relation position. (Posselt found an average 1.25 ± 1 mm with a range of 0.25–2.55 mm) (3).

**Deflective malocclusion** (in Fig. 10.2: the mandible is deflected forward and to the left) is any contact of opposing teeth which guide or direct the mandible away from centric relation, either forward or to one side or both, as the teeth slide together into centric occlusion. Most people have deflective malocclusion to some degree (see Table 10.3, which gives information on 811 dental hygienists) (8). Less than 1% of this group had centric relation occlusion, yet most were asymptomatic.

**Premature or deflective tooth contact** (Figs. 10.2, above and 10.4, *below*) refers to the teeth that contact first as the jaw closes in centric relation (most retruded position). More than likely, you can detect your own deflective tooth contacts and they will not be as severe as those *below* in Fig. 10.4. Compare your first tooth contact in centric relation with those in Table 10.3. Can you determine which direction your premature tooth contacts deflect your mandible? It will almost always be forward, either straight forward or to one side.

**Anterior deprogramming** (33–43) is the process of getting the craniomandibular joints into a relaxed or comfortable neuromuscular position (centric relation) by interrupting or

**Table 10.3.** Deflective Centric Relation Tooth Contact Data from 811 Dental Hygienists

| Location of First Centric Relation Tooth Contact | Number of Hygienists | % | Type and Place of Deflective Contact | |
|---|---|---|---|---|
| | | | Teeth % | Symmetry % |
| Premolars one side | 232 | 28.6 | Only Premolars 39.7 | Unilateral Prematurity 69.2 |
| Premolars both sides | 90 | 11.1 | | |
| Molars one side | 328 | 40.5 | | Bilateral Prematurity |
| Molars both sides | 113 | 13.9 | Only Molars 54.4 | Same Tooth 25.8 |
| Molar one side Premolar one side | 38 | 4.7 | | Premolar-Molar 4.7 |
| Canine | 4 | 0.5 | | |
| Centric relation occlusion (no prematurities) | 6[†] | 0.7 | | |

*Research conducted by Dr. Woelfel at Ohio State University, 1974–1986.
[†]Three of the six recently had an equilibration by their dentists.

negating the proprioceptors surrounding the teeth in the periodontal ligaments. These proprioceptors would otherwise automatically or subconsciously direct the mandible into the maximum intercuspal position (centric occlusion). Anterior deprogramming is usually accomplished in 10–15 minutes by interposing something between the anterior teeth (7, 34, 35, 38, 40, 41) (leaf gauge, Lucia jig, or sliding guide) while the patient retrudes the mandible and squeezes slightly on the centered anterior fulcrum (Figs. 10.3**C** and 10.14**B** and **C**). The posterior teeth must be entirely separated for deprogramming to occur (7, 39). Once it has occurred, the posterior teeth seem to the patient to occlude (contact) improperly or in a strange way (with deflective contacts). In some instances, the deprogramming will not occur until the patient has worn an occlusal splint (orthopedic device) for several weeks and has maintained a stable and comfortable mandibular position for at least 1 week (39). This position would be a neuromuscularly relaxed centric relation to which the natural teeth could, in some cases, be adjusted (equilibrated by eliminating the premature or deflective contacts occurring in the new comfortable mandibular position).

**Fremitus** is the palpable or visible movement of a tooth when subjected to occlusal forces. Fremitus is not necessarily an unhealthy condition, but may be an indication of a premature centric relation tooth contact or an interference during lateral excursions in a dentition that does not have canine protection.

**Mandibular deviation** refers to the direction and movement of the mandible from the first tooth contact (premature) with the jaw in centric relation (Fig. 10.2, *upper row*) to the centric occlusion position (maximum tooth contact, Fig. 10.2, *lower row*). The direction of the deviation is usually upward and forward (1.25 mm) with or without a lateral component (4, 5, 38). In Figure 10.2, there is a lateral shift to the left and forward as the teeth fit maximally together. In Figure 10.4, there is a 2-mm shift forward and to the right.

**Equilibration** is the process by which a dentist corrects or attempts to correct existing premature or deflective tooth contacts or improves the occlusal relationships of a patient by modifying the occlusal and incisal surfaces of the teeth with revolving stones or burs in a dental handpiece (8). An occlusal equilibration should never be attempted without first having the patient wear a maxillary bite plane (occlusal splint) for 1–6 weeks (Fig. 10.10). This permits natural and comfortable repositioning of the mandible and its craniomandibular joints. Thus, the equilibrated teeth will be in harmony with physiologically relaxed joints. The patient should have remained symptom-free during the last several weeks wearing the occlusal splint (8).

**Long centric** is a condition in which the mandibular deviation from centric relation to centric occlusion is only directly forward smoothly in a horizontal plane without interferences. There is no upward or lateral component. It is often the goal during an equilibration to provide the patient with a long centric relationship by relieving all deflective or premature tooth contacts that had previously caused the mandible to deviate either sideways or upward from centric relation to centric occlusion. The patient with a long centric will have a short anteroposterior range (0.5–2.0 mm) of uniform tooth contact occurring at the same vertical dimension.

**Disclusion** refers to the separation of all the posterior teeth on one side as the mandible moves to that side (Fig. 10.10**I**), caused by the opening component produced by a deep vertical overlap of the canines (21, 22). It is generally considered to be a healthy or desirable condition to have. [Dr. Woelfel found it in 37.7% of the natural dentitions of dental hygiene students (Table 10.4)]. These canine protected dentitions were without balancing side interferences. It may be achieved by orthodontics or by adding length or lingual thickness to the maxillary canines (by placing restorations). Compare subjects *A, B,* and *C* in Figures 10.9**B** and 10.10**I** in order to visualize the separation of the posterior teeth produced by steep canine and incisal guidance.

**Canine protected occlusion** is an occlusal relationship in which the vertical overlap of the maxillary and mandibular canines produces a disclusion (separation) of all the posterior teeth when the mandible moves to either side (*B* and *C* in Figs. 10.9**B** and in 10.10**I**). Many dentists consider this to be the best type of relationship to have. One study of 500 persons indicated that there was a lesser tendency toward bruxism with canine protected occlusion (23). Another study found posterior tooth mobility to be higher in dentitions with canine protection than those with group function (24). Comparisons of 30 quadrants with each type of relationship were made using an accurate rigidly mounted periodontimeter (24). Several animal studies using cats have found that canines are more richly represented by neuron units (mechanoreceptors in the periodontal ligament) than any other teeth (19, 25, 26). Another study reported that the periodontal ligament proprioceptors were directionally sensitive to forces of a few grams (27). Such evidence lends credence to the canine protection theory (9,

**Table 10.4.** Eccentric Occlusal Contacts on 342 Hygiene Students*

| Condition | Right Quadrants | Left Quadrants | Total | Percent |
|---|---|---|---|---|
| Working Side Tooth Relationship | | | | |
|   Canine Rise | 207 | 205 | 412 | 60.2% |
|   Group Function | 135 | 137 | 272 | 39.8% |
| Balancing Side Tooth Relationship | | | | |
|   No contact | 250 | 251 | 501 | 73.2% |
|   Interference | 92 | 91 | 183 | 26.8% |

| | Students | Percent |
|---|---|---|
| Bilateral Canine Rise *without* balancing interference[†] | 129 | 37.7% |
| Bilateral Canine Rise with balancing side interference | 29 | 8.5% |
| Bilateral Group Function *without* balancing side interference | 58 | 17.0% |
| Bilateral Group Function with balancing side interference | 34 | 9.9% |
| Different Relationships on each side | 92 | 26.9% |

*Survey conducted by Dr. Woelfel and his carefully trained staff. Doubtful recordings were personally reexamined by him for their validity (1980–1986). More than 30% of these 342 dental hygiene students had undergone orthodontic treatment.

†Considered to be the best type of relationship.

21, 22). Study the uppermost portions of the frontal envelopes of motion in Figure 10.9**B** in order to visualize how the mandible must open at a steep angle before it can move further laterally with canine protection.

**Anterior coupling** (anterior guidance) is a tightly overlapping relationship of the opposing maxillary and mandibular incisors and canines which produces disclusion of the posterior teeth when the mandible protrudes and moves to either side from 1–4 mm (21, 22). Observe the differences in the uppermost portion of the envelopes of motion shown for three subjects in Figure 10.9**B**; subject *B* would necessarily have anterior coupling and canine protected occlusion on both sides.

**Unilateral balanced occlusion** (group function) (Table 10.4) is an occlusal relationship in which all posterior teeth on a side contact evenly as the jaw is moved toward that side. This is much different from disclusion because several posterior teeth contact along with the canines on the working side (9, 17). Subject *A* in Figure 10.9**B** would have a unilateral balanced occlusion, also called group function.

**Balancing side interferences** refers to any tooth contact on the nonworking side, and is considered to be very damaging to both the involved teeth and to the craniomandibular joint on the opposite side. [Of 314 dental hygiene students examined, 26.8% had balancing side interferences in at least one quadrant (Table 10.4).] A balancing side interference can cause craniomandibular joint pain on the opposite side because of the pivoting of the mandible and the stretching of opposite side ligaments and muscles. Poor occlusal relationships of any type can produce a variety of joint problems (10, 11, 14, 17, 28, 29).

**Bilateral balanced occlusion** is an occlusal relationship in which all of the posterior teeth contact on the working side and one or more teeth contact simultaneously on the balancing side. This type of relationship is desirable in a patient who has no teeth and must wear a set of complete dentures. It is considered potentially bad for a patient with natural teeth, however, to have any tooth contact on the balancing side (*balancing side interferences*).

**Crepitus** is the crackling or snapping sound or noise emitted from the craniomandibular joints because of a disharmonious movement of the articular disc and the mandibular condyle, sometimes erroneously thought to be caused by the rubbing together of the dry synovial surfaces of joints. The articular disc snaps in or out of position too quickly or it becomes locked in the wrong position when the crackling noise is heard (9, 10, 17, 20, 28, 29). The frequency of crepitus among 594 dental hygiene students and 505 dental students is given in Table 1.2. Over one-third of these 1099 students had some crepitus while opening widely; it was slightly more prevalent on the right side than on the left side, and was more common in women than in men. As you can see, crepitus is not a rare occurrence. Usually, unless it is accompanied by pain, limited jaw opening, trismus, or locking of the jaw, *treatment is not indicated* (28, 31). The noise may disappear with time, or it may persist for many years being no more than a noisy annoyance.

## I. Accurate Recording of the Centric Relation Jaw Position

The process of obtaining an accurate centric relation jaw registration (checkbite) is seen in Figure 10.3. A leaf wafer (6, 36, 38) is selected, and a leaf gauge or sliding guide (anterior deprogrammer) (4, 8, 33–36, 38, 39) is inserted at an upward angle between the incisors as the patient arcs the mandible open and then closes (hinge type or rotational opening) until the incisors engage the leaf gauge of sufficient thickness so all other teeth separate slightly (Fig. 10.3**C**). In this manner, the *mandible is "tripodized"* (two condyles and leaf gauge) by the patient's neuromusculature, and the patient is unable to aim the jaw into centric occlusion because no signals can be sent to the brain from the proprioceptors (19) in the separated teeth, which would otherwise contact deflectively in the retruded position. The leaf gauge is inserted in the wafer, soft polyether or rubber is thinly spread over tooth indentations (Fig. 10.3**D**), and the entire assembly is carried to the mouth (Fig. 10.3**E**). The patient then retrudes and closes firmly onto the leaf gauge as previously until the recording media sets. The centric relation registration (Fig. 10.3**F**) is assembled on the articulator ready for attaching the lower cast with plaster (Fig. 10.3**G**). The results of a severe unilateral molar prematurity in the centric relation position is seen *below* in Figure 10.4. This patient underwent 2¹/₂ years of orthodontic therapy to correct the enormous error. Other alternatives would have been surgery (intrusion of molars) or possibly root canal therapy on the molars followed by eight cast crowns (reducing molar cusp height). Ordinarily, the very common centric relation prematurities (Table 10.3) are not as severe as this, and often can be corrected when necessary with minimal occlusal alterations or minor orthodontic tooth movement. A diagnostic mounting procedure like this (Fig. 10.3) should always be done prior to attempting any type of equilibrating of teeth in the mouth (4, 6, 8). Harmonizing the tooth contacts with the neuromuscularly relaxed centric relation position recorded can alleviate bruxism, crepitus, and occasional craniomandibular joint pain and/or trismus of the masticatory muscles.

The newest device used for anterior deprogramming of the mandible and for recording centric relation is the sliding guiding inclined gauge or sliding guide (33–35, 39, 43) (Figs. 10.14 and 10.15). It comes in three maximum thicknesses for use, depending on the sever-

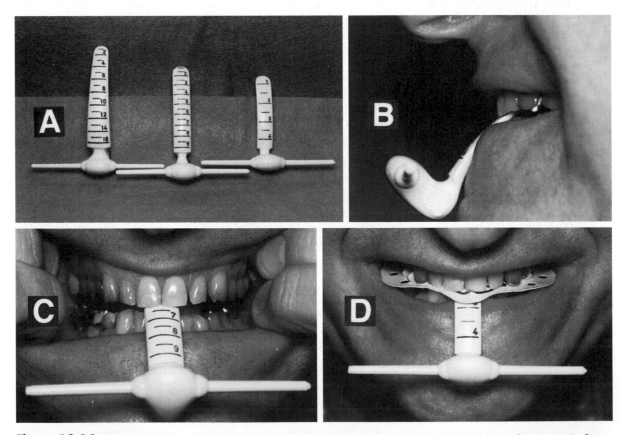

**Figure 10.14. A.** A set of three sliding guiding inclined gauges. The millimeter scales denote the amount of incisal separation between overlapping incisors (left sliding guide 16 mm, center one 9 mm, right one has a maximum thickness of 4 mm). **B.** A 4-mm sliding guide is held between the incisors at a steep angle to the occlusal plane separating them by 2.5 mm, just enough to keep all of the posterior teeth from touching. **C.** A 9-mm sliding guide is placed in the mouth so the incisors are separated by 6.5 mm during the muscular deprogramming period. **D.** A centric relation jaw registration made with a 4-mm sliding guide and a Woelfel leaf wafer. The minimal amount of incisal separation (2.5 mm) was determined prior to the polyvinylsiloxane centric relation registration which was used to mount diagnostic casts of the patient on an articulator.

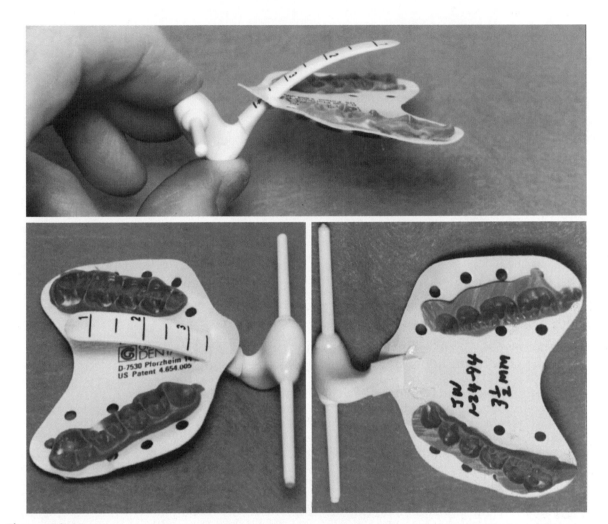

**Figure 10.15.** Three views of a 4-mm sliding guide showing how it is used with the leaf wafer for centric relation jaw registrations made with a semirigid polyvinylsiloxane material. *Above:* The curvature of the sliding guide and its proper angle above the occlusal plane are seen. *Below left:* Maxillary side of registration showing the tooth indentations and the 3.5-mm incisal separation. *Below right:* Inferior view with mandibular tooth imprints in the polyvinylsiloxane registration media and pertinent patient information written with a Sharpie fine point marker. This centric relation registration is seen in the mouth in Figure 10.14**D**.

ity of the malocclusion (Fig. 10.14**A**). The thickness gradually increases from tip to handle and the curvature of the sliding guide is critical so that it can be placed in the mouth between overlapping incisors at a relatively steep angle to the occlusal plane (Fig. 10.14**B**) without injuring the rugae or hard palate. The exact thickness between the incisors is read on the millimeter scale (Fig. 10.14**C**). Minimal incisal separation is the goal for deprogramming so long as no posterior teeth touch, thus avoiding proprioceptive impulses. This is particularly important for the centric relation jaw registration to minimize errors on the articulator (mechanical jaws). The sliding guide is made of a nonbrittle autoclavable plastic, and works well with the Woelfel leaf wafer for centric relation jaw registrations (Figs. 10.14**C** and **D,** and 10.15) (33–35, 39).

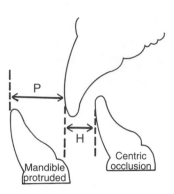

**Figure 10.16.** *H* is the horizontal overlap of central incisors in centric occlusion and *P* is the protrusive overlap with the mandible protruded as far as possible.

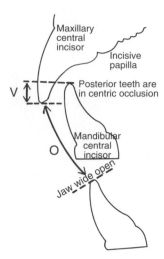

**Figure 10.17.** *V* is the vertical overlap of central incisors in centric occlusion. *O* is the opening distance between incisors which can be measured.

## *LEARNING EXERCISES*

### *EXERCISE ON JAW MOBILITY OR MANDIBULAR MOVEMENT CAPABILITY*

*It should be an educational and interesting experience for you to complete the simple procedures on the next several pages in order to become aware of how one is able to move the lower jaw on command. You should think about which muscles bring about these jaw movements and which ligaments, musculature, and fascia limit the amount of jaw movement. It will take no more than 20 minutes to do this exercise.*

*To measure accurately, it is necessary to use your millimeter ruler (cut off even with the zero mark). Make these measurements while observing your tooth relationship in a mirror. If you have a set of casts of your mouth, measurements H (Fig. 10.16) and V (Fig. 10.17) can be made on them. After finishing, compare all of your measurements with the averages in Table 10.1.*

1.  Measure the horizontal overlap (*H*) (Fig. 10.16) in three places while holding your back teeth tightly closed (in centric occlusion): (a) on the midline between the central incisors, (b) between the labial surfaces of the left canines, and (c) between the labial surfaces of the right canines (use a mirror).

    a.  Horizontal overlap of central incisors: ___ mm

    b.  Horizontal overlap of left canines: ___ mm

    c.  Horizontal overlap of right canines: ___ mm

2.  Measure the protrusive overlap (*P*) (Fig. 10.16) while holding your jaw as described here:

    Lower jaw moved forward as far as possible (like a bulldog), measurement *P* (Fig. 10.16) between the labial surface of the maxillary central incisors to the labial surface of the mandibular incisors: _____ mm (This movement requires contraction of both lateral pterygoid muscles simultaneously.)

3.  Measure the horizontal distance between upper and lower canines during maximum movements in *lateral* excursions.

    a.  Lower jaw moved to the left as far as possible (Fig. 10.18**A**). This is similar to measurement *P* in Figure 10.16 only between the facial surfaces of the maxillary and mandibular left canines: ___ mm (This movement requires contraction of the right lateral pterygoid muscle).

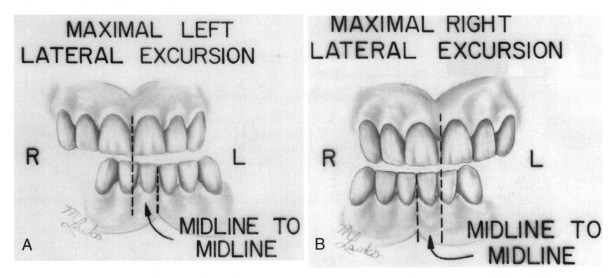

**Figure 10.18.** Lateral jaw movements of the mandibular moved as far as possible to the left (**A**) and to the right (**B**).

    b.   Lower jaw moved to the right as far as possible (Fig. 10.18**B**). Measure between the facial surfaces of the maxillary and mandibular right canines: _____ mm (This movement requires contraction of the left lateral pterygoid muscle). The distance measured is like $P$ in Figure 10.16 but between canines.

4.   Measure the vertical overlap ($V$ Fig. 10.17) on the midline between the central incisors (incisal edge to incisal edge) while holding your back teeth tightly closed:

       Vertical overlap of central incisors: ___ mm

5.   Measure the distance between incisal edges of incisors when opening with hinge-movement only; then after translating into maximum opening.

    a.   Open your jaw slowly as *far as possible while firmly retruding* it (centric relation). Usually one is able to open only half or less than half of the maximal amount on this type of *hinge opening* (Fig. 10.8**B**). Practice doing this, then measure the distance. If you open properly in this manner, there will not be any crepitus because the articular discs and condyles are fixed posteriorly. Hinge opening at incisors (The early part of $O$ in Fig. 10.17). _____ mm

    b.   Measurement $O$ with your jaw opened as widely as possible (usually you can fit four fingers between your incisors). Maximum opening ($O$ in Fig. 10.17): _____ mm

    Did you notice a noise near one or both ears when you opened widely? If you did, this sound is caused by a disharmony between the movement of the jaw and the movement of the disc that fits between the jaw condyle and the skull on either side. It is usually not a serious problem, and many people experience crepitus for a while during their lifetime. The frequency of this noisy phenomenon among 1099 young people is given in Table 1.2. Such noise can be annoying and lead to complications or it often remains innocuous for years. Treatment for complications might involve occlusal splint therapy, an occlusal equilibration, jaw muscle exercise, or possibly orthodontic treatment.

6.   Calculations made from your measurements of the voluntary movements of your mandible:

    a.   Maximum opening at incisors. Add measurements 4 plus *5b*. Total incisor opening: _____ mm

    b.   Maximum hinge opening at incisors (add *4* and *5a*): _____ mm

c. Maximum lateral movement of the mandible toward the left. Add measurements *1b* and *3a.* Total movement to left side: _____ mm

d. Maximum lateral movement of the mandible toward the right. Add measurements *1c* and *3b.* Total movement to right side: _____ mm

e. Maximum protrusion of the mandible. Add measurements *1a* and *2.* Total forward movement of the jaw:    _____ mm

f. Total lateral movement of the mandible (from right side to left side). Add totals *6c* and *6d.* Maximum lateral (side-to-side) movement of the jaw: _____ mm

Are you surprised that you can move your mandible farther from side-to-side than you can move it directly forward? Usually your jaw can move about twice as far sideways (laterally) as it can protrude or move directly forward. Compare the results of your own jaw movement capability with that of 796 dental hygienists and 318 dental students in Table 10.1. With this many young men and women, you would expect to find some real exceptions or extremes. For example, from −5 mm vertical overlap of the incisors (anterior open bite) to 13 mm vertical overlap; a horizontal overlap of 10 mm to one person who had his lower incisors 6½ mm anterior to his uppers when he closed naturally on his back teeth (huge prognathic lower jaw).

# References

1. Williamson EH, Woelfel JB, Williams BH. A longitudinal study of rest position and centric occlusion. Angle Orthod 1975;45:130–136.
2. Winter CM, Woelfel JB, Igarashi T. Five-year changes in the edentulous mandible as determined on oblique cephalometric radiographs. J Dent Res 1974;53(6):1455–1467.
3. Posselt U. The physiology of occlusion and rehabilitation. Philadelphia: F.A. Davis, 1962.
4. Williamson EH, Steinke RM, Morse PK, Swift TR. Centric relation: a comparison of muscle determined position and operator guidance. Am J Orthod 1980;77:133–145.
5. Rosner D, Goldberg G. Condylar retruded contact position correlation in dentulous patients Part I: Three-dimensional analysis of condylar registrations. J Prosthet Dent 1986;56:230–237.
6. Woelfel JB. New device for accurately recording centric relation. J Prosthet Dent 1986;56:716–727.
7. Carroll WJ, Woelfel JB, Huffman RW. Simple application of anterior jig or leaf gauge in routine clinical practice. J Prosthet Dent 1988;59:611–617.
8. Huffman RW. A cusp-fossa equilibration technique using a numbered leaf gauge. J Gnathology 1987;6:23–36.
9. Williamson EH. Occlusion: understanding or misunderstanding. Angle Orthod 1976;46:86–93.
10. American Dental Association. Temporomandibular disorders. JADA Guide to Dental Health Special Issue 1988;45–46.
11. Locker D, Grushka M. The impact of dental and facial pain. J Dent Res 1987;66:1414–1417.
12. Gibbs CH, Mahan PE, Mauderli A, et al. Limits of human bite strength. J Prosthet Dent 1986;56:226–240.
13. Guernsey LH. Biting force measurement. Dent Clin North Am 1966;10:286–289.
14. Gross A, Gale EN. A prevalence study of the clinical signs associated with mandibular dysfunction. JADA 1983;107:932–936.
15. Green CS. A critique of nonconventional treatment concepts and procedures for TMJ disorders. Comp Cont Educ 1984;5:848–851.
16. Pierce CJ, Gale EN. A comparison of different treatments for nocturnal bruxism. J Dent Res 1988;67:597–601.
17. Ramjford SP, Ash MM Jr. Occlusion. Philadelphia: W.B. Saunders, 1966:142–159.
18. Young JL. Successful restorative dentistry for the internal derangement patient. Mo Dent J 1987;67:21–26.
19. Crum RJ, Loiselle RJ. Oral perception and proprioception. A review of the literature and its significance to prosthodontics. J Prosthet Dent 1972;28:215–230.
20. Renner RP. An introduction to dental anatomy and esthetics. Chicago: Quintessence Publishing, 1985:162.
21. Brose MO, Tanquist RA. The influence of anterior coupling on mandibular movement. J Prosthet Dent 1987;57:345–353.

22. Kohno S, Nakano M. The measurement and development of anterior guidance. J Prosthet Dent 1987;57:620–630.

23. Barghi N. Clinical evaluation of occlusion. Tex Dent J 1978;96(Mar):12–14.

24. O'Leary J, Shanley D, Drake R. Tooth mobility in cuspid-protected and group function occlusions. J Prosthet Dent 1972;27(Jan):21–25.

25. Kruger L, Michel F. A single neuron analysis of buccal cavity representation in the sensory trigeminal complex of the cat. Arch Oral Biol 1962;7:491–503.

26. Kawamura Y, Nishiyama T. Projection of dental afferent impulses to the trigeminal nuclei of the cat. Jpn J Physiol 1966;16:584–597.

27. Jerge CR. Comments on the innervation of the teeth. Dent Clin North Am 1965;117–127.

28. Seligman DA, Pullinger AG, Solberg WD. The prevalence of dental attrition and its association with factors of age, gender, occlusion, and TMJ symptomatology. J Dent Res 1988;67:1323–1333.

29. Turrell J, Ruiz HG. Normal and abnormal findings in temporomandibular joints in autopsy specimens. J Craniomandibular Disorders: Facial & Oral Pain 1987;1:257–275.

30. Sicher H, DuBrul EL. Oral anatomy. 7th ed. St. Louis: C.V. Mosby, 1975:174–209.

31. Lindblom G. On the anatomy and function of the temporomandibular joint. ACTA Odontol Scand 1960;17(Supp 28):1–287.

32. Woelfel J, Hickey JC, Allison ML. Effect of posterior tooth form on jaw and denture movement, J Prosthet Dent 1962;12:922–939.

33. Woelfel JB. New device for deprogramming and recording centric jaw relation: the sliding guiding inclined gauge. Advanced Prosthodontics Worldwide, Proceedings of the World Congress on Prosthodontics, Hiroshima, Japan, Sept 21–23, 1991:218–219.

34. Woelfel JB. A new device for mandibular deprogramming and recording centric relation: the sliding guiding inclined gauge. Protesi occlusionone ATM a cura di Giorgio Vogel FDI 1991. Milan, Italy: Monduzzi Editore III, 1991:35–40.

35. Woelfel JB. Sliding and guiding the mandible into the retruded arc without pushing. The Compendium of Continuing Education in Dentistry 1991(Sept);12(9):614–624.

36. Paltaleao JF, Silva-Netto CR, Nunes LJ, Woelfel JB. Determination of the centric relation. A comparison between the wax prepared method and the Leaf Gauge-Leaf Wafer System. RGO 1992;40(5):356–360.

37. Tsolka P, Woelfel JB, Man WK, Preiskel HW. A laboratory assessment of recording reliability and analysis of the K6 diagnostic system. J Craniomandibular Disorders: Facial & Oral Pain 1992;6:273–280.

38. Fenlon, MR, Woelfel JB. Condylar position recorded using leaf gauges and specific closure forces. Intern J Prost 1993;6(4):402–408.

39. Woelfel JB., An easy practical method for centric registration. Jpn J Gnathology 1994;15(3):125–131.

40. Donegan SJ, Carr AB, Christensen LV, et al. An electromyographic study of aspects of "deprogramming" of human jaw muscles. J Oral Rehabil 1990;17:509–518.

41. Carr AB, Donegan SJ, Christensen LV, et al. An electrognathographic study of aspects of "deprogramming" human jaw muscles. J Oral Rehabil 1991;18:143–148.

42. Christensen IV, et al. Observation on the motor control of brief teeth clenching in man. J Oral Rehabil 1991.

43. Yaegashi Y, Tanaka H. An electromyographic study of the effect on masticatory muscle activity applying the leaf guage. J Prosthet Dent 1994.

44. Montgomery RL. Head and neck anatomy with clinical correlations. New York: McGraw-Hill, 1981:202–214.

45. Ricketts RM. Abnormal functions of the temporomandibular joint. Am J Orthod 1955;41:425, 435–441.

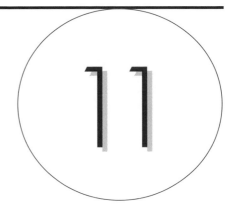

# Dental Anomalies

CONNIE SYLVESTER

**Definition:** An anomaly is a deviation from normal, usually related to embryonic development that may result in absence, excess, or deformity of body parts (1).

Dental anomalies are abnormalities of tooth form that range from such "common" occurrences as permanent maxillary peg-shaped lateral incisors (Fig. 11.1) to such rare occurrences as complete anodontia. Dental anomalies are most often caused by hereditary factors (gene related) or by developmental or metabolic disturbances. While more anomalies occur in permanent than primary dentition, and in the maxilla than the mandible, it is important to remember that their occurrence is rare. Approximately 1–2% of the population have some form of anodontia (missing teeth, Fig. 11.2), while another 1–2% have supernumerary (extra) teeth (2–4). Deformities or abnormal formations of teeth occur slightly more often since it is frequently difficult to determine whether the deviation is a "true" anomaly or simply an extreme variation in tooth morphology.

Familiarity with dental anomalies is essential to the clinical practice of dentistry and dental hygiene. Recognition and correct labeling of anomalies is important for your communication with other dental team members, especially in the case of referral to a specialist. Additionally, your communication with the patient (or, in the case of a child, parent) should reflect knowledge of abnormal oral conditions. Your assurance that the fused front tooth of a 4-year-old child or an adult (Fig. 11.3) occurs with 0.5% frequency and rarely affects the number of teeth in the permanent dentition will go a long way to promote the patient's confidence in you and the office. Likewise, the informed patient who understands why the accessory cusp on the buccal of his maxillary or mandibular molar (Fig. 11.4) is more prone to decay than normal, will likely be more receptive to home care instructions that are specific to his mouth and his needs. Finally, understanding the etiology of the anomaly is important in determining the course of treatment, if any. Additional information related to the etiology of the following anomalies is found in the study of both oral histology/embryology and oral pathology.

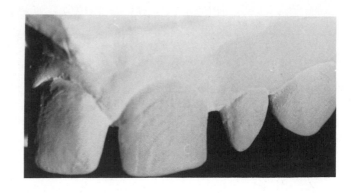

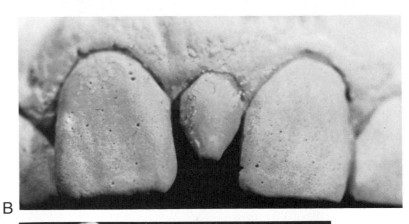

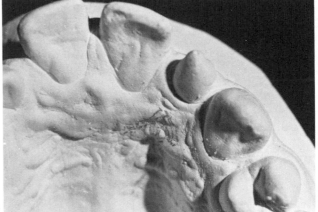

**Figure 11.1.** Peg-shaped maxillary lateral incisors viewed from the facial (in **A**) and from the incisal (in **C**). **B** shows an erupted mesiodens between the central incisors.

# SECTION I. ANODONTIA: ABSENCE OF TEETH

## A. Complete True Anodontia

Complete true anodontia is most often associated with a hereditary disease (sex-linked genetic trait) that is characterized by a large number of missing teeth, usually the entire dentition. Faulty ectodermal development further affects such structures as hair, nails, sebaceous and sweat glands, and salivary glands. The condition of complete true anodontia with absence of the entire dentition is extremely rare.

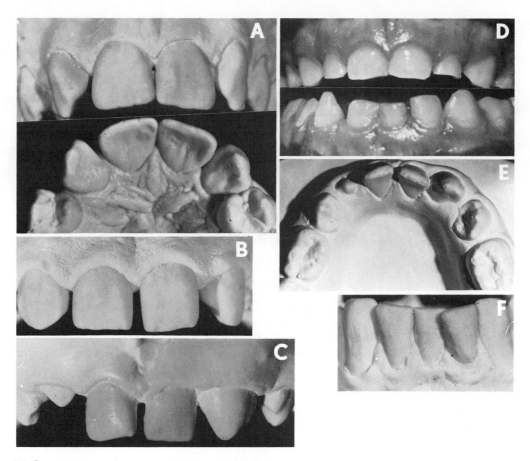

**Figure 11.2.** Congenitally missing teeth (partial anodontia) **A, B,** and **C.** Maxillary lateral incisors. **D.** Deciduous mandibular central incisor. **E.** Both deciduous mandibular central incisors. **F.** Permanent mandibular central incisor.

FUSED TEETH

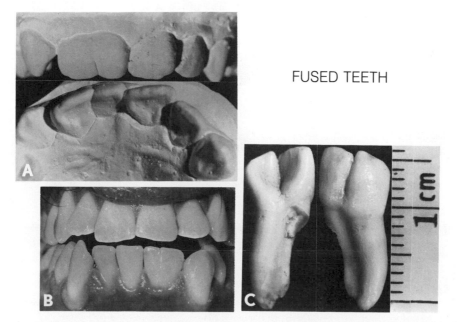

**Figure 11.3.** Fusion. Notice that the number of teeth present from canine to canine is one less than the expected dental formula. **A.** Maxillary central and lateral incisor or central incisor and mesiodens (if lateral incisor is congenitally absent). **B** and **C.** Mandibular central and lateral incisors from different individuals (in **C,** the fused teeth are seen from both lingual and facial aspects).

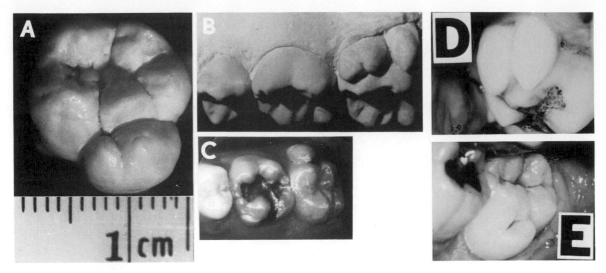

**Figure 11.4.** Extra cusp, cusps, or paramolar fused to mandibular third molar in **A,** to the buccal surfaces of maxillary second molars in **B, C,** and **D,** and to the mesiobuccal cusp of a mandibular second molar in **E.**

## B. Partial Anodontia

Partial anodontia, commonly referred to as congenitally missing teeth, involves one or more missing teeth from a dentition. Though not proven to be a hereditary trait, tendencies toward missing the same tooth do run in families.

1. The most commonly missing permanent teeth are *third molars,* with the maxillary thirds absent from the dentition more often than the mandibular thirds.

2. The *permanent maxillary lateral incisors* (Fig. 11.2A through C) are the next most commonly missing teeth. Approximately 1–2% of the population is missing one or both of these maxillary incisors (4–5). In Figure 9.7, the laterals and second premolars are absent.

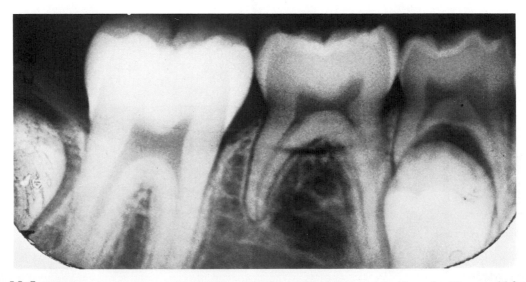

**Figure 11.5.** Missing permanent second premolar. Routine radiographic examination of a 10-year-old female revealed both mandibular right and left permanent second premolars to be missing. The first permanent premolar can be seen situated under the deciduous first molar crown between its roots. Notice the fully erupted permanent first molar and the unerupted second molar (*extreme left*). The deciduous second molar is functional and its roots have not begun to resorb.

3.  The *mandibular second premolar* is the third most frequently missing permanent tooth (Fig. 11.5), with 1% of the population missing one or both (4). [Some studies indicate the order of most commonly missing teeth to be: third molars, maxillary and mandibular premolars, and maxillary lateral incisors (6).]

Some observers state that missing teeth follow evolutionary trends in that the teeth most commonly missing from the dentition (third molars) are those that are most expendable in terms of their role in oral function (4). Conversely, the most stable teeth in the permanent dentition, the canines, are the least likely to be absent from the dentition (6).

## SECTION II. EXCESS, EXTRA, OR SUPERNUMERARY TEETH

Supernumerary teeth occur in 0.3–3.8% of the population (22). They are found in both permanent and deciduous dentitions, *with 90% of all occurrences in the maxilla* (7). "Supernumerary" refers to additional numbers of teeth occurring in the dental arch in excess of the normal dental formulas for each quadrant (deciduous quadrant: I-2, C-1, M-2; permanent quadrant: I-2, C-1, P-2, M-3). Specifically, the most frequent supernumerary specimens are found in one of two locations: maxillary incisor area or maxillary third molar region. One report states that supernumerary teeth occurred eight times more often in the maxillary regions that in the mandibular regions, and twice as frequently in men than in women (29). Another study of 50 patients from 16 months to 17 years of age, found 20% of the supernumerary teeth to be inverted (23). Fourteen percent of these patients had multiple supernumerary teeth, and 80% of the extra teeth were in a lingual position relative to the dental arch (Figs. 11.9**B**, 11.38 and 11.39).

### A. Maxillary Incisor Area

A tooth occurring between the central incisors (Fig. 11.6) is termed a mesiodens (mesial to both central incisors). It may be visible in the oral cavity or remain unerupted. If unerupted, a diastema (space) may be present (8). One study of 375 children with mesiodens reports that they are often in an inverted position and rarely erupt into the oral cavity (29). The prevalence of mesiodens in the permanent dentition in the Caucasian populations is 0.15–1.9% (9). Less frequently, supernumerary teeth may be positioned between central and lateral incisors or between lateral incisors and canines.

The occurrence of supernumerary teeth in the deciduous dentition is low (approximately 0.5%) (9). The most common supernumerary teeth in that dentition, however, are either midline mesiodens or supplemental lateral incisors.

### B. Third Molar Area

The presence of supernumerary teeth distal to the third molars is more common in the maxillary arch but does occur in the mandible (Fig. 11.8). These supernumerary teeth are often called distomolars or paramolars. Extra or fourth molars rarely erupt into the oral cavity and thus are usually discovered through radiographs (Fig. 11.8).

### C. Mandibular Premolar Area

The most common location for supernumerary teeth in the mandible is the second premolar region (Fig. 11.9). Supernumerary teeth appearing in this area generally resemble normal premolars in size and shape (10).

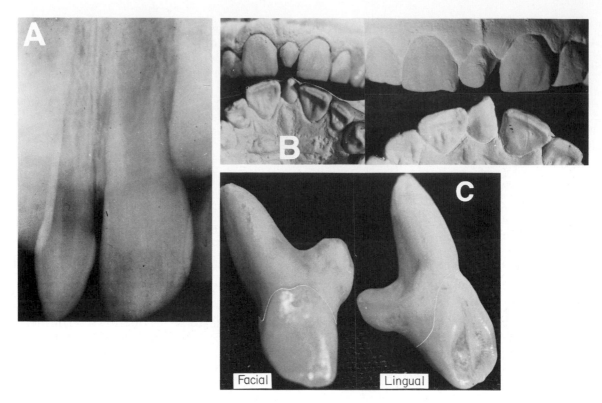

**Figure 11.6.** Mesiodens. **A.** Radiograph. Notice the supernumerary tooth next to the fully erupted maxillary permanent central incisor. The other central incisor has not reached the same occlusal plane due to the eruption of the mesiodens. **B.** Fully erupted mesiodens. One tooth has a similar form to maxillary peg-lateral incisors (Fig. 11.1); the other is more like a normal lateral incisor. **C.** Extracted maxillary central incisor with a fused mesiodens.

# SECTION III. DEFORMITY OR ABNORMALITY IN MORPHOLOGY OF TEETH

## A. Abnormal Crown Formations

These formations may be seen clinically upon visual inspection of the oral cavity.

### 1. THIRD MOLARS

Maxillary third molars have the most variable crown shape of all permanent teeth followed by mandibular thirds. These anomalies can range in shape from a small peg-shaped crown (Fig. 11.7) to a multicusped, malformed version of either the first or second molar (Fig. 11.10).

### 2. PERMANENT MAXILLARY LATERAL INCISORS

The most common anomaly in shape in the anterior of the permanent dentition is the *peg-shaped lateral incisor* (Fig. 11.1**A** and **C**), occurring in 1–2% of the population (4). The tooth is generally conical in shape, broadest cervically, and tapers toward the incisal to a blunt point.

Several studies of identical twins seem to indicate that *missing* and *peg-shaped* lateral incisor teeth may be varied expressions of the same genetic trait (11, 12).

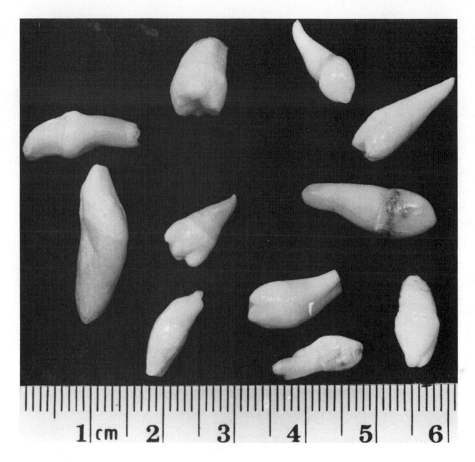

**Figure 11.7.** Supernumerary teeth of various sizes and shapes. Some resemble premolars, some appear like peg-incisors, and others look like very small third molars.

A most unusual occurrence is that of peg-shaped maxillary central incisors (Fig. 11.11).

## 3. GEMINATION OR TWINNING

This appears clinically as double or "fused" teeth. Most commonly seen in the anterior area, gemination is the result of the splitting of a single tooth germ (Fig. 11.12). These teeth generally have a *single root and common pulp canal,* but are notched incisally. Seen in less than 1% of the population, gemination appears in the primary dentition more frequently than in the permanent dentition in the region of the maxillary incisors and canines (3).

The dental arch containing a geminated tooth will generally have the normal (dental formula) number of teeth present, counting the geminated tooth as one (one extra tooth if it is counted as two teeth).

## 4. FUSION

This appears to be clinically similar to gemination except that there is a more observable separation between fused teeth (Fig. 11.13). Fused teeth also occur more commonly in the anterior portion of the mouth and result from the union of two adjacent tooth germs, *always involving the dentin.* Fused teeth usually have separate roots and pulp chambers; thus, a radiograph may be useful in determining whether fusion or gemination has occurred. As with gemination, fusion is evident in less than

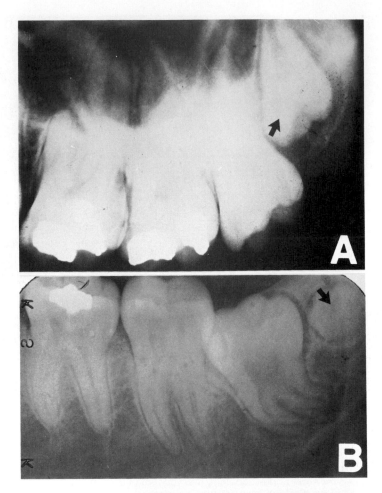

**Figure 11.8.** Supernumerary/fourth molars. **A.** Maxillary. **B.** Mandibular. The extra molar (*arrow*) is just distal to the permanent third molar.

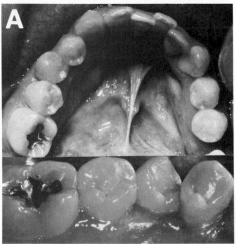

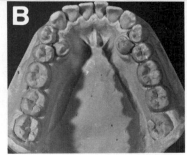

**Figure 11.9.** Supernumerary teeth in mandibular premolar region. **A.** Extra first premolar fully emerged but crowded. (Courtesy of Dr. L. Claman.) **B.** Extra first premolars on each side of the arch in lingual version. The lingual frenum is very prominent on both of these people. The 21-year-old man in **B** also had three unerupted fourth molars (like Fig. 11.8), making a total of 19 teeth in his mandibular dentition, and 18 in the maxillary dentition.

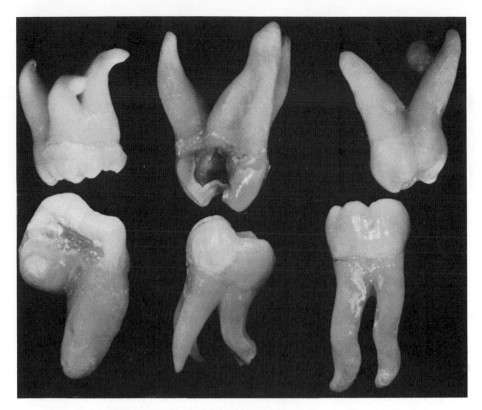

**Figure 11.10.** Unusual maxillary (*top row*) and mandibular third molars.

1% of the population and *affects the deciduous dentition more often than the permanent dentition,* and affects the mandibular incisor area more than it affects the maxilla (Figs. 11.3**C** and 11.14) (2, 3).

Fusion is thought to be caused by *pressure or force* during development of adjacent roots. It follows that many of the reports of fusion involve a supernumerary
tooth joining with an adjacent tooth (e.g., mandibular third and fourth molar fusion,

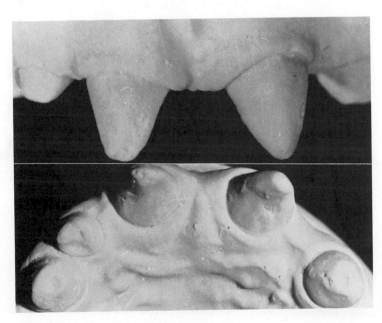

**Figure 11.11.** Peg-shaped maxillary central incisors, a very rare occurrence. *Above:*
Facial view. *Below:* Incisal view showing
both canines and one lateral incisor.

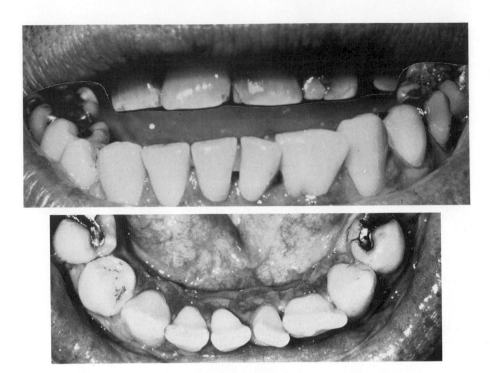

**Figure 11.12.** Gemination. Identify the mandibular canines in this permanent dentition and count the number of teeth present from canine to canine. The mandibular left lateral incisor tooth germ split or divided into two. It will generally have a single root and common pulp canal. There would be the normal number of teeth if the gemination is counted as one, or one extra tooth in this quadrant if it is counted as two teeth.

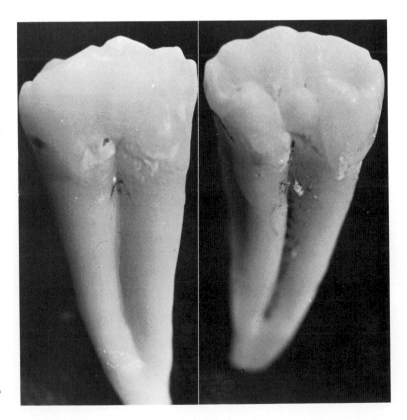

**Figure 11.13.** Fusion. Two mandibular first premolars fused together. Buccal aspect (*left*) and lingual aspect (*right*). Some separation between the roots is visible. There would be two pulp canals.

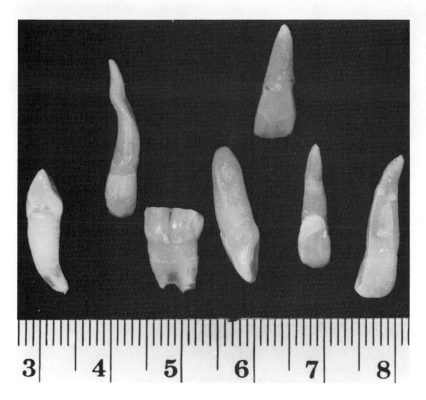

**Figure 11.14.** Unusual maxillary central and lateral incisors (crowns down) and mandibular canine and fused mandibular incisors.

and maxillary lateral incisor and anterior supernumerary fusion) (13–15). The dental arch containing a fused tooth will usually have one less tooth than the normal dental formula, counting the fused tooth as one (Fig. 11.3**A**).

## 5. HUTCHINSON'S TEETH

Unusual teeth may occur in both dentitions as the result of prenatal syphilis. Maxillary and mandibular incisors may be screwdriver shaped, broad cervically and narrowing incisally, with a notched incisal edge. These teeth are often referred to as Hutchinson's incisors (Fig. 11.42). First molars have occlusal anatomy made up of multiple tiny tubercles with poorly developed, indistinguishable cusps. Because of the berry-like shape on the occlusal, these are called *mulberry molars*.

## 6. MANDIBULAR SECOND PREMOLARS

These teeth vary in relation to the number of lingual cusps, ranging from one to three. Occlusal morphology can vary greatly in terms of groove and fossa patterns established by the number of lingual cusps (16). Some variations of these teeth are seen in Figure 6.24. The somewhat rare occurrence of two roots, one mesial and the other distal, is also seen in Figure 11.15.

## 7. ACCESSORY CUSPS OR TUBERCLES

Any tooth may exhibit extra enamel projections (Fig. 11.16), which often result from developmental localized hyperplasia (increase in volume of tissue caused by growth of new cells), or crowded preeruption conditions.

### a. Enamel Pearls

Small nodules of enamel with a tiny core of dentin are found most frequently on the distal of third molars and the buccal root furcation of molars (17) (Figs. 11.17**A** and 8.14). They appear radiographically as small, ground radiopacities.

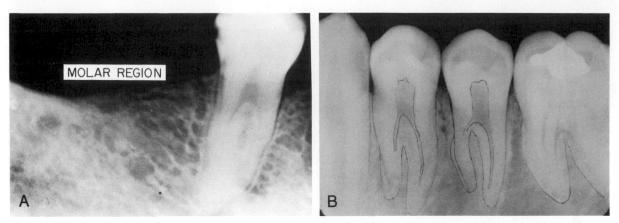

**Figure 11.15. A.** Radiograph of mandibular premolar and molar region showing second premolar with one mesial and one distal root. (Courtesy of Dr. Gary Racey). **B.** Radiograph showing both first and second mandibular premolars with mesial and distal roots. It is a fairly common occurrence for mandibular first premolars to have their root divided buccolingually, unlike this more rare mesiodistal division (root and pulp cavity images have been enhanced). An extracted tooth specimen like this is seen in the *upper row* of Figure 6.24.

Being covered with enamel, they prevent the normal connective tissue attachment and consequently may channel disease (periodontal problems) into this region.

### b. Taurodontia

In taurodontia, or so-called bull or prism teeth (Fig. 11.17**B**), the pulp chamber is very long, without a constriction near the cementoenamel junction. This occurs only in permanent teeth, with a frequency of less than 1 in 1000 among American Indians and Eskimos (24). Taurodontia is caused by a disorganization of the calcified tissues and possibly occurs in dentitions subjected to heavy use.

### c. Talon Cusp

A small enamel projection in the cingulum area of maxillary (Fig. 11.18) or mandibular anterior permanent teeth is a talon ("claw of an animal") cusp. Frequently, the cusp has a pulp horn so that radiographically it may be mistaken for a supernumerary tooth superimposed over an anterior tooth or *dens in dente*.

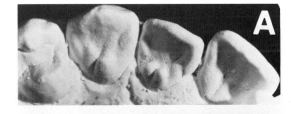

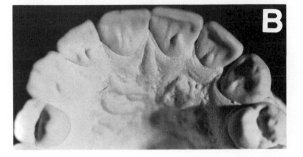

**Figure 11.16.** Maxillary incisors and canines with small tubercles or cusplets on the cingulum. **A.** Two elevations or tubercles on the canine, three on the lateral incisor. The central incisor is shovel-shaped. **B.** Pronounced tubercle on cingulum of central incisor.

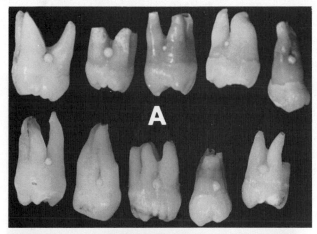

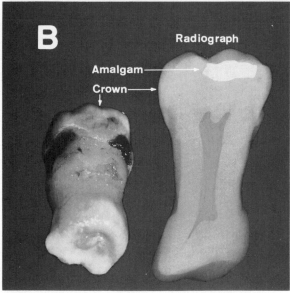

**Figure 11.17. A.** Enamel pearls of various sizes on maxillary third molars. **B.** Taurodontia, photograph of extracted tooth on *left,* radiograph on *right.* (Courtesy of Professor Rudy Melfi, D.D.S.)

Removal of this cusp is often necessary because of its interference in jaw closure with centric occlusion. Since the pulp horn is present, endodontic treatment is usually required when this cusp is removed (2, 18).

## 8. VARIATIONS IN SIZE

Microdontia (very small, but normally shaped teeth) and macrodontia (very large, but normally shaped teeth) may occur as a single tooth, several teeth, or an entire dentition (36). Gigantism most frequently involves incisors and canines and dwarfism affects maxillary lateral incisors and third molars (8, 19, 20). Some examples of variation in size of teeth are shown in Figures 5.11 and 11.19. One report shows a maxillary canine 39 mm long and a maxillary first molar 31 mm long, both removed from a pituitary giant (36).

## 9. SHOVEL-SHAPED MAXILLARY INCISORS

Possibly not a true anomaly, shovel-shaped incisors are a frequently occurring trait that reflect biologic differences between races (4). The lingual anatomy includes a pronounced cingulum and marginal ridges, thus the scoop or "shovel" appearance (Figs. 4.1 and 11.6**B**). These teeth are observed most frequently in the Asian, Mongoloid, Eskimo, and American Indian races.

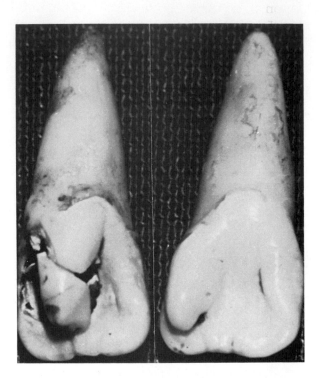

**Figure 11.18.** Lingual view of two maxillary central incisors with talon cusps.

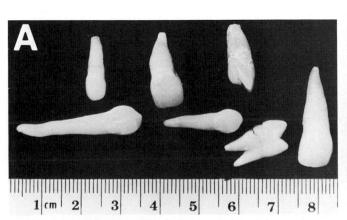

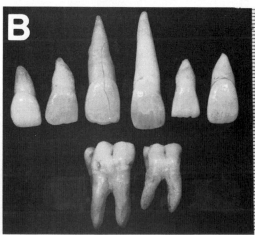

**Figure 11.19.** Variation in tooth size. **A.** *Upper row:* Maxillary lateral incisor, central incisor, and canine. *Lower row:* Two maxillary canines, maxillary first premolar, and central incisors. **B.** *Above:* Three right and three left maxillary central incisors, one 34 mm long, one 16 mm long. The four short central incisors have dwarf roots. *Below:* Two mandibular first molars.

## B. Abnormal Root Formations

These formations are not usually obvious without the aid of radiographs. Close examination of extracted specimens reveals the wide variations that occur. There have been six recent reports (30–35) of contralaterally bifurcated roots on primary maxillary canines: five discovered from routine radiographic examination, the sixth on a routine dental recall examination (Fig. 9.22).

### 1. DILACERATION

A severe bend or distortion of a tooth root and crown, often approximating an angle from 45° to more than 90° is termed dilaceration (Fig. 11.20) (25). This unusual occurrence may be the result of a traumatic injury or of insufficient space for development, as is often the case with mandibular third molars (Fig. 11.10).

### 2. FLEXION

Flexion is a sharp curvature, bend (less than 90°), or twist on a tooth root (Figs. 11.10 and 11.20).

### 3. DENS IN DENTE

This developmental anomaly is the result of the invagination of the enamel organ within the crown of a tooth. Clinically, it appears as a deep crevice primarily in the cingulum area of incisors (Fig. 11.21). Most commonly found in maxillary lateral incisors, it can appear in upper centrals and mandibular incisors.

Radiographically, dens in dente ("tooth within a tooth") appears as a mass of elongated enamel within the dentin of a normal sized tooth (Fig. 11.22). Usually it appears in the coronal third of the tooth, but may extend the entire root length. Often peg-shaped lateral incisors, with failure of mesial and distal lobes to develop, are found to have dens in dente upon radiographic examination. Their occurrence is from 1–5% of the population (2).

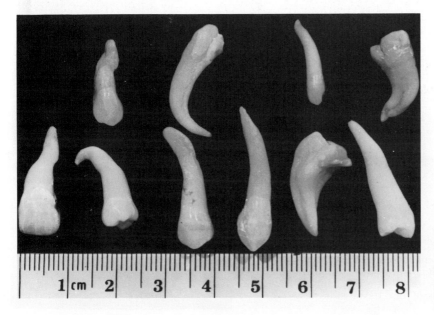

**Figure 11.20.** Dilaceration, root and/or crown twisted severely, and flexion, only the root is distorted (less than 90º). Maxillary teeth crowns are down, mandibular teeth crowns are above the roots. How many of these teeth can you recognize or identify?

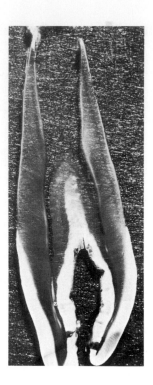

**Figure 11.21.** Faciolingual cross-section of a maxillary lateral incisor with a dens in dente (tooth within a tooth). This tooth section is only 50 micrometers thick. (Courtesy of Professor Rudy Melfi, D.D.S.)

## 4. CONCRESCENCE

Concrescence is a fusion or growing together of two adjacent teeth at the root through the cementum only (Fig. 11.23). Unlike fusion, the teeth involved are originally separate but become joined, usually after eruption into the oral cavity, because of the close proximity of the roots and excessive cementum deposition (6). This anomaly occurs most frequently in the maxillary molar region.

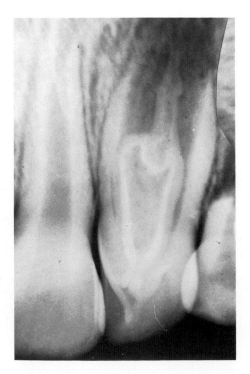

**Figure 11.22.** Radiograph of dens in dente on maxillary right central incisor. It connects with the lingual pit as clearly seen in Figure 11.21. It is caused by an invagination of the epithelium of the enamel organ before the formation of hard tissue. (Courtesy of Professor Rudy Melfi, D.D.S.)

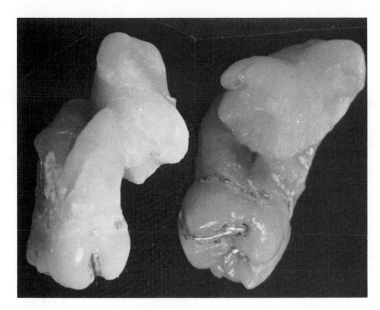

**Figure 11.23.** Examples of concrescence between adjacent maxillary first and second molars. *Left:* Lingual view. *Right:* Disto-occlusal aspect with the buccal toward the right. The emerged maxillary molar has two small amalgam restorations (central and distal fossae).

## 5. SEGMENTED ROOT

A root separated into two parts is thought to be the result of traumatic injury during the formation of the root.

## 6. DWARFED ROOTS

Maxillary teeth often exhibit normal sized crowns with abnormally short roots (Figs. 5.11 and 11.19). The incisal edge is usually displaced lingually as in the mandibular incisors. This condition is often hereditary.

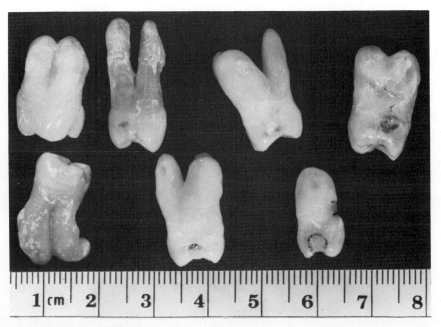

**Figure 11.24.** Hypercementosis. *Top row:* Maxillary third molar, first premolar and two first molars. *Lower row:* Mandibular first molar, maxillary first molar, and second premolar. See Figure 8.32.

Isolated or generalized dwarfing of roots may result when a person has undergone orthodontic movement of the teeth and the movement has occurred too rapidly.

## 7. HYPERCEMENTOSIS

The excessive formation of cementum around the root of a tooth after the tooth has erupted (Fig. 11.24) may be caused by trauma, metabolic dysfunction, or periapical inflammation. The excess amount of cementum may cause webbing of the roots.

## 8. ACCESSORY ROOTS

Usually occurring in teeth whose roots form after birth, accessory roots are probably caused by trauma, metabolic dysfunction, or pressure. Mandibular canines and premolars are the single-rooted teeth most likely affected, while third molars are the multirooted teeth most likely to exhibit accessory roots (mandibular molar in Fig. 7.8 and the deciduous molar in Fig. 9.21) (2). The somewhat rare occurrence of the deciduous maxillary canines with their root divided mesiodistally is shown in Figure 9.22 (30–36). Dilaceration and flexion are often observed in teeth with supernumerary or accessory roots.

## C. Additional Anomalies

Additional anomalies, including those that tend to affect the entire dentition rather than one or two specific teeth, and those related to mechanical retention and injury, should be noted.

## 1. ENAMEL DYSPLASIA

This broad term describes abnormal enamel development. Specifically, *enamel hypoplasia* (Fig 11.25) is any disturbance in the ameloblasts during the enamel matrix formation, while *enamel hypocalcification* is a disturbance in the maturation of

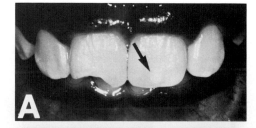

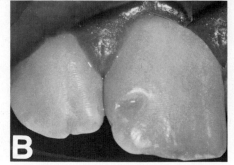

**Figure 11.25.** Enamel hypoplasia caused by a disturbance during the formative stage of the enamel matrix. **A.** Focal hypomaturation (*arrow*). **B.** A defect on the labial surface of the maxillary central incisor because of an abscess on the deciduous central incisor, a so-called "Turner's Tooth." (Courtesy of Professor Donald Bowers, D.D.S.)

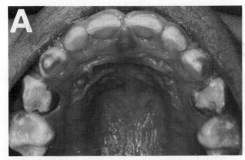

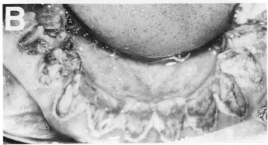

**Figure 11.26.** Amelogenesis imperfecta. **A.** Deciduous maxillary dentition. (Courtesy of Professor Donald Bowers, D.D.S.) **B.** Permanent mandibular dentition. This condition occurs only once in about 15,000 people. Notice the fungiform papillae on the tongue. (Courtesy of Professor Rudy Melfi, D.D.S.)

the enamel matrix. The etiology of enamel dysplasia includes hereditary (amelogenesis imperfecta and Hutchinson's teeth), systemic (drugs, infection, and nutritional deficiencies), or local (trauma and periapical infection) disturbances.

Generally, variations in color (from white to yellow and brown) or morphology (pitted and roughened enamel) can result. Common occurrences include:

### a. Amelogenesis Imperfecta

This hereditary disorder affects the enamel formation of both dentitions (Fig. 11.26). The partial or complete lack of enamel results in yellow to brown rough crowns that are highly susceptible to decay. This disease is extremely rare, with an incidence in the United States of 1 in 15,000 (2).

### b. Fluorosis

Mottled enamel is the result of ingestion of excessively fluoridated drinking water (Fig 11.27). Clinically, all permanent teeth are involved and can exhibit a color change from white to yellow/brown spots and/or a morphologic change of pitted enamel. These teeth are generally very resistant to decay. THE FLUORINE CONTENT OF THE MINERAL WATER CAUSING THIS CONDITION IS MANY

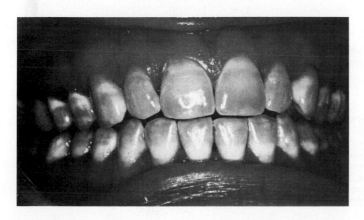

**Figure 11.27.** Fluorosis. This case of mottled enamel is generalized in a 25-year-old female and consists of a chalky white coloration in the cervical and/or middle third of all permanent teeth. Some pitting of the enamel surface is also visible.

TIMES GREATER THAN THE ONE PART PER MILLION THAT IS ADDED TO DRINKING WATER IN MANY CITIES TO REDUCE THE PREVALENCE OF DECAY.

### c. High Fever

Pitted enamel on permanent teeth is often the result of early childhood fever from such diseases as measles (4). Usually, the specific crowns that are developing at the time of the fever are affected (Fig. 11.28). Thus, there are identifiable patterns, such as the pitting of enamel in all permanent first molars, as well as the permanent incisors.

### d. Focal Hypomaturation

A localized chalky white spot on a tooth may be the result of trauma or some other interference in enamel matrix maturation (Fig. 11.25**A**). Unlike decalcification (predecay), which usually forms around the cervical thirds of teeth or occlusal surfaces of posterior teeth, hypomaturation generally appears in the middle third of the smooth crown surfaces (facial and lingual surfaces). The underlying enamel is usually soft, and thus the area is susceptible to decay.

## 2. DENTAL DYSPLASIA

Anomalies of the dentin include those with hereditary and systemic causes:

### a. Dentinogenesis Imperfecta

This hereditary disorder affects the dentin formation of both dentitions. Clinically, all teeth have a light blue-gray to yellow, somewhat opalescent appearance (Fig. 11.29). Radiographically, there is partial or total absence of pulp chambers and root canals. These teeth are weak because of a lack of support in the dentin and, as with amelogenesis imperfecta, are aesthetically displeasing. Dentin dysplasias occur twice as often as those in enamel (1 in 8000) (28).

### b. Tetracycline Stain

This condition has been erroneously blamed on community fluoridated drinking water which, of course, has been only highly beneficial for both teeth and general health. Antibiotic tetracyclines, taken either by a pregnant woman, an infant, or a child, can become incorporated in developing dentin. Clinically, the staining is generalized in the deciduous dentition, ranging in color, depending on the dose of the

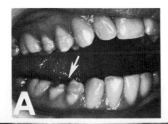

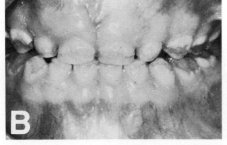

**Figure 11.28.** Dysplasia of the enamel due to high fever. **A.** Permanent dentition. Patient reported a history of high fever between the ages of 2 and 3 years. Notice that the teeth whose enamel matrix was forming at the time of the fever are affected: mandibular first and second premolars and second molar, and maxillary second premolar and second molar. **B.** Deciduous dentition. Patient had a high fever during the first 6 weeks after birth. (Courtesy of Professor Donald Bowers, D.D.S.)

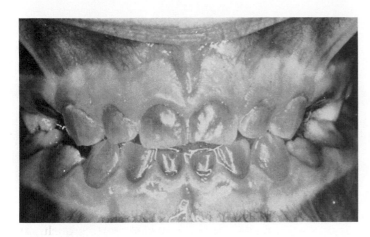

**Figure 11.29.** Dentogenesis imperfecta (opalescent dentin), a hereditary disorder that affects the dentin and external appearance of all teeth. This condition occurs only once in 8000 people. (Courtesy of Professor Donald Bowers, D.D.S.)

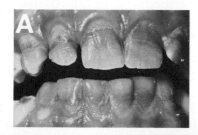

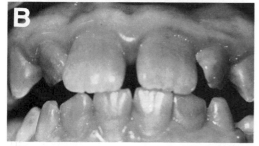

**Figure 11.30.** Tetracycline staining in permanent dentitions resulting from the administration of this antibiotic during the time that these crowns were forming. In **A,** the horizontal bands in the enamel are a result of a high fever that required antibiotic therapy. In **B,** the staining is again evidenced but the antibiotic controlled the fever sufficiently to prevent the deeply grooved bands seen in **A.** (Courtesy of Professor Donald Bowers, D.D.S.)

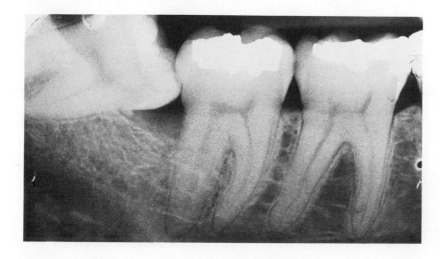

**Figure 11.31.** Impacted mandibular third molar. Because of its horizontal position, it is mechanically locked beneath the distal bulge on the second molar.

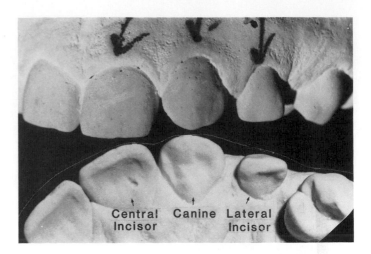

**Figure 11.32.** Misplaced left maxillary lateral incisor and canine.

drug, from yellow to gray-brown. The permanent dentition may also be affected, depending on the age at which tetracycline was prescribed (Fig. 11.30). To determine the age at which which the tetracyclines were administered, refer to the chronology chart listing the ages for hard tissue formation and calcification (Table 9.3).

## 3. UNERUPTED TEETH

Unerupted teeth are embedded teeth that fail to erupt into the oral cavity because of a lack of eruptive force. *Impacted teeth*, on the other hand, fail to erupt due to mechanical obstruction, often related to the decreasing size of modern man's jaw. At least 10% of the population have impacted teeth (Fig. 11.31), which most often include maxillary and mandibular third molars and maxillary canines (2, 4, 21).

## 4. MISPLACED TEETH (TRANSPOSITION)

Occasionally, toothbuds seem to get out of place, causing teeth to emerge in peculiar locations. Two interesting examples of this are seen in Figures 11.32 and 11.33. The most common tooth involved is the maxillary canine (20 of 25 cases reported) (26), followed by the mandibular canine. Maxillary canines can even be transposed to the central incisor region (37, 38).

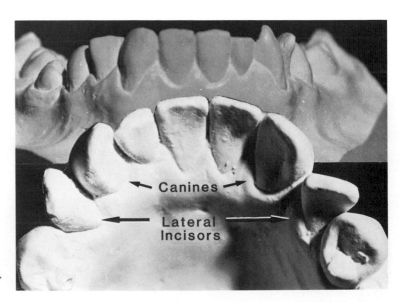

**Figure 11.33.** Bilaterally misplaced mandibular canines and lateral incisors, a rare occurrence.

ABRASION

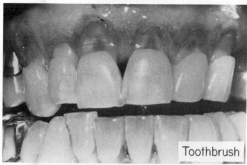

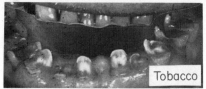

**Figure 11.34.** Abrasion. *Above:* From incorrect horizontal toothbrushing. *Below:* From chewing tobacco over a 30-year span. (Courtesy of Professor Rudy Melfi, D.D.S.)

## 5. ROTATION

Rotation is a rare anomaly, most common for the maxillary second premolar, sometimes the maxillary incisor, first premolar, or mandibular second premolar (27). A tooth may be rotated on its axis by as much as 180° (see rotated maxillary second premolar in Fig. 6.25).

## 6. REACTIONS TO INJURY

### a. Abrasion

The wearing away of tooth structure by mechanical means is called abrasion. Toothbrush abrasion most often results in worn enamel on the facial surfaces of premolars and canines at the cementoenamel junction (Fig. 11.34). It is caused by use of a hard toothbrush and/or a horizontal brushing stroke and/or a gritty dentifrice. Occlusal abrasion, from chewing or biting hard foods or objects or chewing tobacco (Fig. 11.34), results in flattened cusps on all posterior teeth and worn incisal edges. An unusual type of abrasion, caused by the use for many years of a toothpick between the maxillary central incisors, has been reported by Melfi (39). The same type of proximal abrasion has been reported from the use of a straight pin for the same purpose over many years.

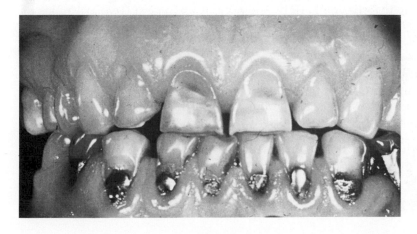

**Figure 11.35.** Erosion from an unknown cause (idiopathic). Restorations have been placed in the cervical regions of the mandibular teeth, but the erosion process continues beyond the amalgam margins and is evidenced on the maxillary central incisors.

# ATTRITION
## Deciduous Dentition

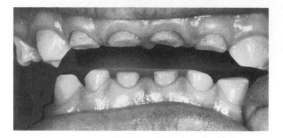

## Secondary Dentition

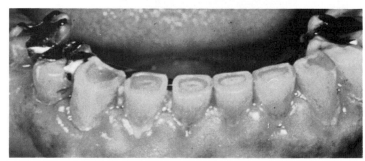

**Figure 11.36.** Attrition from prolonged bruxism or grinding of the teeth. The deciduous maxillary central incisors have been worn down almost to the gingival sulcus. The secondary mandibular incisors are worn down to a level where the pulp chamber was at one time many years previously (note the circular and oval regions on the incisal ridges).

### b. Erosion

Erosion is the loss of tooth structure from nonmechanical means (Fig. 11.35). Affecting smooth and occlusal surfaces, erosion can be the result of excessive intake or use of citric acid (lemons), carbonated beverages, industrial acids, or the result of regurgitated stomach acids (seen in bulimic individuals who habitually induce vomiting, as in the "binge and purge" syndrome) (2). Erosion can also occur from an unknown cause (idiopathic), as seen in Figure 11.35.

### c. Severe Attrition

This is not an anomaly, but it must be recognized and distinguished from abrasion (foreign substances) and erosion (unknown cause). Attrition is the wearing away of enamel and dentin from normal function or, more commonly, from excessive grinding or gritting together of teeth by the patient (bruxism). Two examples of severe attrition are shown in Figure 11.36. Stress greatly increases bruxism.

### d. Ankylosis

Teeth that erupt into the oral cavity but fail to reach occlusion with the opposing arch appear submerged or "ankylosed." Ankylosis may be initiated by an infection or trauma to the periodontal ligament. The ankylosed tooth has lost its periodontal ligament space and is truly fused to the alveolar process or bone.

Deciduous mandibular second molars most often fail to continue erupting as the jaw grows. Many times, the ankylosis occurs when the permanent successor is missing. Consequently, the ankylosed tooth will be 2–4 mm out of occlusion.

# A MOST UNUSUAL MANDIBULAR DENTITION

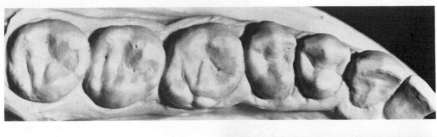

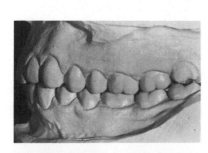

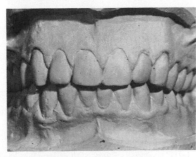

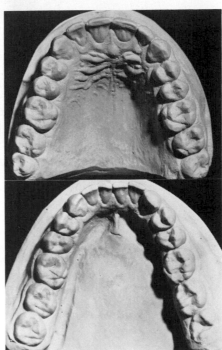

**Figure 11.37.** Mandibular dentition of 23-year-old man that has maxillary premolars and apparently maxillary molars, particularly on the left side. Both dentitions are seen from the occlusal aspect and on the left as they fit together well in centric occlusion. The lower premolar crowns do not resemble mandibular premolars in any fashion. The six mandibular anterior teeth are truly mandibular, however. The mandibular right first molar has three buccal cusps, but otherwise seems to be a mixture of both maxillary and mandibular first molars, oblong mesiodistally like a lower, but with a much larger mesiolingual cusp and Carabelli cusp like an upper first molar. The mandibular left three molars seem to have only morphologic characteristics of maxillary molars. This man's maxillary dentition seems entirely normal. It is most interesting to note that the lower left posterior teeth have the morphology of maxillary right side teeth. Likewise, the lower right teeth belong in the upper left quadrant (transposed sides and arches).

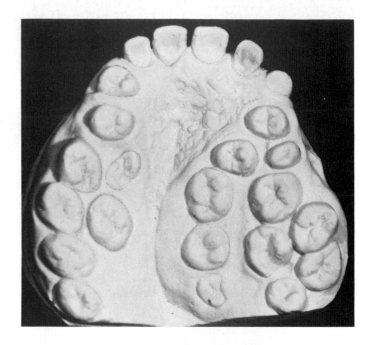

**Figure 11.38.** Permanent maxillary dentition with 24 teeth, including 13 molars. This cast was furnished courtesy of J. Andrew Stevenson (D.T.L.) and Dr. Robert Stevenson, Dayton and Columbus, Ohio.

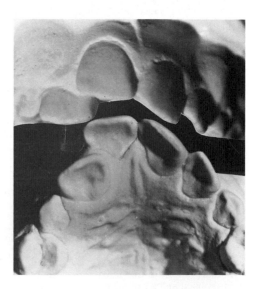

**Figure 11.39.** Maxillary dentition with three central incisors of similar size and shape.

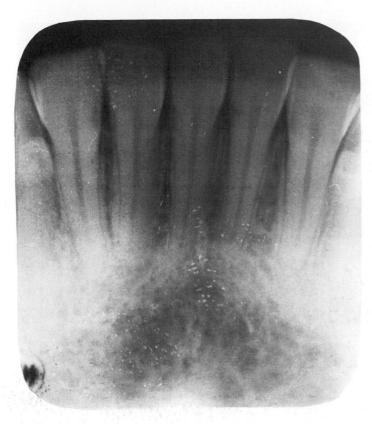

**Figure 11.40.** Radiograph of the mandibular incisor region depicting three central incisors and two lateral incisors, all nonfused and with normal pulp cavities.

## 7. UNUSUAL DENTITIONS

During a routine check of a dental hygiene student's completed oral prophylaxis on a 23-year-old man, the instructor noticed what appeared to be an oblique ridge and cusp of Carabelli on the left mandibular first molar. Alginate impressions were made and casts poured (Fig. 11.37). Careful examination of the casts by both the instructor and Dr. Woelfel revealed not only that the mandibular left first molar closely resembled a maxillary first molar, but also that first and second mandibular premolars and first, second, and third mandibular molars on both sides were remarkably similar morphologically to maxillary posterior teeth. The mandibular six anterior teeth were unquestionably mandibular anteriors. The occlusion of the young man's teeth was remarkably good considering the fact that maxillary posterior teeth were occluding against practically identical maxillary teeth on both sides!

A most unusual maxillary dentition with a total of 24 erupted or partially erupted teeth is seen in Figure 11.38. This was the maxillary dentition of a foreign exchange student from Africa. There are four incisors, one canine, six premolars, and 13 molars (five of which somewhat resemble mandibular molars).

An upper dentition with three maxillary central incisors is seen in Figure 11.39, and a mandibular dentition with five incisors is seen in a radiograph (Fig. 11.40). Other examples of morphologically unique teeth are seen in Figure 11.41.

## Acknowledgments

This chapter was contributed by Connie Sylvester, R.D.H., B.A., M.S. Formerly on the faculties of the Ohio State University and the University of Texas Schools of Dental Hygiene, Ms. Sylvester is presently involved in the clinical practice of dental hygiene.

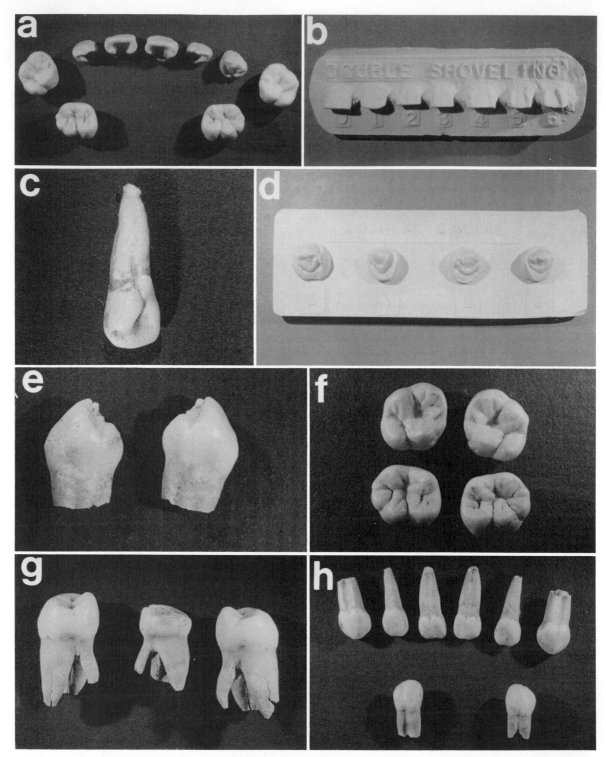

**Figure 11.41.** Unique Morphological characteristics of teeth. **A.** Shovel-shaped permanent incisors from a young Native American dentition (occlusal view). Note the prominent marginal ridges on the lingual surface (see also Fig. 4.1). The labioproximal margins are also reinforced for greater strength, making these double-shoveled. The lingual surface of the maxillary right canine has a distal accessory ridge that appears as an oblique ridge between the lingual ridge and the distal marginal ridge. On the mandibular first molars, there is a sixth cusp on the distal marginal ridge called the tuberculum sextum. **B.** The range of double shoveling from barely discernable labial ridges on the *left* of the figure to prominent ridges on the *right*. **C.** Lingual view of a maxillary left lateral incisor shows an incisor interruption groove at the junction of the prominent mesial and distal marginal ridges. The groove continues across the cervical line onto the root. **D.** Mesial accessory ridge appears as an oblique ridge

**Figure 11.41.** (*continued*) between the lingual ridge and the mesial marginal ridge in San and Hottentot canines. This incisal view shows the range of expression of this canine trait. **E.** Proximal views of contralateral first premolars from a young Native American showing odontomes emanating from the buccal triangular ridges, just lingual to the buccal cusps. **F.** All four first molars from a young Native American. The Maxillary molars illustrate Carabelli's complex and the mandibular molars illustrate the Y shape and + shape groove patterns and tuberculum sextum. The lower right mandibular molar also displays a deflecting wrinkle, which is an enlarged mesiolingual triangular ridge running from the ML cusp first toward the central developmental groove and then distally toward the central pit. **G.** Three examples of distolingual accessory roots in a young Native American; two permanent contralateral first mandibular molars and a deciduous second molar. **H.** Deep labial grooves on maxillary central incisors and on all four canines in the deciduous dentition of a Native American. Note the notching of the cervical line where the labial groove extends across the cervical line.

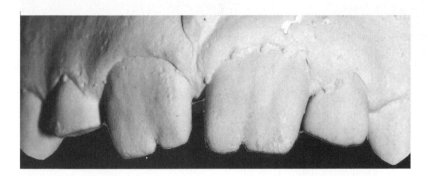

**Figure 11.42.** Hutchinson's (notched) incisors (maxillary) of a 9-year-old female. (Model courtesy of Dmitri J. Haralampopoulos, D.D.S.)

Special thanks to Drs. C.C. Dollens, Rudy Melfi, and Donald Bowers for their gracious assistance in obtaining several of the photographs and radiographs used in this chapter. Also, special thanks to the first-year dental hygiene students at Ohio State University (1977–1987), who brought in numerous anomalies and casts depicting such unusual teeth.

# References

1. Dorland's pocket medical dictionary. Philadelphia: W.B. Saunders, 1965.
2. Smith RM, Turner JE, Robbins, ML. Atlas of oral pathology. St. Louis: C.V. Mosby, 1981
3. Croll TP, Rains JR, Chen, E. Fusion and gemination in one dental arch: report of case. ASDC J Dent Child 1981;48:297.
4. Rowe AHR, Johns RB, eds. A companion to dental studies: dental anatomy and embryology. Vol. 1, Book 2. Boston: Blackwell Scientific Publications, 1981.
5. McDonald TP. An American Board of Orthodontics case report. Am J Orthod 1981;80:437–442.
6. Fuller JL, Denehy GE. Concise dental anatomy and morphology. Chicago: Year Book Publishers, Inc, 1984:264–5.
7. Jones AW. Supernumerary mandibular premolars. Report of a case in a patient of mongoloid origins. Br J Oral Surg 1981;19:305–306.
8. Robinson HB, Miller AS. *Colby, Kerr and Robinson's Color Atlas of Oral Pathology*. Philadelphia: J.B. Lippincott Comp., 1983, p.38.
9. Primosch RE. Anterior supernumerary teeth—assessment and surgical intervention in children. Pediatr Dentistry 1981;3:204–215.
10. Ranta R, Ylipaavalniemi P. Developmental course of supernumerary premolars in childhood: report of two cases. ASDC J Dent Child 1981;48:385–388.
11. Rubin MM, Nevins A, Berg M, Borden B. A comparison of identical twins in relation to three dental anomalies. Multiple supernumerary teeth, juvenile periodontosis, and zero caries incidence. Oral Surg 1981;52:391–394.
12. Zvolanek JW. Maxillary lateral incisor anomalies in identical twins. Dent Radiogr Photog, 1981;54:17–18.
13. Hemmig SB. Third and fourth molar fusion. Oral Surg 1979;48:572.
14. Good DL, Berson RB. A supernumerary tooth fused to a maxillary permanent central incisor. Pediatr Dentistry 1980;2:294–296.
15. Powell RE. Fusion of maxillary lateral incisor and supernumerary tooth. Oral Surg 1981; 51(3):331.
16. Speiser AM, Bikofsky VM. Premolars with double occlusal surfaces. JADA 1981;103:600–601.

17. Melfi, RC. Permar's Oral embryology and microscopic anatomy. Philadelphia, Lea and Febiger, 1988, pp 79–82.
18. Myers CL. Treatment of a talon-cusp incisor: report of case. ASDC J Dent Child 1980;47:119–121.
19. Hayward JR. Cuspid gigantism. Oral Surg 1980;49:500–501.
20. Ruprecht A, Singer DL. Macrodontia of the mandibular left first premolar. Oral Surg 1979;48:573.
21. Becker A, Smith P, Behar, R. The incidence of anomalous maxillary lateral incisors in relation to palatally-displaced cuspids. Angle Orthod 1981;51:24–29.
22. McKibben DR, Brearley LJ. Radiographic determination of the prevalence of selected dental anomalies in children. J Dent Child 1971;28:390–398.
23. Nazif MM, Ruffalo RC, Zullo T. Impacted supernumerary teeth: a survey of fifty cases. JADA 1983;106:201–204.
24. Hamner JE, Witkop CJ, Metro PS. Taurodontism. Oral Surg 1964;18:409–418.
25. Pindborg JJ. Pathology of the dental hard tissues. Philadelphia: W.B. Saunders, 1970:15–73.
26. Schachter H. A treated case of transposed upper canine. Dent Rec 1951;71:105–108.
27. DeJong TE. Rotatio dentis. Gegenbaurs Morphologisches Jahrbuch 1965;108:67–70.
28. Schulze C. Developmental abnormalities of the teeth and jaws. In: Gorlin RJ, Goldman HM, eds. Thoma's oral pathology. 6th ed. St. Louis: C.V. Mosby, 1970, 138–140.
29. Rothberg J, Kopel M. Early versus late removal of mesiodens: a clinical study of 375 children. Comp Cont Educ Pract 1984;5:115–120.
30. Paulson RB, Gottlieb LJ, Sciulli PW, et al. Double-rooted maxillary primary canines. ASDC J Dent Child 1985;52: 195–198.
31. Bimstein E, Bystrom E. Birooted bilateral maxillary primary canines. ASDC J Dent Child 1982;49:217–218.
32. Kelly JR. Birooted primary canines. Oral Surg 1978;46:872.
33. Brown CK. Bilateral bifurcation of the maxillary deciduous cuspids. Oral Surg 1975;40:817.
34. Kroll SO. Double rooted maxillary primary canines. Oral Surg 1980;49:379.
35. Bryant RH Jr, Bowers DF. Four birooted primary canines: report of a case. ASDC J Dent Child 1982;49:441–442.
36. Goldman HM. Anomalies of Teeth (Part 1). Comp Cont Educ Pract 1981;2:358–367.
37. Jackson M, Leeds, LD. Upper canine in position of upper central. Brit. Dent. J 1951;90:243.
38. Curran JD, Baker CG. Roentgeno-oddities. Oral Surg 1973;41:906–907.
39. Dr. Rudy Melfi, Columbus, Ohio, personal communication

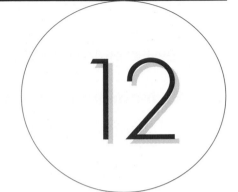

# Operative Dentistry

Rickne C. Scheid

This chapter presents a brief overview of operative and restorative dentistry as it is taught at the Ohio State University College of Dentistry. After studying this chapter, students should be able to identify and classify dental caries and understand the philosophy regarding tooth preparations, type of restorations, related terminology, and appropriate preventive measures.

## SECTION I. DEFINITIONS

### A. Operative Dentistry

Operative dentistry may be defined as that aspect of dentistry that is involved in the prevention and treatment of defects in the enamel and dentin of individual teeth (1). The most frequently occurring defects are the result of dental caries, attrition or abrasion, erosion, fracture, and the breakdown of old restorations. Dental caries and the resultant intracoronal restorations needed to replace the lost tooth structure are the aspects of operative dentistry discussed in this chapter.

In a 1979–80 survey representing 45.3 million United States school children between the ages of 5 and 17 years, the estimated prevalence of breakdown in permanent dentition was 4.77 decayed, missing, or filled surfaces per child (2). Although reports have shown a worldwide decrease in the incidence of coronal caries, especially in children and adolescents, ranging from 10–60% depending on the article cited, it is estimated that the number of hours required to meet all needs for operative dental treatment will increase by the year 2000 (3). This increase is due primarily to the greater number of older patients and the number of dentulous adults. The prevalence of root caries in the elderly is increasing (4), with one study reporting 75% of elderly women with clinically detectable root caries (5).

Many texts on operative dentistry include discussions on the construction of crowns, which are actually extracoronal restorations.

## B. Intracoronal Restorations

Intracoronal restorations (within the crown of the tooth) involve restorative material such as amalgam, composite, and cast metal for inlays or onlays (covering the cusps) that are placed into preparations within the tooth. The details of intracoronal preparations and restorations on individual teeth comprise much of what is taught in operative dentistry courses.

## C. Extracoronal Restorations

Extracoronal restorations (surrounding and covering the tooth) include crowns of gold, semi- or nonprecious metal, or porcelain, which surround or cover the entire tooth in a relatively thin outer shell, gaining retention from the encompassing shape, nearly parallel walls, accurate fit, and the cement. Retention of large onlays or crowns may be enhanced through mechanical bonding by etching the tooth or crown, and chemical bonding utilizing a glass ionomer or polycarboxylate cement.

## D. Restorative Dentistry

Restorative dentistry includes not only the prevention and treatment of defects of individual teeth, as in operative dentistry, but also the placement of extracoronal restorations (crowns) to restore badly broken down teeth or to attach or anchor a fixed bridge to replace missing teeth. Thus, restorative dentistry involves the restoration of lost tooth structure and/or lost teeth with the ultimate goal of reestablishing a healthy, functioning, and comfortable dentition. Patient education and preventive treatment are included in the discussion and are important aspects of patient care. Prevention and treatment should be based on personalized risk-based assessment of each patient's caries history and status (6).

## E. Dental Caries

Dental caries, known more commonly as tooth decay, is the breakdown or softening of enamel and dentin that results from the destructive process of an acid-producing bacteria layer (called dental plaque) located on the tooth surface. Bacterial action is greatly accelerated by the presence of certain carbohydrates in the diet, especially those found in sugar-containing food items such as candy, soft drinks, honey, pastries, and so forth (7). *Streptococcus mutans* is a type of bacteria known to contribute to the caries process.

# SECTION II. CLASSIFICATION OF CARIOUS LESIONS

There are two major classifications of tooth decay based on the anatomy of the surface involved: smooth surface and pit and fissure carious lesions.

## A. Pit and Fissure Carious Lesions

Pit and fissure carious lesions, also classified by Dr. G.V. Black as Class I caries (8), begin in the depth of pits and fissures in enamel which may occur due to incomplete fusion of enamel lobes during tooth development (Fig. 12.1**A**). These areas are nearly impossible to keep clean. Recalling the location of pits and fissures, this type of decay is most likely to occur on the occlusal surfaces of posterior teeth (molars and premolars), including the ends of the buccal and lingual grooves, which may terminate in pits (found most frequently on the lingual surface of maxillary molars and the buccal surface of mandibular molars). This type of decay is also frequently found in the lingual fossae of maxillary incisors where distinct pits or fissures occur.

Small pit and fissure caries can be detected at the surface as an almost undetectable area externally, and, as it progresses deeper into the tooth, it follows the direction of the enamel rods, widening as it approaches the dentinoenamel junction (occlusal surface in Fig. 12.1). Once into dentin, it spreads out widely at the dentinoenamel junction due to decreased mineral content in the dentin (occlusal surface in Fig. 12.1**B**).

## B. Smooth Surface Carious Lesions

Smooth surface carious lesions occur on the smooth surfaces of the anatomic crown of a tooth, in the areas that are most inaccessible to the natural cleansing action of the lips, cheeks, and tongue. These areas include the proximal surfaces of teeth just cervical to the proximal contact, and the facial and lingual surfaces just cervical to the crest of curvature of the crown in the gingival one-third). Smooth surface lesions include G.V. Black's Classifications II, III, IV, and V, which are discussed individually in Section V of this chapter.

Smooth surface caries spreads within enamel differently than the pit and fissure type. Smooth surface caries begins as a broad area on the external surface, and then narrows as it progresses deeper toward the dentinoenamel junction. Once it reaches dentin, it spreads out wider, just like pit and fissure caries (mesial surface in Fig. 12.1**B**).

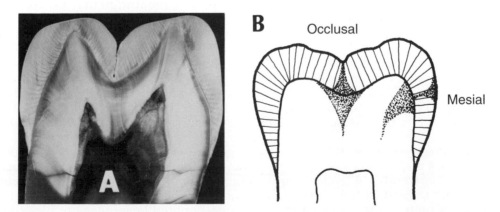

**Figure 12.1.** **A.** Photomicrograph of a thinly ground section of a mandibular molar prepared by the late Professor Dorothy Permar. Notice the very deep fissure beneath the central groove (no decay) and that a considerable amount of attrition has flattened both cusps. A large amount of reparative dentin has formed and just about filled in the buccal and lingual pulp horns. **B.** Cross-section of a mandibular molar showing the usual pattern of spreading decay. The occlusal lesion (Class I, pit and fissure) is small externally, widening towards the dentinoenamel junction. Once within dentin, the caries spreads out laterally as well as progressing toward the pulp. The mesial lesion (Class II, smooth surface) is broad externally, narrowing toward the dentinoenamel junction. Once within dentin, this lesion spreads out laterally (like the Class I), as well as progressing toward the pulp.

Root caries is yet another type of smooth surface caries that occurs on cementum, most frequently in older patients who have had gingival recession resulting in exposure of root surfaces to the oral environment. This type of caries is a softening destructive process (9) that may not require a restoration if there is only minimal cavitation. Treatment in these cases may include polishing the root, which then should then be kept clean by the patient, treated by the dentist regularly with fluorides, and by the daily use of fluoride-containing paste at home.

## SECTION III. PRINCIPLES OF CAVITY PREPARATION

These principles have been modified from G.V. Black's original principles (8).

A successful cavity preparation for a restorative material such as dental amalgam, composite, resin, or cast metal is designed to allow placement and maintenance of the restorative material and, at the same time, to ensure the preservation of remaining tooth structure. To accomplish this, the dentist must simultaneously apply several basic principles of cavity preparation.

## A. Establish an Outline Form

An outline form of a cavity preparation developed by the dentist is established by removing the least amount of tooth structure possible, yet adhering to these principles:

### 1. EXTEND FOR PREVENTION

The dentist enlarges the preparation in enamel beyond the specific area of decay in order to include adjacent tooth structure prone to developing future decay. This may involve enlarging a preparation for a pit and fissure lesion to include adjacent deep pits and fissures, even though the adjacent pits and fissures have not yet become carious (Fig. 12.7). Similarly, when developing the cavity preparation for smooth surface carious lesions, the outline of the preparation may be extended to include adjacent smooth surface areas likely to become carious. That is, if one small area of tooth next to the gingiva has decay, the preparation might be enlarged to include more of the tooth adjacent to that caries-prone area (especially if the adjacent area shows signs of early decay such as white decalcified areas). Because of improved fluoride treatment (in community water, toothpastes, rinses, and topical applications applied periodically by the dentist) and increased efforts to educate the population regarding oral hygiene, present day conservatism generally minimizes the need for preventive extension on smooth surface lesions (see Figs. 12.12 and 12.27).

The degree of extension for prevention depends on the patient's susceptibility to new caries and involves such factors as the age of the patient, his or her rate of caries activity, personal oral hygiene, and dietary habits (Fig. 12.7). Tooth preparations on a younger patient with multiple areas of active decay, poor oral hygiene, and frequent intake of high sugar snacks and popular carbonated beverages are likely to require more extension for prevention than a preparation for an older patient with a lower caries rate, better eating habits, and good oral hygiene.

### 2. EXTEND TO SOUND ENAMEL

The dentist enlarges the preparation outline so it extends to enamel that has no signs of beginning (incipient) or active caries, and is supported by, or resting on, sound dentin (i.e., not undermined by the spread of caries within the dentin). Since enamel is brittle, if it is not supported by sound dentin, the unsupported enamel rods may fracture off, leaving a gap between tooth and the restorative material (Fig. 12.2).

## 3. EXTEND FOR ACCESS

A restoration outline must be large enough for the dentist to assure that all caries are removed, and that instruments required to place the filling material will fit. A small narrow initial cut through the enamel might not allow the detection of all of the lateral spread of caries since it spreads laterally when it reaches the dentinoenamel junction (Fig. 12.2). Further, even when the removal of all caries can be visually or tactually verified, a very small initial preparation might be too small for the instruments to fit into the preparation as required to place the restorative material without voids.

## 4. RESISTANCE FORM

The dentist must design a preparation to ensure room for an adequate thickness of restorative material for strength, and sufficient remaining solid tooth structure to withstand occlusal forces. If depth is inadequate, the restoration could break. If the remaining tooth is too thin, it could fracture. One solution to protect thin remaining tooth structure is to cover it with cast onlays or crowns, as discussed in Section VI of this chapter. Another is to acid etch and bond a sleeve of composite material over the thin enamel (Fig. 12.24).

## B. Provide Retention Form

Retention form is the internal design of a preparation that prevents the restoration from falling out or becoming dislodged. The methods for providing retention differ depending on the restorative material and on the location of the carious lesion. Methods for establishing appropriate retention form for various restorative materials are described in Section V.

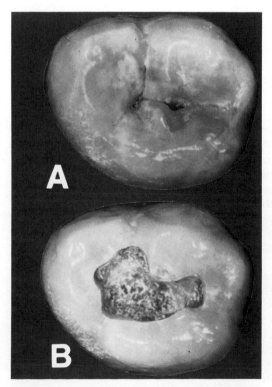

**Figure 12.2.** Extending the preparation for access and extending to sound enamel. **A.** A Class I lesion seen as small pits on the occlusal surface. **B.** The same tooth after preparation showing the extension necessary to obtain access (convenience form) to remove decay, which spread out laterally beneath the dentinoenamel junction (Fig. 12.1). This outline form is also necessary to end the preparation on sound enamel walls, which are supported by sound dentin (not softer caries).

## C. Remove Caries and Treat the Pulp

All principles of the cavity preparation described up to this point assume that caries has spread minimally, just into the outer 0.5 mm of dentin. The dentist usually prepares these conservative cavity preparations with a high-speed dental handpiece using carbide or diamond burs that cut quickly, reducing potentially damaging heat by using an effective water coolant spray. When removing carious lesions that have progressed deeper than 0.5 mm into dentin, the dentist selects slowly rotating round burs (in slow-speed handpieces) or hand instruments. The slow-speed handpiece permits the dentist to differentiate softer carious dentin from the harder, sound dentin.

When tooth structure has to be removed deeper than 0.5 mm into dentin, it is advisable to replace this lost dentin with a dental cement prior to placing the permanent restoration. Various dental cements have been developed for this purpose. When used in the appropriate combination and in the correct order, they can provide thermal insulation, sedation of the pulp, and stimulation producing secondary dentin.

## D. Finish the Walls

This refers to using a slow-speed handpiece with appropriate burs, discs, and hand instruments (chisel type) designed to smoothly plane the walls while removing unsound enamel (i.e., enamel that is crazed or cracked or not supported by sound dentin).

## E. Clean the Preparation and Evaluate

The operator removes all crumbs of tooth debris, old cement bases, hemorrhage, and saliva from the walls of the preparation so the restorative material will contact only sound, clean tooth structure. The preparation is then evaluated to ensure that all of the principles of cavity preparation have been addressed.

# SECTION IV. RESTORATIVE MATERIALS (OR FILLING MATERIALS)

**AMALGAM** is the most widely used restorative material owing to its ease of placement and relatively low cost. It is silver in color and is packed into a preparation in successive small increments that eventually cohere and become hard enough to withstand chewing forces. Therefore, it is used for restorations on the chewing (or occlusal) surfaces of posterior teeth and other restorations when maintenance of proximal and occlusal contacts is important but when aesthetics is not a factor (Figs. 12.3 and 12.4).

**AESTHETIC RESTORATIVE MATERIALS,** such as composite resin and glass ionomer, are being increasingly used due to patients' demands for aesthetic restorations.

Composite resin is a tooth-colored restorative material that is applied as a plastic-like mass into a preparation. It can be hardened quickly. Due to initial concerns about the strength and abrasion resistance of composite resins (10, 11), it was historically used primarily for restoring the proximal surfaces of anterior teeth and the facial surfaces of teeth on which aesthetics is a chief concern (Figs. 12.18, 12.27**B,** and 12.28). As composite resin properties and placement techniques improved, it is now being used more often in posterior occlusal surfaces. One recent longitudinal study rated composite restorations after 10 years (using an United States Public Health system of evaluation) to be over 90% satisfactory for

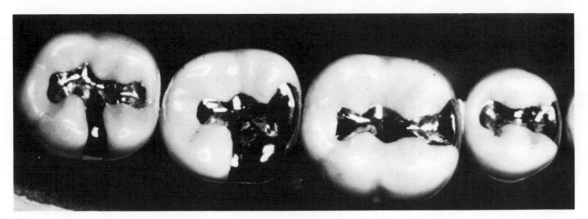

**Figure 12.3.** Class I and II amalgam restorations, mandibular arch. *Left:* Class I OBA (occlusobuccal amalgam) on tooth number 32. *Left-center:* A Class II MOBA (mesio-occlusobuccal amalgam) with a mesiobuccal cusp buildup or replacement on tooth number 31. *Right-center:* A Class II MOA (mesio-occlusal amalgam) on tooth number 30. *Right:* A Class II MOA on tooth number 29.

color stability, surface smoothness, anatomical form, lack of recurrent caries, and pulp response (12). Only marginal adaptation was below 90%, with a score of 81%. With recent physical property improvements (13) and a new generation of dentin bonding agents that can withstand contraction shrinkage (14), composite restorations may be used even more widely in the future.

Preliminary studies in the 1980s using glass ionomer cements to restore erosion lesions showed a high degree of success after 1–3 years. These materials bond to dentin chemically, are reasonably aesthetic and contain fluoride, which reduces the possibility of recurrent caries (15, 16).

**CAST GOLD** or semiprecious alloys, when used for inlays, onlays (or even full crowns), are constructed on accurate models (dies) of the patient's teeth (Figs. 12.11, 12.30, and 12.33). These cast metal restorations require considerably more time to construct than composite resin or amalgam restorations because of the laboratory procedures. Consequently, they are more expensive for the patient.

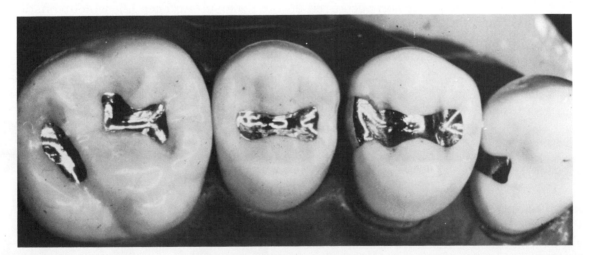

**Figure 12.4.** Class I, II, and III amalgam restorations, maxillary arch. *Left:* Class I OA (occlusal amalgams) on tooth number 3 with two parts separated by a strong intact oblique ridge. *Left-center:* A Class I OA (occlusal amalgam) on tooth number 4. *Right-center:* A Class II DOA (disto-occlusal amalgam) on tooth number 5. *Right:* A Class III DA (distal amalgam) on tooth number 6. These are all very conservative restorations, extended only as wide as necessary for access and prevention.

An inlay is a cast restoration that fits within the prepared tooth cavity but does not overlay the cusps, in contrast to an onlay, which overlays or replaces cusps (Fig. 12.11). Onlays (as well as full crowns) are recommended when the tooth structure remaining after tooth preparation is frail and needs to be protected from occlusal forces. The greater strength of the cast metal versus amalgam permits optimum protection and strength with less bulk of metal, resulting in less occlusal reduction of tooth structure. Further, cast metal restorations can be contoured more perfectly and are more inert in the mouth (i.e., cast restorations have better marginal stability over time). For these reasons, an inlay may be selected over amalgam for patients who desire and can afford the cast restoration, even when the restoration will be quite conservative and will not require onlaying.

Ceramic inlay/onlays are becoming an aesthetic alternative to cast inlay/onlays due to advanced processing methods and bonding techniques which improve fit (17).

# SECTION V. G.V. BLACK'S CLASSIFICATION OF DECAY, CAVITY PREPARATION, AND RESTORATION

The discussion of tooth restoration that follows assumes that the tooth to be prepared is periodontally sound (stable alveolus and healthy gingiva) and that the maintenance of the tooth is an integral part of the overall treatment for that patient. The five classifications of decay devised and published by Dr. G.V. Black in 1908 are still appropriate (8), although the principles of cavity preparation are now applied uniquely for each class of decay and each new restorative material.

## A. Class I Type of Dental Caries, Cavity Preparation, and Restoration

### 1. DEFINITION

The Class I lesion (Figs. 12.2**A** and 12.5) is a pit and fissure lesion that is found wherever pits and fissures occur; that is, on the occlusal surfaces of posterior teeth, on the occlusal two-thirds of the buccal and lingual surfaces of molars (buccal or lingual pits and grooves), and on the lingual surface of maxillary incisors (cingulum pits or grooves). In a 1979–80 survey of United States school children aged 5 to 17 years, 54% of all carious lesions occurred on the occlusal surfaces (2), which constitute one-fifth of the surfaces of any premolar or molar.

### 2. CLINICAL DETECTION

Carious pits or fissures may or may not be discolored and may be filled with food debris, so that it is necessary to clean the tooth, use a good light, and dry the tooth

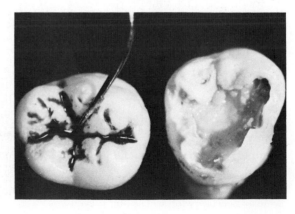

**Figure 12.5.** Class I carious lesions. On the *left* is a lesion on tooth number 18 at the depth of stained grooves, which must be detected with a sharp explorer by feeling for tugback. On the right is an enormous, clinically obvious lesion on tooth number 2 that has resulted in the collapse of most of the occlusal enamel by the undermining spread of the decay in dentin (Fig. 12.1). Both teeth appear to be restorable, but the larger one would probably require endodontics (root canal therapy) and an inlay-onlay or crown.

with air in order to properly examine the suspect areas. Pits or fissures that appear deep or wide and are surrounded by enamel that is chalky or more opaque (less translucent) than the rest of the enamel, are areas that should be investigated. The presence of caries at the depth of these suspicious defects is confirmed by probing with a very sharp explorer. If, after pressing the explorer into the defect with moderate to firm pressure, there is *tug-back,* or *resistance* to removing the explorer, this confirms the presence of softness or caries in the defect. Even in the absence of obvious *tug-back,* if an area of enamel around a pit or fissure is less translucent, this condition may be considered to be reliable evidence of attack (18). It is important to avoid undue pressure with the explorer point, especially in larger, frank lesions (Fig. 12.5, *right*), because injudicious probing may cause pain.

## 3. RADIOGRAPHIC DETECTION OF DENTAL CARIES

Refer to Figure 12.6.

Class I caries appears as a radiolucency or darkening through enamel and spreads out in dentin. Detection of a Class I lesion is usually not possible on the radiograph until it is quite deep into dentin because the lesion is superimposed between the thick buccal and lingual surfaces of enamel which show up whiter (radiopaque), thereby masking the darker caries. By the time the cavity is visible on the radiograph, the size of the preparation required to remove all of the decay would be considerably deeper (toward the pulp) than if the decay had been detected earlier during a good clinical examination. Thus, early Class I decay can be best diagnosed during a thorough clinical examination (i.e., clean tooth, good lighting, dry field, and a sharp exploring point).

## 4. INDICATIONS FOR RESTORING

Some Class I lesions are difficult to differentiate from noncarious, deep enamel defects. If tug-back occurs with a sharp explorer in a deep pit or fissure, and the surrounding enamel is chalky or less translucent, a restoration is indicated. Certainly, by the time caries is obvious on the radiograph, it would be evident clinically and

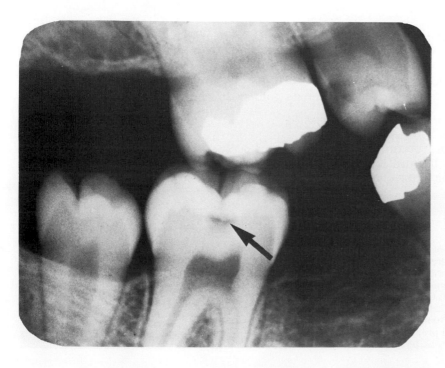

**Figure 12.6.** Radiographic evidence of a Class I lesion on tooth number 31. By the time it appears this deep on the radiograph, the caries has destroyed dentin to such a depth that a thermal-insulating base of some type of dental cement will be needed to protect the pulp from thermal conductivity through the metal filling. This pit and fissure caries could probably have been detected earlier with a good clinical examination. There is also a large distal Class II lesion on tooth number 4, which appears to be rotated (*top right*).

should be restored. However, if tug-back is minimal and without the accompanying evidence, the dentist might consider periodically reevaluating the area during recall appointments, especially if the patient is older and has a low caries rate.

## 5. RESTORATION OF CHOICE

Amalgam is frequently chosen for stress-bearing Class I restorations on occlusal surfaces. For small Class I pits or fissures on posterior teeth where aesthetics are important, composite resins may be used. Pit and fissure sealants can be used as a preventive measure, especially for the young patient. A sealant is a flowable resin that is applied over the unprepared pits and fissures of noncarious, but caries prone, teeth like the one in Figure 12.1**A.** These sealants have been shown to be an effective alternative to amalgam and composite resin which require cavity preparation for each tooth treated (19–21). An initial sealant application for all permanent molars and premolars requires only 15–20 minutes per child (22). A transitional restoration involving composite in a very conservative preparation within enamel, and a sealant, is called a preventive resin restoration.

Cast gold would only be considered for Class I restorations if there were few restorations in the mouth with a low evidence of new decay, or the size of the restoration necessitated onlaying cusps.

## 6. PREPARATION

Certain of G.V. Black's principles of cavity preparation are uniquely applied when restoring the Class I cavity as described here.

### a. Extension for Prevention

Refer to Figure 12.7.

Extension for prevention, to include those pits and fissures adjoining the defects with active decay, should be considered when the patient is young, has a high caries rate, and/or exhibits poor oral hygiene.

### b. Resistance Form

When amalgam is used on a stress bearing surface, a minimum depth of 2.5–3 mm is recommended due to the brittleness of amalgam in thinner layers; whereas, if cast metal is used, a thickness of 1 mm may be sufficient to withstand occlusal forces. Ideally, amalgam meets the unprepared tooth surface at right angles to provide resistance form, whereas gold ends in an overlapping bevel.

### c. Retention

For amalgam, retention is provided in an occlusal preparation by converging the buccal and lingual walls of the preparation towards the occlusal surface, which, due to the slope of the triangular ridges, is coincidentally accomplished by

**Figure 12.7.** Several examples of Class I amalgam preparations showing various degrees of extension for prevention. *Left:* Tooth number 3 with an occlusal and an occlusal-lingual preparation. The preparations are separate since in this case, there was no need to cross the oblique ridge. *Center:* An occlusal amalgam preparation of tooth number 31. *Right:* An occlusobuccal amalgam preparation on tooth number 30.

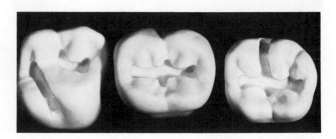

ending the buccal and lingual cavity walls at right angles to the unprepared surface (Fig. 12.8**C**).

For composite preparations, retention is provided by converging opposing walls towards the external surface, and/or by acid etching the enamel to produce microscopic irregularities or undercuts on the surface. Then, flowable resins can form retentive resin tags that mechanically lock into the microscopic retentive features of the etched enamel (Fig. 12.21**B**). Layers of the stronger composite resins can then be chemically bonded to this flowable resin layer.

For cast gold inlays or onlays, retention is provided by preparing the opposing internal walls of the preparation with a slight (5–7°) divergence toward the occlusal (Fig. 12.15), thus allowing the solid casting to be seated snugly within the tooth, somewhat like a glass stopper fitting into the opening of a decanter (Fig. 12.11). The dental cement used between the inlay and tooth provides the permanent retention by sealing the beveled margins and by setting to hardness at the interface between the slight irregularities of the enamel walls of the preparation and those of the casting. Some dental cements chemically bond to the calcium of the tooth and can be mechanically attached to the etched surface of the metal casting (glass ionomer and polycarboxylate types).

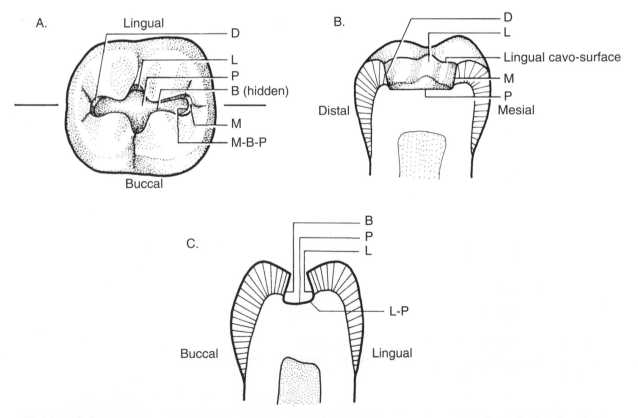

**Figure 12.8.** A conservative Class I cavity preparation for amalgam on tooth number 31. **A.** Occlusal surface showing extension for prevention into the major grooves. **B.** Mesiodistal cross-section of the same tooth showing the ideal depth of the pulpal floor, just into dentin (about 0.5 mm). The lingual cavosurface is also identified where the lingual wall of the preparation joins the unprepared surface of the tooth. **C.** Buccolingual cross-section of the same tooth showing the convergence of the vertical buccal and lingual walls toward the occlusal for retention and resistance form. Key for nomenclature: *B* = Buccal wall; *L* = Lingual wall; *M* = Mesial wall; *D* = Distal wall; *P* = Pulpal wall or floor. Example of a line angle: *L-P* is the linguopulpal line angle. Example of a point angle: *M-B-P* is the mesiobuccopulpal point angle in *A, above left.*

### 7. CAVITY NOMENCLATURE

Refer to Figure 12.8.

The occlusal preparation is like a room with four walls and a *pulpal* floor or wall, so-called because it is over the pulp. The four walls are named after the most closely related tooth surface, namely, *buccal, mesial, lingual,* and *distal.*

A line angle in the preparation is the angular region where two walls join. There are eight internal line angles in the Class I preparation. These are named by combining the terms for the two walls that join to make up each line angle, changing the suffix of the first word from "al" to "o." It makes no difference which wall is named first. For example, the junction of the pulpal floor and distal wall is the distopulpal or pulpodistal line angle. All possible line angles include four horizontal ones—distopulpal, mesiopulpal, buccopulpal, and linguopulpal—and four vertical ones—mesiobuccal, distobuccal, mesiolingual, and distolingual.

The term that describes the junction of any wall of the preparation with the un-prepared tooth structure is called the cavosurface. The cavosurface, therefore, is the outline that encircles the preparation and restoration. An occlusal restoration where the buccal wall of a preparation meets the uncut surface is the buccal cavosurface; where the lingual wall ends is known as the lingual cavosurface, and so on (Fig. 12.8**B**).

Finally, there are four *point angles* in a Class I preparation, each formed by the *junction of three walls.* Point angles are named after the three walls that form them: *mesiolinguopulpal, mesiobuccopulpal* (Fig. 12.8**A**), *distolinguopulpal, distobuccopulpal.* Since the junction of walls in a preparation is often rounded, line angles and point angles may be small, general areas rather than sharp angles or points.

A Class I restoration is properly identified by naming the *surfaces involved* and *material used.* For example, an amalgam on tooth #14 involving the occlusal surface with a lingual extension would be abbreviated OLA, #14. A lower left first molar with an occlusal amalgam and buccal extension would be an OBA, #19 (Fig. 12.3). A buccal or lingual pit restored with composite would be a BC or LC, followed or preceded by the tooth number.

## B. Class II Type of Dental Caries, Cavity Preparation, and Restoration

### 1. DEFINITION

A Class II lesion (Fig. 12.9) is one that forms on the smooth proximal surface of posterior teeth just cervical to proximal contact. It results from inadequate plaque removal in these hard to reach interproximal surfaces.

### 2. CLINICAL DETECTION

Refer to Figure 12.9.

Detection of small Class II lesions in the mouth without the aid of radiographs is often difficult due to the inaccessible areas where they form. As the carious lesion increases in size, it may appear as a dark, cavitated area that can be detected by a thin probe (explorer) in the buccal or lingual embrasure. Often, there is a loss of translucency of the enamel seen when examining the overlying marginal ridge. A very large Class II lesion may actually undermine the marginal ridge, causing this ridge of enamel to break off during mastication (Fig. 12.9**B**).

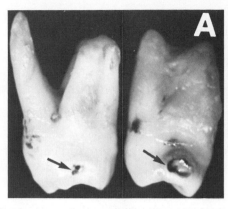
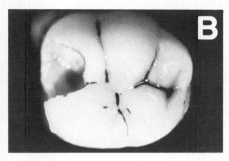

**Figure 12.9.** Class II lesions. **A.** *Left:* An incipient (beginning) lesion without cavitation on the mesial surface of tooth number 14, probably visible only on a radiograph if an adjacent tooth were present. *Right:* A larger Class II lesion with cavitation on the mesial surface of tooth number 15, with color changes to the enamel that would be evident beyond the proximal contact area in the mouth. **B.** A Class II lesion on the mesial surface of tooth number 30 that resulted in the collapse of the entire mesial marginal ridge of enamel.

## 3. RADIOGRAPHIC DETECTION OF DENTAL CARIES

Refer to Figure 12.10.

Radiographic detection of an incipient Class II lesion is readily accomplished using bitewing radiographs. A Class II lesion is seen as a triangular shadow within the enamel just cervical to the proximal contact and within the dentin. A typical spread of a smooth surface lesion is seen on the mesial in Fig. 12.1**B.** The Class II lesion is often visible on the radiograph before it can be detected clinically.

## 4. INDICATIONS FOR RESTORING

Clinically obvious Class II lesions, when cavitated (with a break or hole in the surface) or soft to the explorer, should be restored. The radiographic indication for restoring small lesions is when the lesion begins to spread out into dentin. If the lesion is small enough to be confined to enamel on the radiograph, the dentist must

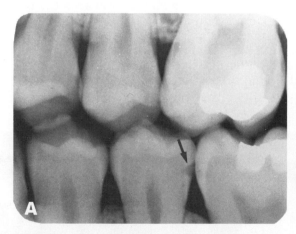
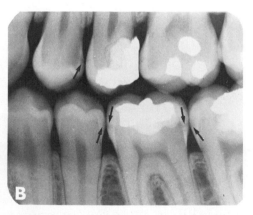

**Figure 12.10. A.** Radiographic evidence of a Class II lesion on the distal surface of tooth number 20 that has barely spread into dentin. Note, the lesion is wider at the surface of enamel than at the *D-E* junction. **B.** Several Class II lesions (*arrows*), some of which are confined to enamel and two that have spread out in dentin. Note the existing Class II amalgam on tooth number 13 with a deep base and large overhang (i.e., excess bulk of amalgam beyond the gingival cavosurface margin).

consider the patient's caries activity, oral hygiene, and age in order to decide whether to restore now or reevaluate at subsequent recall intervals. A young patient with a small carious lesion only two-thirds of the way through enamel, but with many deeper lesions and poor oral hygiene, should probably have this tooth restored, especially since a lesion extends deeper in the tooth than it appears on the radiograph (9).

## 5. RESTORATION OF CHOICE

The Class II restoration of choice includes both amalgam and cast metal inlays or onlays. The larger the preparation (and, therefore, the thinner the remaining tooth structure), the more appropriate a cast metal onlay would be to protect the remaining thin tooth and provide adequate resistance form (Fig. 12.11). Recent improvements in composite restorative materials and techniques have resulted in increased use of this material for Class II restorations, especially when aesthetics is a factor (10).

## 6. PREPARATION

Refer to Figures 12.12 through 12.15.

Usually the Class II preparation includes a Class I portion and therefore the principles for restoring a Class I lesion apply, but the proximal extension (box) adds these new features:

### a. Extension for Prevention

Since to reach the Class II lesions the approach is to cut a "box" apically through the marginal ridge, the preparation is often extended over some of the occlusal surface to include adjacent occlusal pits and fissures as in a Class I preparation. Also, the buccal and lingual walls of the proximal box of Class II preparations are placed beyond the proximal contact areas just into the buccal and lingual embrasures. In this way, the margins can be better evaluated by the dentist and kept clean by the patient.

### b. Retention Form

For amalgam cavity preparations, the buccal and lingual walls of the occlusal portion and the proximal box are made to converge slightly towards the occlusal to prevent the restoration from dislodging occlusally as in the Class I preparation (Figs. 12.12**B** and 12.13**B**). Further, retentive grooves are prepared as internal extensions of the axial wall (buccally and lingually) to prevent the amalgam restoration from dislodging in a proximal direction (*A-B*, or axiobuccal, and *A-L*, or axiolingual, in Fig. 12.13**C** denote the line angles where the retentive features are located).

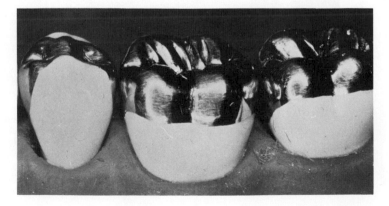

**Figure 12.11.** Class II cast-metal restorations. *Left:* An MODI (mesio-occlusodistal inlay) on tooth number 20. *Center* and *Right:* MODOs (extensive mesio-occlusodistal onlays) on teeth numbers 19 and 18. Onlays are often indicated when remaining tooth structure is thin and requires occlusal protection. Inlays may be recommended for smaller restorations as an option to amalgam for patients with a low caries rate, but due to a much higher expense relative to amalgam, inlays are rarely recommended.

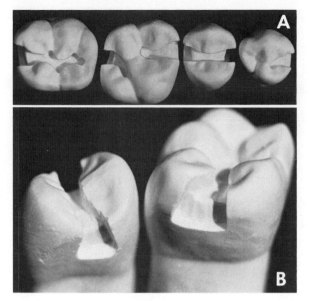

**Figure 12.12.** Models of conservative Class II amalgam preparations. **A.** Occlusal views: *Left:* An MOA (mesio-occlusal amalgam) preparation on tooth number 30. *Left-center:* An MOA, DOA (mesio-occlusal and disto-occlusal amalgam) preparation on tooth number 3 with the oblique ridge intact. *Right-center:* An MODA (mesio-occlusodistal amalgam) preparation on tooth number 5. *Right:* A DOA (disto-occlusal amalgam) preparation on tooth number 28. **B.** Proximal views of Class II amalgam preparations. *Left:* An MODA preparation on tooth number 4. *Right:* An MOA preparation on tooth number 30. Note the convergence of the buccal and lingual walls toward the occlusal for retention and resistance form. When the decay process has progressed deeper or wider, the prepared walls by necessity will be farther apart than these.

For cast metal inlays, opposing buccal and lingual walls must diverge slightly toward the occlusal. The two axial walls in a mesio-occlusodistal inlay preparation must converge slightly towards the occlusal so that an accurate wax model (pattern) and subsequent casting can be seated within the preparation and then removed while constructing and refining the casting (Figs. 12.14 and 12.15). Bevels are formed at the cavosurface so the margins of the casting are thin enough to be more perfectly adapted to the tooth, minimizing the cavosurface gap between tooth and metal. The goal is to minimize the gap between the casting and tooth since this gap is filled with a dental cement, which is not as strong nor as durable as the metal.

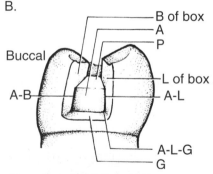

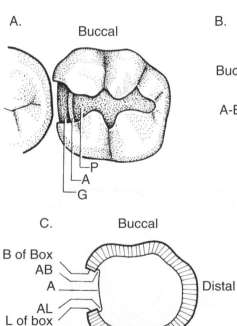

**Figure 12.13.** Conservative Class II preparation for amalgam on tooth number 30. **A.** Occlusal view showing the proximal box extending just through the proximal contact buccally and lingually. **B.** The mesial view showing the slight convergence towards the occlusal of the buccal and lingual walls of the box and axiobuccal and axiolingual line angles where retentive grooves are placed. An example of a point angle: *A-L-G* for Axiolinguogingival is seen. **C.** A cross-section of **B** in the middle third of the crown showing the placement of the retentive grooves entirely within dentin at the axiobuccal and axiolingual line angles. Key for nomenclature: Walls, *B* = Buccal; *P* = Pulpal; *L* = Lingual; *A* = Axial; *G* = Gingival. Example of line angles: *A-B* = Axiobuccal; *A-L* = Axiolingual (location of retentive grooves).

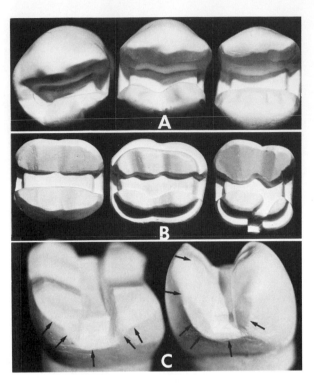

**Figure 12.14.** Models of Class II inlay and onlay preparations. **A.** Three inlay preparations. *Left:* An MOI (mesio-occlusal inlay) preparation on tooth number 21. *Center:* An MODI (mesio-occlusodistal inlay) preparation on tooth number 20. *Right:* An MODI preparation on tooth number 13. **B.** Three onlay preparations. *Left:* A conventional MOD-O (mesio-occlusodistal onlay) preparation on tooth number 18. *Center:* An MOD-O preparation (for ledge-onlays) on tooth number 19. *Right:* An MODL-O (mesio-occlusodistolingual onlay) with conventional onlayed lingual cusps on tooth number 14. **C.** Proximal views of an onlay (*left*) and inlay (*right*) preparation showing the continuous bevel that surrounds the preparation and the divergence of the buccal and lingual walls towards the occlusal. The cavosurface, or outline of the preparation (*marked with arrows*) is at the outer end of the prepared bevels.

## 7. CAVITY NOMENCLATURE

Refer to Figure 12.13.

A Class II preparation such as a mesio-occlusal can be divided into an occlusal portion (which has the same terminology already discussed in the section on Class I preparations) and a proximal box. This proximal box has a buccal and a lingual wall, an axial wall (along the long axis of the tooth), and a gingival wall or floor. For the mesio-occlusal preparation, the mesial wall of the occlusal portion is not present because of the extension of the occlusal preparation, which removed some of the mesial surface of the tooth.

The line angles that are present in the proximal box are *axiopulpal, axiogingival, buccogingival, linguogingival, axiobuccal,* and *axiolingual.*

The axiobuccal and axiolingual line angles are where the retentive grooves for an amalgam preparation are placed. In a mesio-occlusodistal preparation, each line angle is differentiated by stating whether it is in the mesial or distal box. For example, there are two axiopulpal line angles in the mesio-occlusodistal amalgam preparation:

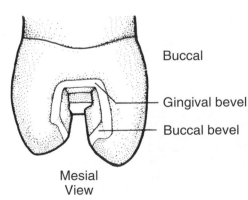

Buccal

Gingival bevel

Buccal bevel

Mesial View

**Figure 12.15.** Diagram of a conservative Class II MOD inlay preparation on a maxillary premolar. Note that the buccal and lingual walls of the preparation diverge toward the occlusal, allowing the casting to be seated. Notice also that the preparation ends with continuous bevels that allow a thin overlap of the metal, which can be burnished or adapted more closely to the enamel with a blunt instrument.

one is the axiopulpal line angle of the mesial box and the other is the axiopulpal line angle of the distal box. The point angles in each box include buccoaxiogingival, linguoaxiogingival, buccoaxiopulpal, and linguoaxiopulpal.

The Class II preparation for amalgam may involve only two surfaces, such as mesio-occlusal or disto-occlusal, abbreviated MOA or DOA. A mesio-occlusodistal amalgam preparation is abbreviated MODA. For inlays (I), or onlays (O), the abbreviation would be MOI, DOI, MODI and MO-O, DO-O and MOD-O, respectively.

## C. Class III Type of Dental Caries, Cavity Preparation, and Restoration

### 1. DEFINITION

The Class III lesion (Fig. 12.16) is a smooth surface lesion that is found on the proximal surface of anterior teeth, just cervical to the proximal contact, but *not involving the incisal angle* (or corner) of the tooth.

### 2. CLINICAL DETECTION

An incipient Class III lesion can usually be detected clinically by carefully examining the enamel facially or lingually for changes in translucency (increased opacity). These changes are most evident when a source of light (such as fiber optics) is placed lingually against the proximal of the tooth, revealing the change in translucency facially. An area of caries appears more opaque than sound enamel.

### 3. RADIOGRAPHIC DETECTION OF DENTAL CARIES

Refer to Figure 12.17.

Periapical radiographs of the anterior teeth (and the bitewing radiographs for the distal of the canines) may be used to detect Class III lesions. The location (just cervical to the proximal contact) and pattern of spread is typical of smooth surface lesions (Fig. 12.1**B**).

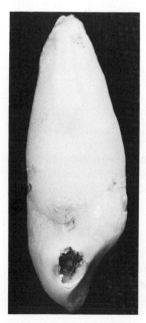

**Figure 12.16.** Class III smooth surface lesion on the mesial of tooth number 6 with an area of obvious cavitation or break in the enamel surface. If this lesion involved any more of the mesial incisal angle, it would become a Class IV, rather than a Class III.

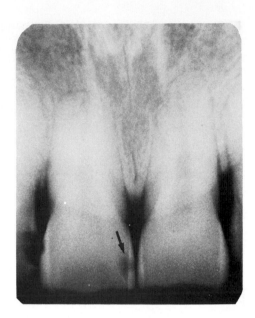

**Figure 12.17.** Radiographic evidence of a Class III lesion on the mesial of tooth number 8. Note the characteristic smooth surface spread or widening of the decay at the dentinoenamel junction.

## 4. INDICATIONS FOR RESTORING

The indications for restoring a Class III lesion are the same as for a Class II lesion: i.e., if the surface is cavitated or soft to the explorer, or has reached the dentin as seen on the radiograph or through transillumination (directing a bright fiberoptic light source through the proximal tooth enamel to detect the changes in translucency inherent in a carious lesion) (Fig. 12.17).

## 5. RESTORATIONS OF CHOICE

Since the Class III lesion occurs in a nonstress-bearing area that is often of aesthetic concern to the patient, a composite resin (tooth-colored plastic modified resin) is usually the restoration of choice. The distal proximal surface of canines serves to preserve the arch form of the posterior teeth, however, and composite in this area could wear flat over time, permitting mesial drift of the premolars. Therefore, on the distal of canines, a conservative Class II amalgam might be used (Figs. 12.4 and 12.18**B**).

## 6. PREPARATION

Refer to Figures 12.19 and 12.20.

### a. Class III Lesions: Approach to the Decay

For all Class III lesions, the approach to the decay, whenever possible, is from the lingual of the tooth so the facial enamel is preserved for maximum aesthetic effect (Figs. 12.19**A** and **C**, and 12.20**A** and **B**). Extension for prevention is minimal in the Class III preparation since the dentist wants to preserve as much enamel as possible for aesthetic reasons, and because the anterior teeth may be easier to keep clean.

### b. Retention

Retention form may be obtained by simply removing the decay that has spread out at the dentinoenamel junction, resulting in a preparation that is wider internally than externally. Retentive pits or grooves may also be used as extensions of the axial wall in order to improve retention for either a composite or amalgam Class III preparation (Fig. 12.20).

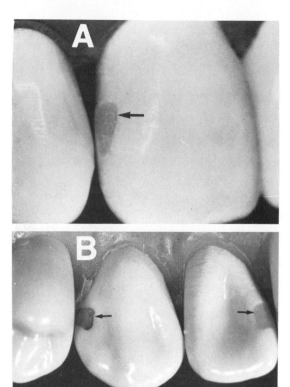

**Figure 12.18.** Class III restorations. **A.** A DC (distal composite) with labial approach on tooth number 8. **B.** *Left:* The DA (distal amalgam) with lingual approach on tooth number 11; metal is used here to maintain the distal contact. *Right:* The MC (mesial composite) with lingual approach on tooth number 10. (The dark shade of the composite was used to improve visibility in the photograph.)

Another means of affording retention and reducing leakage at the cavosurface margin involves etching the surrounding enamel with an acid prior to the insertion of the composite resin material into the cavity preparation, to produce a microscopically irregular surface (Fig. 12.21**B**). The resin can flow into these irregularities and harden, thus locking the restoration in place.

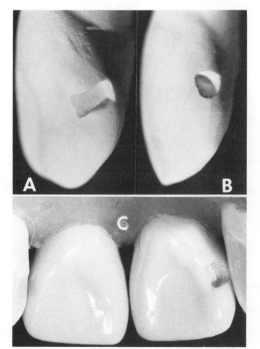

**Figure 12.19.** Class III cavity preparations. **A.** A model of a DA (distal amalgam) preparation with lingual approach on tooth number 6. Note the box-like shape and axioincisal retentive groove in the shadow (the axiogingival retentive groove is hidden). **B.** A model of the DC (distal composite) preparation with facial approach on tooth number 10. Note the generally triangular form. **C.** A DC (distal composite) preparation with lingual approach on tooth number 8. Note the axioincisal retentive feature. (The axiogingival retentive feature is less visible here.)

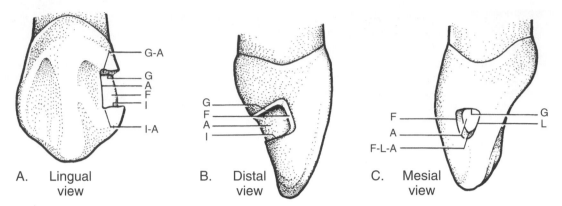

A. Lingual view

B. Distal view

C. Mesial view

**Figure 12.20.** Several Class III preparations. **A.** The lingual view of the Class III amalgam preparation, lingual approach, on the distal of the canine, tooth number 6. Retentive grooves are evident at the cavosurface of the gingivoaxial and incisoaxial line angles. **B.** The distal view of a Class III composite preparation, lingual approach. Note the slight convergence of the incisal and lingual wall toward the lingual for retention. This preparation also has retentive grooves (or pits) at the incisoaxial and gingivoaxial line angles, but they do not extend to the cavosurface. The gingivoaxial groove is in the shadow between *G* and *A*. **C.** The mesial view of a Class III composite preparation, labial approach. Note the triangular shape. Retentive features are found internally at the axiogingival line angle and the faciolinguoaxial point angle. Key for nomenclature: For lingual approach (Diagrams **A** and **B**): *G* = Gingival; *A* = Axial; *F* = Facial or Labial; *I* = Incisal. Example of the angles are the retentive features *G-A* and *I-A* for the gingivoaxial and incisoaxial line angles. For the labial (or facial) approach (Diagram **C**): *F* = Facial or Labial; *A* = Axial; *G* = Gingival; and *L* = Lingual.

## 7. CAVITY NOMENCLATURE

Refer to Figure 12.20.

The preparation for the *lingual approach* for a Class III composite has the same terminology as the lingual approach for a Class III amalgam (Fig. 12.20**A** and **B**). There are four walls: *gingival, labial, incisal,* and *axial.* There are only five internal line angles: *gingivolabial, incisolabial, gingivoaxial, labioaxial,* and *incisoaxial.* There are only two internal point angles: *gingivolabioaxial* and *incisolabioaxial.*

The preparation for a composite with a labial approach tends to be more triangular in shape with three walls and a floor (Fig. 12.20**C**). The three walls are the *labial, lingual,* and *gingival walls,* and the fourth wall (or floor) is the *axial.* Subsequently, this preparation has six internal line angles: *labioaxial, linguoaxial,*

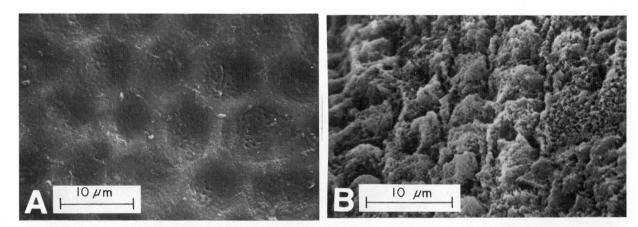

**Figure 12.21. A.** Magnified view of a nonetched enamel surface (x3260). **B.** Magnified view of etched enamel surface (x3600) after application of 50% phosphoric acid. This etched surface allows the resin bonding agent of the composite systems to flow into the irregular microscopic undercuts, thus affording mechanical retention for the material. (Courtesy of Dr. Ruth Paulson, Ohio State University).

*gingivoaxial, labiolingual, linguogingival,* and *gingivolabial.* There are only three internal point angles: *labiolinguoaxial, linguogingivoaxial,* and *gingivolabioaxial.*

Class III amalgam or composite restorations may be abbreviated by identifying the surface and the material and by noting the approach. For example, a composite on the mesial surface of tooth #7 with access to the decay through the lingual enamel would be identified as MC, #7, lingual approach, or MLC, #7.

## D. Class IV Type of Dental Caries, Cavity Preparation, and Restoration

### 1. DEFINITION

The Class IV lesion (and resultant preparation) is one that involves the proximal surface of an anterior tooth (as in a Class III), but also involves the incisal angle (or corner) of the tooth (Figs. 12.22, 12.23, and 12.24**A**).

### 2. CLINICAL DETECTION

Refer to Figure 12.22.

The Class IV lesion is plainly visible upon clinical examination.

### 3. RADIOGRAPHIC DETECTION OF DENTAL CARIES

Refer to Figure 12.23.

Radiographs are not needed to detect the Class IV lesion but may be useful to determine the depth of the lesion and its proximity to the pulp chamber.

### 4. INDICATIONS FOR RESTORING

The Class IV restoration is indicated when active caries is detected. Many Class IV restorations are indicated, however, not because of caries but because the corner

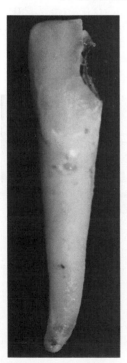

**Figure 12.22.** An enormous Class IV carious lesion involving the mesioincisal angle of tooth number 26.

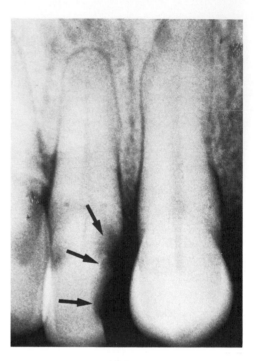

**Figure 12.23.** Radiographic evidence of a Class IV lesion involving the distoincisal angle of tooth number 10.

of the tooth has fractured off in an accident. In these instances, the extent of the fracture, the proximity of the exposed tooth structure to the pulp chamber, hypersensitivity to temperature changes, and the patients' concern for aesthetics are important in determining whether or not to restore the tooth. If the fracture is not into the dentin and the patient is not concerned about the appearance of the tooth, smoothing the rough edges of the tooth may suffice. If, however, dentin is involved, or if there is evidence of decay, a restoration is indicated to prevent discomfort from the exposed dentin and to stop the spread of decay.

## 5. RESTORATION OF CHOICE

If the preparation is conservative, a composite, particularly one that utilizes an acid-etching technique, is the restoration of choice (Fig. 12.24). If the preparation is extensive, or if the whole incisal edge of the tooth and both proximal surfaces are involved, but there is sufficient remaining tooth structure, it may be better to recommend a full cast crown with facial porcelain, or a full porcelain crown for the best aesthetics and longevity.

## 6. PREPARATION

Caries removal and smoothing extremely rough or unsupported enamel may be all that is needed to prepare the tooth for a Class IV composite. The occlusion, as al-

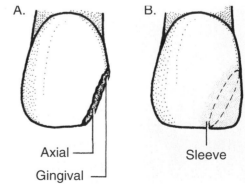

**Figure 12.24.** Facial diagrams of a Class IV area of carious lesion or fracture on tooth number 8 and the resultant restoration. **A.** View of the lesion or fracture showing the gingival and axial portions of the break. **B.** After smoothing the preparation and acid-etching the enamel, the restored tooth with a sleeve (thin film of bonded resin that extends beyond the original cavosurface margin) of composite overlaps the etched enamel surface, thus establishing maximum retention and enhancing (blending) the color match.

ways, must be analyzed to be sure that there is occlusal clearance for the restoration (i.e., to be sure there is room for the restoration when the patient chews and incises). Retention is most commonly achieved by acid-etch techniques that allow resin tags to bond the composite to the tooth (Fig. 12.21). A thin sleeve or skirt of excess composite material can cover beveled enamel that is acid-etched to maximize retention (Fig. 12.24**B**) and to improve aesthetics by blending the color differential between composite and enamel.

## 7. CAVITY NOMENCLATURE

Depending on the degree of involvement, this preparation may have only one flat wall (as in a fracture; see Fig. 12.24), or may be made up of two main surfaces: a gingival surface and a more axial surface. If these two portions join at an angle, the resultant line angle is axiogingival. There are no point angles.

This composite restoration may be abbreviated as either an MIC or DIC, to denote the involvement of either the mesioincisal or the distoincisal angle of the tooth. If both proximal surfaces are involved, the restoration would be designated as MIDC.

# E. Class V Type of Dental Caries, Cavity Preparation, and Restoration

## 1. DEFINITION

The Class V lesion (Fig. 12.25) is one that occurs in and involves the cervical one-third of the buccal or lingual surface of any tooth. It is a smooth surface lesion that results from poor hygiene in the area of the tooth just cervical to the buccal or lingual crest of curvature. It is next to the gingiva where the natural cleansing action of the lips, tongue, and cheeks is ineffective. This area of the tooth is, therefore, more susceptible to plaque accumulation and resultant caries. Root caries may also be called Class V.

## 2. CLINICAL DETECTION

Refer to Figure 12.25.

The Class V lesion is best detected by carefully examining the smooth, gingival portion of the teeth with good lighting to determine a chalky white or stained appearance with a break in the enamel surface. These lesions may occur at, or slightly apical to, the level of inflamed gingiva, so that the use of the tactile sense obtained through the explorer is critical for detection of cavitation. Care should be taken not to break through an early area of decay that has not yet cavitated, since excellent oral hygiene and fluoride has been shown to reverse the caries process. Also, it is

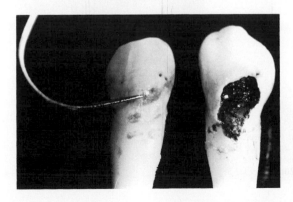

**Figure 12.25.** Class V lesions. *Left:* Incipient (beginning) buccal lesion that is seen as chalky and discolored and is flaking away. *Right:* An obvious, cavitated Class V buccal lesion that has destroyed much of the enamel on the buccal surface of the crown and adjacent cementum and dentin of the root, and may have progressed deeply enough to involve the pulp.

necessary to distinguish these lesions (which are cavitated) from a calcified buildup of calculus (which is felt as a bump on the surface of the tooth).

## 3. RADIOGRAPHIC DETECTION OF DENTAL CARIES

Refer to Figure 12.26.

By the time Class V lesions are evident on radiographs, the lesion has progressed far beyond the incipient stage and will require a much larger restoration. Therefore, the examiner should not depend on radiographs for detection of these lesions. When a gingival radiolucency is suspected of being a Class V lesion, this area on the tooth in question should be carefully evaluated clinically to prove or disprove the presence of caries.

## 4. INDICATIONS FOR RESTORING

Class V lesions require restorations when there is an area of cavitation that cannot be kept clean. Not all areas that are white or darkly stained require a Class V restoration, since some of these areas of discoloration may be either areas of arrested (old, inactive) decay or noncarious developmental defects.

## 5. RESTORATION OF CHOICE

Refer to Figure 12.27.

Since a Class V lesion occurs in nonstress-bearing areas, when aesthetics is a factor a composite may be used, even though it may be less resistant to abrasion than amalgam. In gingival abrasion lesions, the dentist may use a glass ionomer that bonds to dentin and contains fluoride. Amalgam may be used when the aesthetics are not of prime concern. In rare cases, primarily at the patient's request, a cast metal inlay could be used to replace lost tooth contour.

## 6. PREPARATION

Refer to Figures 12.28 and 12.29.

The preparation for a Class V restoration is usually kept as conservative as possible, with little or no extension for prevention. Prevention of future caries occurs through patient education in oral hygiene techniques and from periodic application

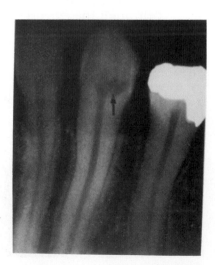

**Figure 12.26.** Radiographic evidence of a Class V defect on tooth number 22. It is impossible to tell from the radiograph whether it is on the buccal or lingual surface or whether it is decay or a radiolucent composite restoration. Caries in this region on the lingual surface of anterior teeth is an uncommon occurrence.

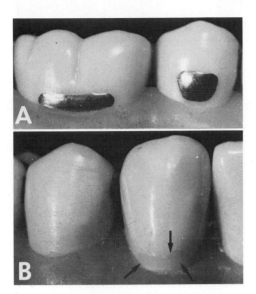

**Figure 12.27.** Class V restorations. **A.** Two BAs (buccal amalgams) on teeth number 29 and 30. The extent of these amalgams is usually dictated by the extent of the caries. **B.** Class V BC (buccal composite) on tooth number 27. If the shade of the material is good, these restorations are difficult to detect, and their surface grittiness felt by an explorer or scaler might be confused for incipient calculus formation. (Restorations by Gregory Blackstone, second-year dental student.)

of topical fluoride. The retention of amalgam restorations is obtained by preparing retentive grooves that are extensions of the axial wall in an occlusal and cervical direction (*AO* and *AG* in Fig. 12.29**B**). When using composite, similar retentive grooves could be used, but more often, retention is dependent on beveled enamel surfaces that have been acid etched (see the discussion under Class III preparations). A glass ionomer restoration in an area of deep (V-shaped or notched) cervical abrasion may require no preparation, only a treatment with a dentin conditioner or primer that aids in the chemical bond between dentin and the glass ionomer. A Class V inlay must have walls slightly divergent toward the crown surface to allow the wax model (pattern) removal from the tooth model (die) and, like all gold castings, should have short bevels at the cavosurface margins.

## 7. CAVITY NOMENCLATURE

Refer to Figure 12.29.

The Class V preparation is box shaped and consists of four walls and a floor: mesial, gingival, distal, occlusal, and axial. There are eight line angles: *mesioaxial, gingivoaxial, distoaxial, occlusoaxial, mesiogingival, distogingival, mesio-occlusal,* and *disto-occlusal.* There are four point angles: *mesiogingivoaxial, distogingivoaxial, mesio-occlusoaxial,* and *disto-occlusoaxial.*

The restoration is identified by surface and material. For example, a buccal amalgam on tooth #19 is BA, #19. A facial composite on tooth #7 is FC#7, and a glass ionomer on the facial surface of tooth #11 would be FGI #11.

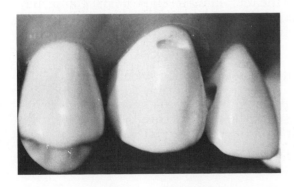

**Figure 12.28.** *Center:* A Class V labial composite preparation on tooth number 6. *Right:* A Class III DC (distal composite) preparation with labial approach on tooth number 7. (Preparations by Gregory Blackstone, second-year dental student.)

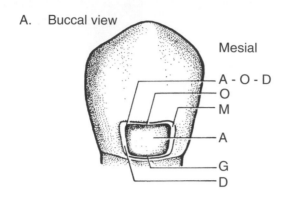

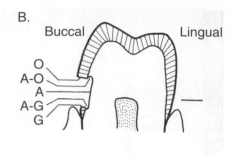

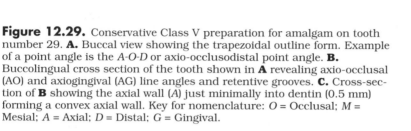

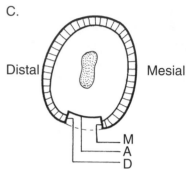

**Figure 12.29.** Conservative Class V preparation for amalgam on tooth number 29. **A.** Buccal view showing the trapezoidal outline form. Example of a point angle is the *A-O-D* or axio-occlusodistal point angle. **B.** Buccolingual cross section of the tooth shown in **A** revealing axio-occlusal (AO) and axiogingival (AG) line angles and retentive grooves. **C.** Cross-section of **B** showing the axial wall (*A*) just minimally into dentin (0.5 mm) forming a convex axial wall. Key for nomenclature: *O* = Occlusal; *M* = Mesial; *A* = Axial; *D* = Distal; *G* = Gingival.

## F. Class VI Type of Dental Caries or Restoration

A Class VI type of dental caries or restoration is not one of Black's original classifications. It is defined differently in different texts. In Baum's text (9), it is defined as the cavity or defect found on the tips of cusps or along the biting edges of incisors. The resultant preparation conservatively follows Black's principles of cavity preparation, and the restoration of choice depends on size and location of the lesion and the need for strength and aesthetics.

# SECTION VI. CROWNS AND VENEERS

Refer to Figures 12.30 through 12.33.

When a tooth is too badly broken down to be restored with an operative restoration because only a thin shell of enamel remains, it may be necessary to remove decay and replace some or all of the lost tooth structure with amalgam or composite to develop a "core" around which a cast crown can be constructed. Sometimes the remaining tooth is almost completely gone, so this core must be designed with a metal post that fits snugly into one of the root canals which has been treated with appropriate endodontic therapy. The post is necessary to provide retention. This restoration is called a cast post and core.

On posterior teeth, a crown will often be made of cast metal. To accomplish this, the anatomic tooth crown or restored "core" is externally reduced uniformly with burs to make room for the metal casting. The preparation usually extends gingivally beyond the core filling material so that the crown margins end on sound tooth structure. Full metal crown preparations end at the gingival cavosurface with a rounded shape called a chamfer (Figs. 12.30 and 12.31**A**).

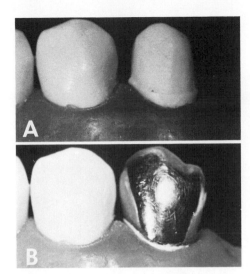

**Figure 12.30. A.** Crown preparation on tooth number 21 for a full cast-metal crown that will eventually support the framework of a removable partial denture with clasps. **B.** The resultant solid metal, cast crown in place. The facial surface of a crown like this can be veneered with porcelain if visible when speaking or laughing.

When aesthetics are a factor, especially on anterior teeth and maxillary premolars, further reduction of tooth structure is necessary on the facial surface to make room for not only the cast metal, but also an additional veneer of porcelain over the metal to visually resemble a natural tooth. This restoration is called a porcelain crown veneer, or a metal ceramic crown (MCC). The preparation for this type of crown ends at the gingival margins with a ledge that has a bevel (Fig. 12.31**B**). Photographs of a crown with a porcelain facing used to improve the aesthetics of severely fractured tooth #9 is shown in Figure 12.32**B.**

Even when little or no caries or breakdown are evident, a crown may be recommended if the tooth is cracked, or when needed to support an adjacent false tooth that replaces a missing tooth. The crowned teeth and the replaced tooth or teeth together are called a fixed partial denture (FPD) (commonly called a fixed bridge). The false tooth is called a pontic, and the teeth that are crowned on either side that support the pontic are called the abutment teeth covered by the FPD retainers. An FPD replacing tooth #4, with abutment metal ceramic crowns on teeth #3 and #5, is shown in Figure 12.33. Recently, techniques for replacing lost teeth with dental implants (titanium alloy roots surgically embedded into the bone) have been perfected (Fig. 12.34). Three to 6 months after surgical placement, these implants can be used to provide retention for crowns or stability for removable dentures.

Groups of lost teeth can also be replaced with multiple implants, removable partial dentures (RPD) or even with complete dentures (CD) when all natural teeth have been lost.

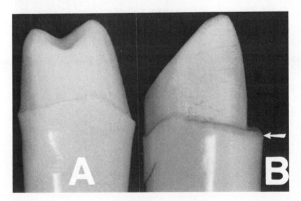

**Figure 12.31.** Proximal views of two types of full-crown preparation with their buccal surface toward the right. **A.** Full metal crown (no veneer) preparation on a mandibular premolar with chamfer finish lines. **B.** Preparation on a maxillary canine that will have baked-on porcelain covering the facial surface for aesthetics. The finish line on the lingual is a chamfer, but on the facial, to make room for porcelain, a ledge with bevel (*arrow*) is necessary.

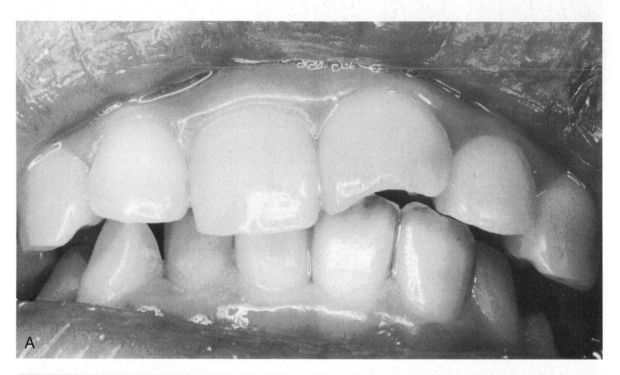

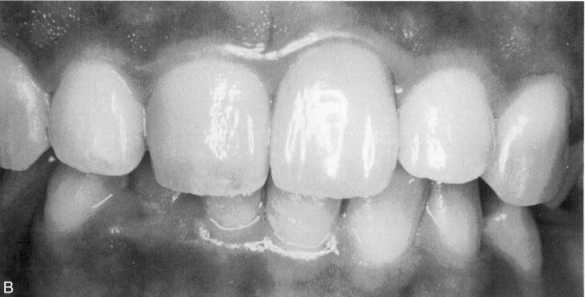

**Figure 12.32. A.** Tooth 9 with a fracture that includes the entire incisal edge. A large Class IV composite could be used to restore this defect but would be more susceptible to fracture and discoloration than a crown with a porcelain facing. **B.** The same patient with an esthetic cast metal crown and porcelain facing on tooth 9. (Reproduced by permission from and courtesy of Rosenstiel SF, Land MF, Fujimoto J. Contemporary fixed prosthodontics. St. Louis: C.V. Mosby Co., 1995.)

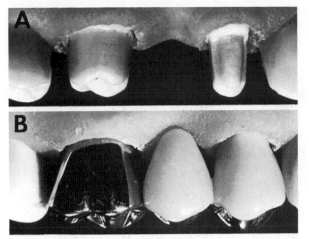

**Figure 12.33.** **A.** Buccal view of full-crown preparation on tooth 3 (on *left*) and a crown-veneer preparation on tooth 5 for the attachment of a bridge to replace tooth 4. **B.** The completed three-tooth fixed partial denture (bridge) for replacing tooth 4. The veneer and pontic (replacement tooth) in the photograph are porcelain veneered to metal.

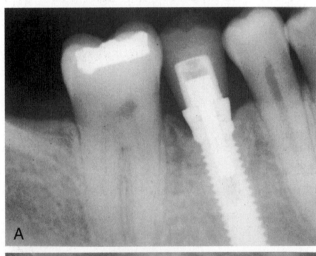

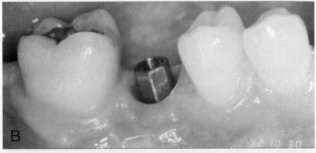

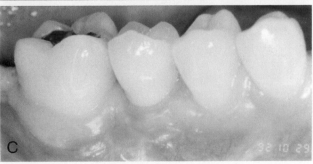

**Figure 12.34.** Tooth 29 has been extracted and replaced with a dental implant. It supports a crown veneered with porcelain. **A.** A bitewing radiograph of the implant with the screw-retained component and crown. **B.** The screw-retained component (crown support) attached to the implant and extending above the tissue prior to placement of the crown. **C.** The crown cemented on the screw-retained component of the implant. (Photographs courtesy of Ed McGlumphy, D.D.S., M.S., Associate Professor, Ohio State University, College of Dentistry.)

## SECTION VII. RECENT ADVANCES IN AESTHETIC DENTISTRY

In recent years, the number of aesthetic restorative materials and techniques for restoring anterior and posterior teeth has increased tremendously. These include tooth-colored inlays or onlays such as cast ceramic (23, 24), fired porcelain (25), indirect resins (26), direct resin inlays (27), and advancements in bonding amalgam, and advancements in implants (28).

Conservative techniques for veneering the labial surfaces of anterior teeth to improve aesthetics include direct resin and porcelain veneers that require minimal or no tooth reduction and fees that are generally less than for a crown with a porcelain veneer. An example of composite veneers to close an anterior diastema is shown in Figure 12.35. Porcelain veneers used to improve the aesthetics of anterior teeth with old, unaesthetic composite restorations are shown in Figure 12.36.

### LEARNING EXERCISE

*Without looking at the key to each photograph of restorations in this chapter, identify the material used, the surfaces involved, and the abbreviation that could be used to denote the restoration.*

*Do the same with extracted teeth that have existing restorations.*

*Looking in your mouth using a mirror or in a friend's mouth, identify the classification of the restorations (according to Dr. G.V. Black). Note that some restorations are extended over more of the tooth than others. Could this be because the dentist extended the preparations or was it due to the spread of caries? Do you suspect any areas of decay? (If so, check with a dentist.)*

## Acknowledgments

This chapter was written entirely by Rickne C. Scheid, D.D.S., M.A., for the 4th edition and has been updated.

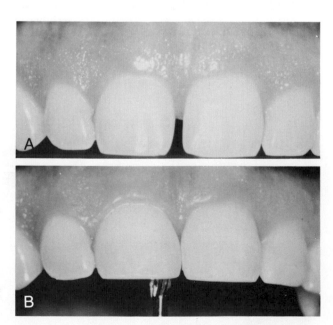

**Figure 12.35. A.** Teeth numbers 8 and 9 with diastema. **B.** Same teeth during final finishing stages after placement of composite veneers used to close the diastema. No tooth preparation was necessary. (Courtesy of Dr. Roland Pagniano, D.D.S.)

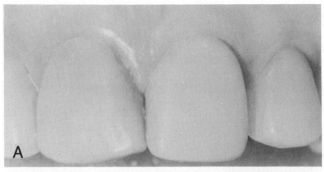

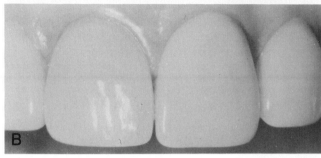

**Figure 12.36. A.** Teeth numbers 8, 9, and 10 with old composite resin veneers that have chipped and exhibit a loss of translucency. **B.** These same teeth after placement of esthetic porcelain veneers that cover the entire facial surfaces. (Courtesy of Dr. Roland Pagniano, D.D.S.)

Dr. Scheid wishes to acknowledge the help of the Section of Restorative and Prosthetic Dentistry, Ohio State University College of Dentistry, for contributing departmental slides and models for incorporation into this chapter. The late George C. Paffenbarger, D.D.S., assisted with editorial changes and acted as consultant on the composite, acid-etch portion.

## References

1. Gilmore HW. Textbook of operative dentistry. St. Louis: C.V. Mosby, 1967.
2. National Caries Program. The prevalence of caries in U.S. children, 1979–80. NIH Publication No. 82–2245, December 1981.
3. Douglass CW, Gammon MD. The epidemiology of dental caries and its impact on the operative dentistry curriculum. J Dent Educ 1984;48:547–555.
4. Hicks MJ, Flaitz CM. Epidemiology of dental caries in the pediatric and adolescent population: a review of past and current trends. J Clin Pediatr Dent 1993:18:43–49.
5. Heinrich R, Heinrich J, Kunzel W. Prevalence of root caries in women. Z Stomatol 1989:86:241–247.
6. Newbrun E. Problems in caries diagnosis. Int Dent J 1993:43:133–142.
7. DiOrio LP. Clinical preventive dentistry. East Norwalk, CT: Appleton-Century-Crofts, 1983.
8. Black GV. A work on operative dentistry. Vol.1 Chicago: Medico-Dental Publishing Company, 1908:203–234.
9. Baum L, Phillips RW, Lund MR. Textbook of Operative Dentistry. Philadelphia: W. B. Saunders, 1985, p28.
10. Leinfelder KF. Posterior composite resins. JADA 1988;11(Special Issue):21E-26E.
11. Roulet JF. The problems associated with substituting composite resins for amalgam: a status report on posterior composites. J Dent 1988:16:101–113.
12. Ishikawa A. 10-year clinical evaluation of a posterior composite resin [Abstract 2178]. J Dent Res 1996;75:290.
13. Leinfelder KF. Posterior composite resins: the materials and their clinical performance. JADA 1995;126(May):663–676.
14. Jordan RE, Suzuki M, Davidson D. Clinical evaluation of a universal dentin bonding resin. JADA 1993;124(Nov):71–76.
15. Ngo H, Earl A, Mount GJ. Glass ionomer cements: a twelve-month evaluation. J Prosthet Dent 1986;55:203.
16. Matis BA, Cochran MA, Carlson TJ, Phillips RW. Clinical evaluation and early finishing of glass ionomer restorative materials. Oper Dent 1988;13:74.

17. Nathanson D, Riis D. Advances and current research on ceramic restorative materials. Curr Opin Cosmetic Dent 1993;34–40.

18. Radike AW. Criteria for diagnosis of dental caries. In: Proceedings of the Conference on the Clinical Testing of Cariostatic Agents. Chicago: ADA, 1972.

19. Simonsen RJ. The clinical effectiveness of a colored sealant at 36 months. J Dent Res 1980;59:406.

20. Simonson RJ. Preventive resin restorations: three-year results. JADA 1980;100:535.

21. Craig RG, O'Brien WJ, Powers JM. Dental materials properties and manipulation. 3rd ed. St. Louis: C.V. Mosby, 1983:34–44.

22. Harris NO, Cristen G. Primary preventive dentistry. Reston, VA: Reston Publishing, 1982.

23. Cavel WT, et al. A pilot study of the clinical evaluation of castable ceramic inlays and a dual-cure resin cement. Oper Dent 1988;19:257–262.

24. Boyajian GK, Hart RI, Sausen RE. The "Dicor" inlay/onlay case report and summary of advantages. WV Dent J 1988;62:6.

25. Telglani M, Leinfelder KF, Lane J. Posterior porcelain bonded inlays. Comp Cont Educ Dent 1987;8:410.

26. Christensen GJ, Christensen RP. Comparison of veneer types. CRA News 1986;10:1.

27. Christensen GJ, Christensen RP. Resin inlay, direct. CRA News 1987;11:1–2.

28. Frommer HH. Radiology in dental practice. St. Louis: C.V. Mosby, 1981.

29. Christensen GJ. 1993 in review: a look back on a year of advancement. JADA 1993;124:69–70.

## General References

Chandler HH, Dagefoerde RO, Huffman RW, Pagniano RP, Postle HH, Metzler J. Operative manual: a laboratory clinic manual of operative dentistry. Ohio State University, 1983.

Downes R, Vessels R. Fixed prosthodontics laboratory manual. Ohio State University, 1983.

# Directions for Drawing and Carving Teeth

# 13

## SECTION I. DRAWING TEETH

### A. Materials Needed

Graph paper ruled 8 squares to the inch

Drawing pencil, 3H or 4H, sharpened to a fine point

Eraser

Ruler with millimeter scale

Boley gauge

Teeth or tooth model

Chart with dimensions of tooth to be drawn (such as Table 3.2 on page 107)

### B. How to Draw a Tooth

To make an accurate drawing of any object, you must not only *look* at the object, you must also *see* or visualize it. A carefully drawn, accurate outline of a tooth is a good indication that you have clearly seen and understood its external morphology. Rarely is there a person, however lacking in artistic skill, who cannot make a reasonably good drawing of a human tooth. Those who are not skilled in *accurate* drawing (extensive art training does not necessarily result in accuracy of outline) may find a solution in using graph paper ruled 8 squares to the inch. The tooth specimen is measured in millimeters with a Boley gauge, and the measurements are transferred to the graph paper, allowing 1 square to equal 1 mm. Drawings may be made to scale of each type of tooth: maxillary and mandibular incisors, canines, premolars, and molars. Draw maxillary teeth with crowns down and mandibular teeth with crowns up, the same orientation they have in the mouth.

Using an undamaged extracted tooth or tooth model for a specimen, make the following six measurements with the Boley gauge (Figs. 13.1 and 13.2).

Crown length

Mesiodistal crown

Faciolingual crown

Root length

Mesiodistal cervix

Faciolingual cervix

On anterior teeth, measure the crown length on the facial side from the cervical line to the incisal edge. On posterior teeth, measure the crown length on the facial side from the cervical line to the tip of the buccal cusp on premolars, and to the tip of the mesiobuccal cusp on molars. In drawing, make the other cusps their proper length relative to the measured cusp, i.e., either longer or shorter. Using a consistent method of measurement avoids confusion. With more than one buccal cusp, crown length is always to the mesiobuccal cusp. With more than one root, the overall tooth length will be from the mesial or mesiobuccal root apex to the mesiobuccal cusp (Table 3.2).

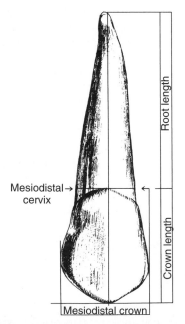

**Figure 13.1.** Facial side of a maxillary right canine tooth model showing how measurements of a tooth may be made to assist in drawing and carving.

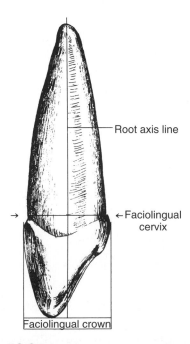

**Figure 13.2.** Mesial side of the maxillary canine depicted in Figure 13.1 showing how tooth measurements can be made and how the incisal portion is compared to the root axis line.

Plan how you want to place your drawings on the graph paper. One convenient arrangement is facial aspect, upper left corner; lingual aspect, upper right; mesial aspect, lower left; distal aspect, lower right; and incisal aspect, center (Figs. 13.3 and 13.4). These views will be centered nicely if you allow a four-square border on all sides as shown in the same illustrations.

## C. Example: How to Draw a Maxillary Central Incisor

### 1. FACIAL SKETCH

Use the measurements you have made of the tooth specimen you intend to draw. In the upper left corner of the page, count down from the upper four square border the number of squares and fraction thereof equal to the root length in millimeters and draw a horizontal line. From this line, count down the number of squares equal to the crown length in millimeters and draw a second horizontal line. From the left four square border, count to the right the number of squares equal to the mesiodistal crown measurement and draw a vertical line. Inside this box, you will draw the facial aspect of the tooth. Make your lines *very light* at first, so that corrections can be made easily. Remember to begin from the four-square margin (top and side) as seen in Figure 13.3.

Before you start to draw, make a light dash mark at the locations of the mesial and distal contact areas of the crown. (A pencil or straight-edge held against the side of the tooth parallel to the root axis line will help you determine where to put the small marks.) Also, mark the location of the apex of the root. Estimate the location mesiodistally of the cervix of the tooth. When you fit the crown into the box, if you remember to keep the root vertical, the axis may not be an equal distance from the mesial and distal sides because the crowns of some teeth are tilted distally. Mark off the mesiodistal cervical measurement very lightly.

Now draw in the curvature of the crown at the contact areas (you marked the location), and draw in a portion of the cervical line and a portion of the incisal edge. Draw the root apex and the cervical part of the root. Correct any errors in location or shape, and then connect the lines you have drawn. You have a drawing of a tooth. You may be pleasantly surprised how natural and morphologically correct this first sketch appears. Many professional artists are unable to depict natural teeth accurately because they are unfamiliar with tooth morphology, and they do not have the proportions that were dictated by your measurements.

### 2. LINGUAL SKETCH

In the upper right corner of the page (Fig. 13.3) use the same set of measurements to make the box in which to draw the lingual aspect of the tooth. Remember that almost all teeth are narrower on the lingual than on the facial surfaces, but this narrower sketch must be made within the same size facial dimensions (general labial outline), which, of course, would be in the background as viewed from this aspect. The cingulum is narrower than the cervical portion on the labial sketch, and it should be drawn a little off-center toward the distal.

### 3. MESIAL AND DISTAL SKETCHES

Draw these two boxes in the lower left and right corner of the page (Fig. 13.3) using the same root and crown lengths, but use the *faciolingual* crown measurement instead of the mesiodistal measurement. Before you start to draw the tooth, lightly mark the locations of the incisal edge, the labial crest of curvature (i.e., where the curve or greatest convexity of the labial surface will touch the line of the box), and

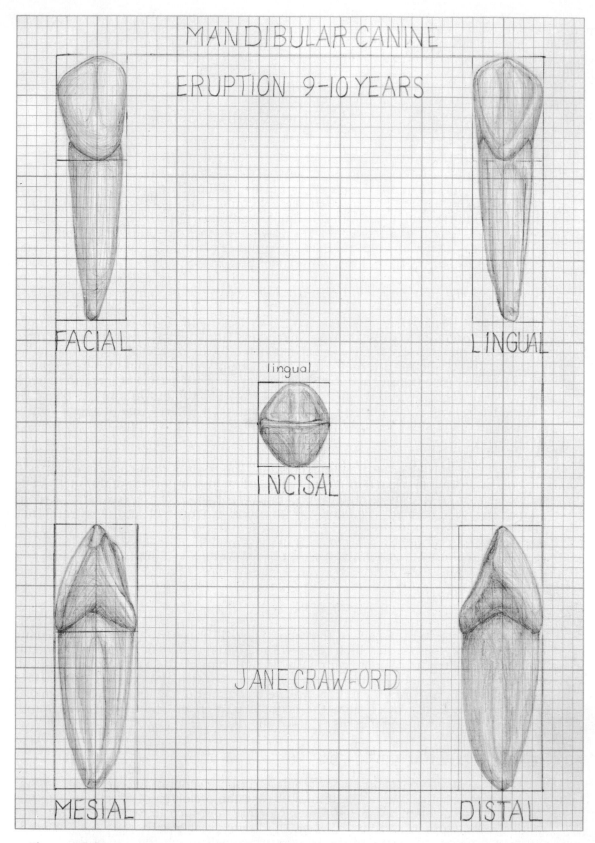

**Figure 13.3.** An oversized model of a mandibular right canine, drawn by a first-year hygiene student.

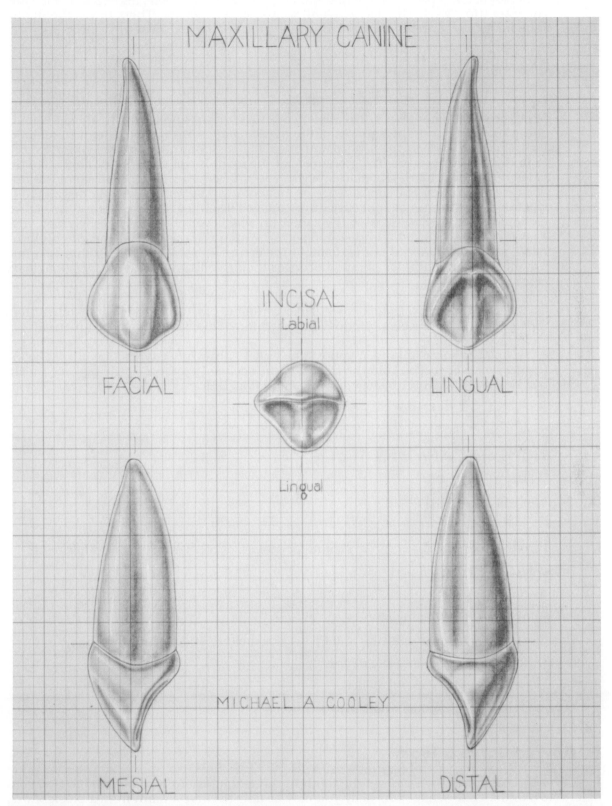

**Figure 13.4.** Professional drawing (by medical artist) from an oversized model of a maxillary canine, based on dimensions given in Table 3.2.

the crest of curvature on the cingulum (Figs. 13.2, 13.3, *below*, and 13.4, *below*) and the root tip. Mark the faciolingual width of the cervix. Then draw the tooth. Remember the four-square border at each side and below these views.

## 4. INCISAL SKETCH

Near the center of the page draw a box with the distance between the upper and lower horizontal lines the exact number of squares for the *faciolingual* measurement of the crown in millimeters. The distance between right and left vertical lines should equal the number of the squares of the *mesiodistal* crown measurement in millimeters. Hold the tooth facial side up and in such a position that you are looking exactly in line with the root axis line. Be sure that the tooth is not tilted up or down. On the sides of the box, mark the places where you are going to put the mesioincisal and distoincisal angles. The incisal edge of the tooth will be approximately horizontal (it will have a slight mesiodistal curvature) and will lie either in the center of the box faciolingually or slightly facial to the center (in whichever position it is shown on your drawings of the mesial and distal aspects). Watch the position of the cingulum on maxillary central incisors. It is distal to the center of the lower line in this box; and the mesial marginal ridge should be longer than the distal marginal ridge (maxillary central incisor).

Do you find any straight lines (ruler-straight, that is) on any tooth other than those lines that have been produced by attrition? This would be most unusual.

Using the same approach you will be able to draw other types of teeth. Labeling the grooves, the fossae, and the ridges on the occlusal surfaces of the posterior teeth will help to fix the morphology in your mind (Fig. 3.9).

# SECTION II. CARVING TEETH

## A. Materials Needed

Blocks of carving wax (34 × 17 × 17 mm for molars or 32 × 12 × 12 for other teeth)

Boley gauge (Vernier caliper)

Millimeter ruler

Office knife and sharpening stone

Roach carver, No. 7 wax spatula, and PKT-1 (for melting and adding wax)

No. 3, No. 5-6, 6C, and PKT-4 carvers

Sharpened 3H or 4H drawing pencil

Large or small tooth model and its measurements

## B. How to Carve a Tooth

Carving a tooth helps you to see the tooth in three dimensions and also to develop considerable manual skill. While eventually you may be able to carve a tooth from a block of wax without preliminary measurement, the beginner can only do well by approaching the carving systematically in the same way you approached the drawing: first, by outlining a box on the wax block; second, by sketching an outline of the tooth in the box; and third, by carving around the sketch or outline, one view or aspect at a time (sequence is shown in Fig. 13.6).

Perhaps, after all, it is encouraging rather than ridiculous to approach the task of carving a tooth with the thought in mind that Michelangelo conceived of his task of producing a marble statue as "liberating the figure from the marble that imprisons it." And remember that he, too, sometimes made mistakes and had to discard a half-finished statue of St. Matthew, which appears to the casual observer to be all right from the front, but from the side, the leg, bent at the knee, is seen to be hopelessly out of position.

The same can happen to your tooth carving. As you cut away, repeatedly examine your carving from all sides; turn it round and round and compare it with your specimen. Where it is too bulbous, the fault is easily correctable by further reductions. Where too much wax has been removed, you have one of three choices: add molten wax to the deficient region, make the entire carving proportionally smaller, or start with a new block of wax.

## C. Example: How to Carve a Maxillary Central Incisor

Refer to Figures 13.5 and 13.6.

1. Use the measurements you used for drawing. (Again, use the measurement of the buccal cusp on premolars and of the mesiobuccal cusp and mesiobuccal or mesial root on molars.) This consistency of method prevents confusion. Allowance is made for the greater length of some lingual cusps, which are longer than the measured buccal cusp.

2. Shave the sides of the block flat, and make all angles right angles.

3. Measure 2 mm from one end of the block and draw a line at this level encircling the block (on all four sides). (This end of the block will be the incisal or occlusal end of the tooth and the 2-mm allowance here is to provide for the extra length of the lingual cups on molars that are longer than the cusp measured to establish crown length. Although it is convenient to allow the 2 mm on all carvings, it is essential only for molars.)

4. From the 2-mm line, measure the crown length and draw a line around the block at this level. This second line is the location of the cervical line on the facial, mesial, distal, and lingual sides of the tooth (Fig. 13.6**A**).

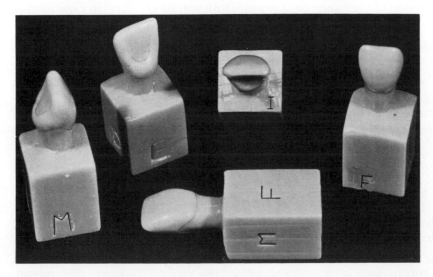

**Figure 13.5.** Maxillary central incisor wax carvings by first-year dental hygiene students as seen from the mesial (*M*), lingual (*L*), incisal (*I*), mesial-facial (*M*, *F*), and facial (*F*) aspects. The crown and half of the root were carved to specific dimensions that were proportional to the large plaster tooth model (5½ times larger) that was viewed during the carving. These excellent carvings were each done in less than 3 hours as a required skill test.

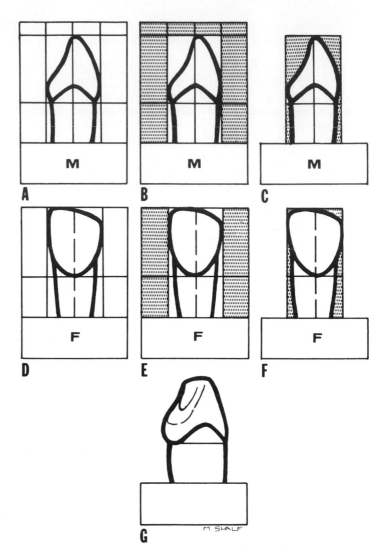

**Figure 13.6.** The sequential method described in this chapter for carving a tooth from a block of wax. The final product (your very nice carving) should look like those shown in Figure 13.5. The large letter *M* denotes the mesial aspect of the carving. Likewise, *F* indicates the facial side of the block.

5. From this cervical line, measure one-half of the length of the root and draw a line around the block. (The end of the block beyond this line will be referred to now as the *base*.)

6. On the base of the block, carve, on appropriate sides, *F* (facial), *L* (lingual), *M* (mesial), and *D* (distal). Be sure to put M and D in the proper relation to F and L so that you will carve a *right* or a *left* tooth, whichever you intend.

7. Draw a light line lengthwise on the block in the *center* of the mesial surface. Do the same on the distal surface, and BE SURE THAT THESE LINES ARE EXACTLY OPPOSITE.

8. Add 0.5 mm to the faciolingual measurement of the crown. Divide this number by 2. Using this measurement, draw a line this distance on either side of the center line on the mesial and distal sides of the block (Fig. 13.6**A**). These two lines are to be parallel to the center line and extend from the top of the block to the line located at one-half of the root length (Fig. 13.6**A**). These two lines box in the faciolingual crown dimension plus 0.5 mm. The extra 0.5 mm is an allowance for safety in carving. *Do not make trouble for yourself by allowing more than this extra 0.5 mm.*

9. On the surface of the block marked *M*, draw, within the box, an outline of the mesial side of the tooth as you drew it on the graph paper. Be careful to place the incisal

edge and the labial and lingual crests of curvature accurately. Your carving will probably be no better than this drawing.

10. Draw a similar outline on the distal side of the block. Be sure that on both sides, the drawings are oriented so the facial surface of the tooth is toward the side of the block you have marked *F*. (It is easy to make a mistake here.) These drawings or sketches of the crown may appear slightly fat due to the extra 0.5 mm width allowance confining the crown size faciolingually.

11. Carve away the gross excess wax from the facial, lingual, and incisal sides of the block so it is exactly like Figure 13.6**C.** *At this time, do not carve around the outline of the tooth, but rather carve in to the vertical lines that form the box in which the tooth picture is drawn* (Fig. 13.6**B**). **The shaded portion in B is removed.**

12. Check the distance between the two parallel carved surfaces carefully with your Boley gauge. *Be sure they are perfectly flat and smooth. Be sure the thickness of the column of wax between these parallel surfaces exactly equals the given faciolingual crown dimension plus 0.5 mm.*

13. Now carve around and down to the outline of the tooth. Follow the drawing carefully, making the tooth shape the same all the way through the block (Fig. 13.6**C**). *Do not leave a bulge in the center.* Keep the carving surface smooth; if it becomes chopped up, it will be impossible to smooth it without losing both the shape and the size of the carving. **Carve away the shaded regions seen in Figure 13.6C.**

14. Draw center lines, *very lightly,* on the curved facial and lingual surfaces of the carving. Be sure they are exactly opposite.

15. Add 0.5 mm to the mesiodistal crown measurement and draw two lines one-half this distance on either side of the center line. This makes a box on the curved surface as wide as the greatest mesiodistal crown measurement plus 0.5 mm (Fig. 13.6**D**).

16. Draw the facial outline of the crown and half of the root on the curved facial side of the block (Fig. 13.6**D**) after redrawing a horizontal cervical line the exact crown length distance from the incisal edge. This drawing is on the curved surface.

17. On the lingual surface of the block, draw an outline the same shape as the one on the facial surface except, of course, that it is a mirror image; the distal side of the tooth must be toward the same side of the block in each case. Check the crown length on the lingual surface too. So the crown won't be too long.

18. Carve away all the wax outside the drawing box, **removing all the dark shaded portions as shown in Figure 13.6E.** On some first molars their spreading roots may extend beyond the box lines, and these roots should be carved accordingly. Check your measurements again.

19. Shape the tooth by carefully carving into the curved mesial and distal contours so that it resembles your tooth specimen from the facial and lingual sides. **Remove dark shaded portions shown in Figure 13.6F.**

20. Now it is time to round off the corners, narrow the lingual surface, shape the cingulum (it is distal to the center line, and the mesial marginal ridge is longer than the distal), and carve out the lingual fossa. Be sure to look at all aspects of the tooth as you are finishing the carving. These include, of course, the incisal (occlusal) aspect (Figs. 13.5 and 13.7, *upper right center*). Four nice carvings of maxillary canines, made by dental hygiene students at Ohio State University, are shown in Figure 13.7. Five aspects of another very fine carving by a dental student are seen in Figure 13.8.

21. Carve your initials on the bottom of the base of the block. Be an honest critic of your work, constantly looking for regions where the carving can be improved.

The best carvings from a 45-minute carving test are seen in Figure 13.9. These carvings were done entirely with an ordinary flat-bladed office knife with a wood handle. Many measurements had to be properly sketched on these blocks to facilitate such accurate results.

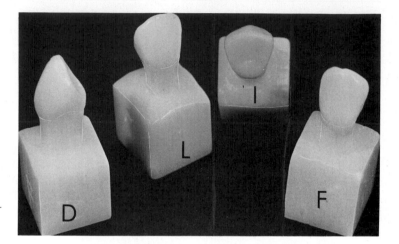

**Figure 13.7.** Maxillary canine wax carvings viewed from the distal (*D*), lingual (*L*), incisal (*I*), and facial (*F*) aspects. These were done by first-year dental hygiene students during a skill test (2 hours, 50 minutes time limit).

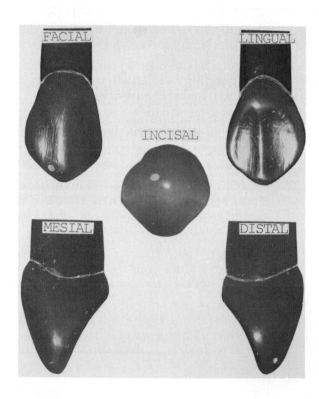

**Figure 13.8.** Maxillary right canine carving done by dental student Keith Schmidt. Observe the nearly perfect contours from all aspects and that the root is not becoming narrower as it joins the crown (a very common carving error in attempting to refine the cervical line).

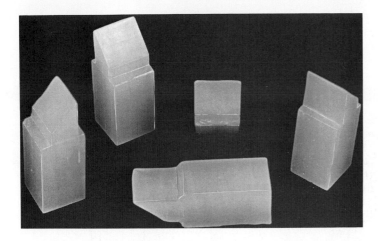

**Figure 13.9.** Wax block carvings with flat surfaces instead of curved surfaces so typical on teeth. All five carvings are the same shape and size, but viewed from several perspectives. These carvings were made from a solid block during a 45-minute skill test by first-year dental hygiene students. These carvings were made from specific measurements and a three-dimensional drawing.

All of the surfaces on the carvings in Figure 13.9 are flat. Tooth surfaces should never be flat. Nature makes all tooth contours convex to varying degrees. A facet (flat, shiny spot from attrition) is usually a sign of excessive wear.

You can work toward becoming proficient in drawing teeth by sketching in outlines (lightly at first) in the blank boxes which are proportionally the correct size for the view and tooth listed in Figures 13.10, 13.11, and 13.13. You should have a tooth model or extracted tooth specimen to view as you make these sketches. One example of how to sketch teeth into the blank boxes is shown in Figure 13.12. The large tooth models seen in Figure 3.1 were the guides for these drawings.

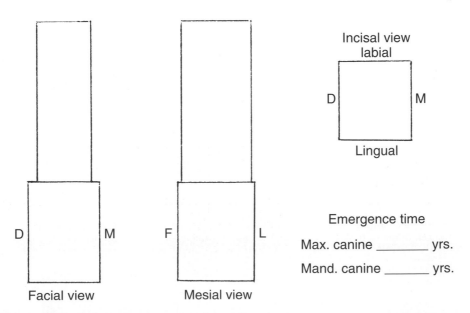

**Figure 13.10.** Outlines within which you may draw three views of a maxillary canine. The boxes are proportional to the natural teeth measured in Table 3.2. The widest portions of the crown (mesial and distal contacts) should touch the sides of the wider lower box. Only the widest part of the root should touch the sides of the narrower box above with the root apex touching the top of this box. On the incisal view, be sure to position the incisal ridge just labial to the faciolingual middle of this box. Drawing these three views will be helpful to you when you outline similar contours on a block of wax for carving a maxillary canine like the ones seen in Figures 13.7 and 13.8. An illustration of maxillary premolar drawings framed inside boxes like this is seen in Figure 13.12.

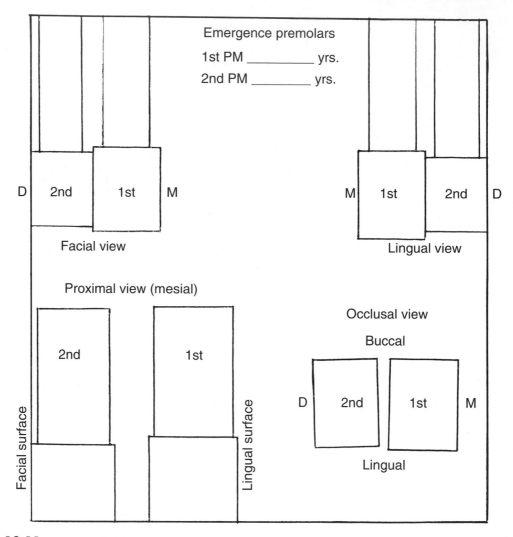

**Figure 13.11.** Outlined proportional boxes for drawing several views of the maxillary first and second premolars in their usual relationship to each other. Use the same guidelines given in the legend for Figure 13.10. A dental hygiene student's drawing of these two teeth within the outlined boxes is seen in Figure 13.12.

Maxillary premolars

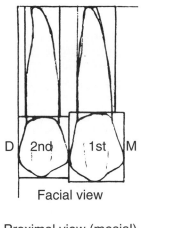

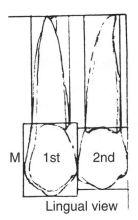

Facial view

Lingual view

Proximal view (mesial)

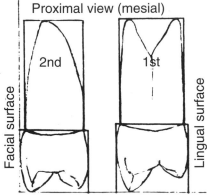

Facial surface

Lingual surface

Occlusal view
Buccal

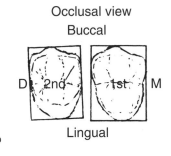

Lingual

**Figure 13.12.** A dental hygiene student's drawings within the outlined boxes is an example for your own drawings in the blank boxes in Figure 13.11. Study these and perhaps you can make even better drawings. For example, in the lingual view, the maxillary first premolar's lingual cusp is too long. It is the correct length in the drawing of the mesial aspect. The oversized tooth models seen in Figure 3.1 were viewed from each aspect for perspective as these drawings were made.

## D. Notes

Practice makes perfect, or at least you will see pronounced improvement in your later carvings. Therefore, do not discard your first ones, but keep them for future comparisons. The most difficult task is to begin for the very first time. We have found from many years of experience, however, that the inexperienced people who follow these or similar directions and proceed step by step, often end up with some of the best carvings in the class. Do not be afraid to begin. Make your measurements from center and end lines, draw in boxes for the crown and root portions and then you are ready to start shaving off wax. You may find a very nice looking tooth within your block (just do not make it too skinny or fat, or too tall or short). Perfect it from one view prior to rotating it and shaping another side or aspect.

When you become skillful at carving teeth, it may surprise you that it is possible to carve a tooth from memory alone of the contours, possibly aided only be several important dimensions. Average measurements from 4572 extracted teeth are given in Table 3.2. Should you draw or carve a tooth to these average dimensions, it might surprise you how normal it looks.

Really, you can both draw and carve a tooth. Don't develop a mental block to the contrary. Save your early drawings and carvings. They will serve as nice mementoes of your early and serious (time-consuming, yes) endeavors in your chosen field.

You may find the following books helpful in perfecting your carving techniques.

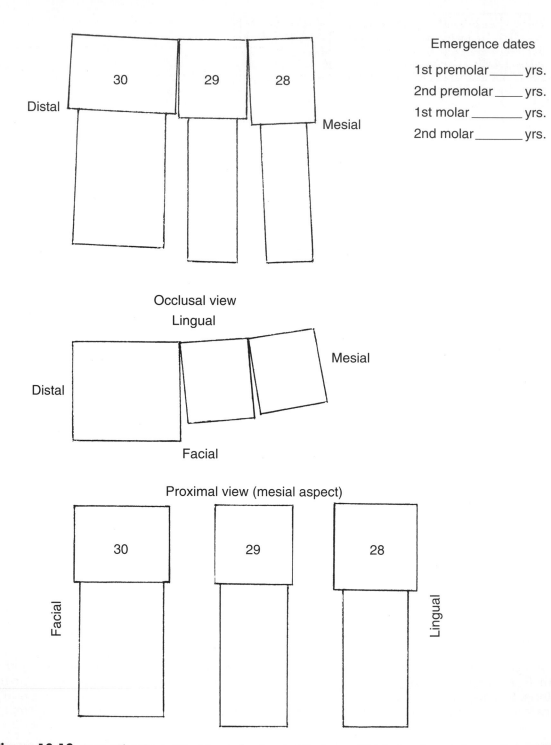

Emergence dates

1st premolar_____ yrs.

2nd premolar_____ yrs.

1st molar_____ yrs.

2nd molar_____ yrs.

Occlusal view

**Figure 13.13.** Proportionally outlined boxes for drawing the lower right first and second premolars and first molar in their usual relationship to one another. Select three nice tooth specimens or oversized tooth models and go to work.

## General References

Ash MM Jr. Wheeler's atlas of tooth form. Philadelphia: W.B. Saunders, 1984.

Beaudreau DE. Tooth form and contour. JASPD 1973;3:36–37.

Burch JG. Coronal tooth contours: didactic, clinical and laboratory. 3rd ed. Worthington: James G. Burch, 1980.

Grundler H. The study of tooth shapes: a systematic procedure. Berlin: Buch-und Zeitschriften-Verlag "Die Quintessenz," 1976.

Linek HA. Tooth carving manual. Pasadena, CA: Wood and Jones, Printers, 1948.

# 14

# Forensic Dentistry

Theodore Berg, Jr.

*Forensic dentistry* is an investigative aspect of dentistry that analyzes dental evidence for human identification. The forensic dentist plays an important role in our justice system. This field of dentistry is divided into forensic odontology and jurisprudence (the science of law). *Forensic odontologists* study and identify teeth, jaws, prostheses, dental appliances, bite marks, dental injuries, and dental records in the interest of justice.

This chapter provides an overview and introduction to forensic dentistry, while illustrating its elemental dependence on dental anatomy. This textbook is cited as the prime dental anatomy reference in the American Socity of Forensic Odontology Manual on this subject.

Forensic dentistry is one of a number of forensic sciences. Other forensic sciences include:

1. **FORENSIC ANTHROPOLOGY** examines and interprets skeletal evidence with methods used by archaeologists and with knowledge of human biological variation. This evidence includes bones, teeth, hair, clothing, artifacts, and scene analysis. The examination considers time of death, aging, sexing, race, body size and weight, individualization, and the cause and manner of death.

2. **FORENSIC PATHOLOGY AND BIOLOGY** utilizes autopsy, tissue study, and review of medical records in the investigation of injury or death as a result of accident, homicide, or suicide. Legal responsibility usually resides with a medical examiner or coroner. The criteria for death is irreversible cerebral function. The forensic pathologist attempts to determine and report on the (a) cause, (b) manner (homicide, suicide, accident, or unknown), and (c) mechanism of death.

3. **CRIMINALISTICS** includes fingerprints, ballistics, tool marks (chisel, hammer, etc.), and scene investigation to identify and analyze physical evidence in order to reconstruct the crime and to connect or eliminate suspects and victims.

4. **TOXICOLOGY** utilizes chemistry, photography, and biology to identify harmful substances within a body. These include medications, poisons, and illegal drugs.

5. **FORENSIC PSYCHIATRY** examines and testifies about the aspects of legal sanity, human motivation, and possible personality profile.

6. **FORENSIC ENGINEERING** uses engineers to investigate incidents such as airplane crashes, auto accidents, and structural collapse.

7. **QUESTIONED DOCUMENTS** technicians study and report about printing, typewriting, handwriting, ink, paper, and other features of documents.

8. **GENERAL FORENSICS** involves other specialists who are qualified to analyze specific evidence such as designers, photographers, and technical experts. They might report, for example, in a case of product liability associated with death or injury.

9. **FORENSIC JURISPRUDENCE** involves criminal and civil lawyers using the earlier described specialists, reports, and testimony to pursue their case in our system of justice.

Forensic dentistry as a science is represented in the United States of America by numerous forensic dentistry teams on local levels, including the Odontology Section of the American Academy of Forensic Sciences, the American Board of Forensic Odontology, and the American Society of Forensic Odontology. Each year more dentists become involved as law enforcement becomes increasingly aware of dentistry's potential contribution.

## DENTISTRY AND HUMAN IDENTIFICATION

Dentistry often has much to offer in identification since teeth are the most durable parts of the body and dentitions are as individual as fingerprints. Situations involving decomposition and skeletal remains will yield no recognizable facial features or fingerprints. *Postmortem* (after death) teeth, jaws, prostheses, and appliances can yield a positive identification, given *antemortem* (before death) records (Figs. 14.1 and 14.2).

Erroneous suspected identifications are often eliminated. The benefits of this are such that even with the lack of antemortem records, the effort is worthwhile to aid investigators with information from dental aging, sexing, and estimated socioeconomic grouping derived from restorative materials, attrition patterns, periodontal status, eruption patterns, skeletal features, and serology (Figs. 14.3 and 14.4).

Forensic dental techniques most commonly include collection and preservation of dental and jaw remains, dental radiology, photography, impressions and casts, antemortem and postmortem charting, and the comparison of these records. Features are referred to as Points of Comparison and include (a) the number and identity of teeth, (b) tooth rotation, spacing, and malposition, (c) anomalies, (d) restorations and prostheses or appliances, (e) caries, (f) endodontic treatment, (g) implants and surgical repairs, (h) pathology, (i) bone patterns, and (j) occlusion, erosion, and attrition (Figs. 14.3 and 14.4).

A well-organized approach results in accurate comparisons and minimizes the chance of error. The examiner should record each feature of the postmortem teeth and jaws and the radiographs on a standardized dental chart (Fig. 14.5). The same is done for antemortem records, radiographs, casts, and pictures on a separate, but identical, chart. Great caution must be exercised with antemortem record interpretation. Records vary widely in quality and completeness. Some dentists mount radiographs as viewed from the front (film bump out) and others prefer mounting them as viewed from the lingual (film bump inward)! Charting tooth identification is not always done in the Universal System (see Chapter 3 for other tooth

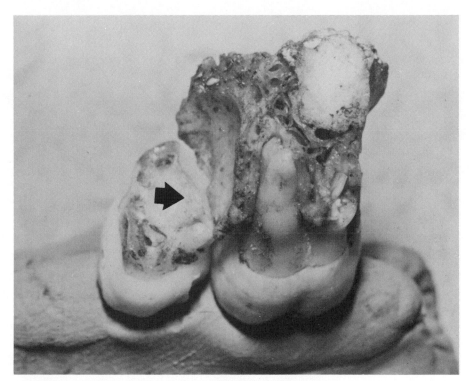

**Figure 14.1.** Deciduous tooth J and permanent tooth 14 were recovered in an air crash involving many adults and several children. The fully erupted position and root completion of tooth 14, the resorbed roots of J (deciduous second molar), and the crypt for tooth 13 (*arrow*) suggest that this specimen is from a person in the 10–14-year-old age group. The victim was identified by dental records and the radiographs in Figure 14.2. Modeling clay is often useful to position postmortem specimens for radiographic survey.

identification systems such as Palmer and International). The forensic dentist must carefully organize all evidence so that it is analyzed in a systematic manner using consistent and standardized methods.

## MASS DISASTERS

Forensic dentists have made many contributions in the identification of bodies involved in air crashes, mass homicides, structural collapses, floods, and similar disasters. The large volume of specimens and records demands a team approach with excellent organization. The coroner's or medical examiner's office commonly develops a mass disaster medical/dental team, with a Center Team Chief. The *dental team* has a chief who both organizes and schedules the

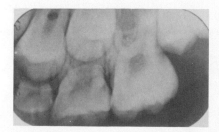
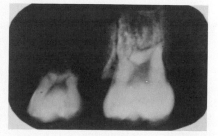

**Figure 14.2.** The postmortem radiograph of the specimen in Figure 14.1 (at *right*) shows consistent points of comparison to one of the antemortem radiographs (at *left*) gathered in the investigation of an air crash and subsequently led to the victim's identification.

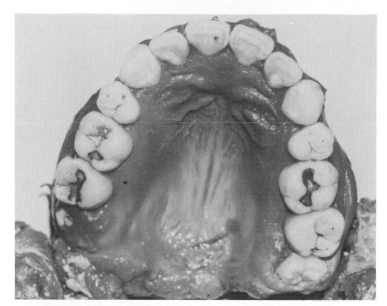

**Figure 14.3.** The maxillae and teeth offer many clues to age, origin, and identity, including a missing premolar on each side, erupting third molars, type of restorations, arch form, morphology of incisors, and the occlusal and incisal attrition in an otherwise young-appearing specimen.

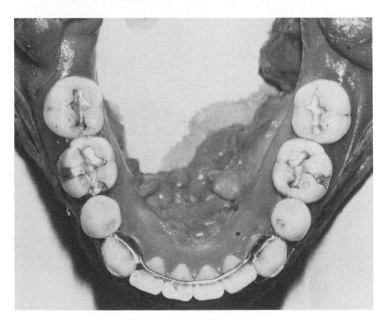

**Figure 14.4.** A mandible, teeth, restorations, and orthodontic arch wire offered a high probability for the eventual identification of a victim. Positive identification depends on adequate antemortem records. Postmortem radiographs will define the unique internal configurations of restorations and the status of the third permanent molars.

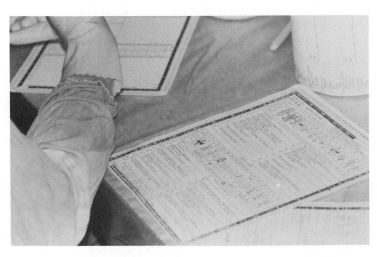

**Figure 14.5.** Separate, standardized dental charts are carefully completed during examination of both antemortem records and radiographs and postmortem specimens and radiographs.

team members and provides a consistent communication link with the Center Team Chief and the other teams, including those working in radiology, autopsy, and fingerprints.

The ground search teams are organized with a *site grid chart*. These teams collect bodies and body parts while carefully charting locations. Remains are sent to storage and examination sites with adequate security, lighting, and support equipment for preservation and study.

The *dental team* is best organized into antemortem and postmortem teams of *two examiners* per team. One person handles the specimen and examines the radiographs while the other person charts findings (Fig. 14.5). The examining pair then reverses roles and checks each other's efforts. Ideally, a third person, usually the Dental Team Chief, reviews the work of the team. Antemortem charting will usually come later as records arrive. Antemortem charting and records must be done separately and stored separately from postmortem evidence during the investigation. An air crash investigation, for example, can result in dozens to hundreds of records, and take days to weeks to complete. Long hours of work are involved, as authorities and families seek answers and identifications quickly. There must be organization to avoid errors and oversights from fatigue and to provide the numbers of team members required to complete a project.

In mass disasters and in single human identifications, success at the task goes to the undaunted and determined examiner. Knowledge of dental anatomy as represented in this text is a basic. The examiner refers to texts such as this book for calcification and eruption tables, charting systems, and suggestions for rare or anomalous tooth identifications or relationships. Dental forensic examiners also use close-up photography systems and commonly used equipment, as suggested in the forensic dentistry books referenced at the end of this chapter.

What may seem of no value, or what may actually be overlooked by site searchers who are not dentists or anthropologists, may be the key to an identification (Figs. 14.6 through 14.9). Even a removable partial denture (Fig. 14.6) or a piece of a denture (Fig. 14.7) may be useful and critical. A lay person might not imagine that one or two teeth could be useful, but nothing should be overlooked if possible (Fig. 14.8). An edentulous jaw, which might seem useless at casual glance, may be correlated with a prosthesis or with dental casts and radiographs, and offers unique trabecular bone patterns and, perhaps, impactions, old fracture sites, implanted metals, foreign bodies, and pathologic disorder (Fig. 14.9). Often identifications are established by comparing unique features of restorations that show up on both antemortem and postmortem radiographs (Fig. 14.10).

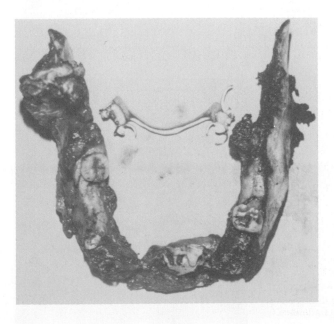

**Figure 14.6.** A mandible broken in three pieces with several teeth and a removable partial denture was recovered from a crash and burn accident. The survivors directed investigators to the suspected victim's dentist. The dentist provided antemortem records and a working cast for the partial denture that permitted identification.

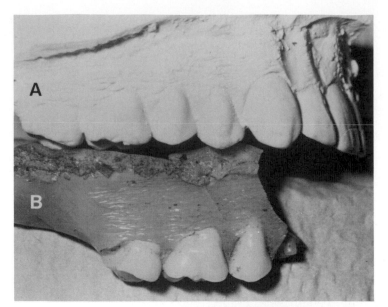

**Figure 14.7.** The dental stone cast of an upper denture (**A**) was obtained in evidence collection for investigation of an airliner crash. A denture fragment (**B**) recovered from the crash site, with teeth numbers 2, 3, and 4 present, matches the antemortem cast. The impact broke off a distal piece of tooth 2. Unique horizontal grooves in the buccal resin of the denture precisely match those seen in the antemortem cast.

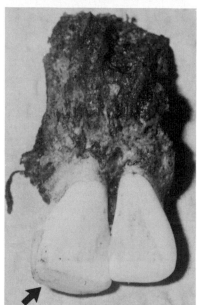

**Figure 14.8.** Although one or two teeth might seem scant evidence for identification, they should be thoroughly examined and radiographed. The labial laminate bonded veneer (*arrow*) made this specimen especially unique since this was in the early period of such technique. Also useful can be crown, root and pulp shape, tooth positions, other restorations, pin and base buildups, endodontic therapy, posts, and bone trabecular patterns.

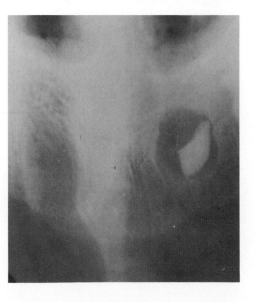

**Figure 14.9.** Even an endutulous jaw might provide a big clue to identification with some unique feature such as the dentigerous cyst shown in the maxillary canine region. Each case challenges the investigator to carefully consider all possibilities and to make no premature assumptions.

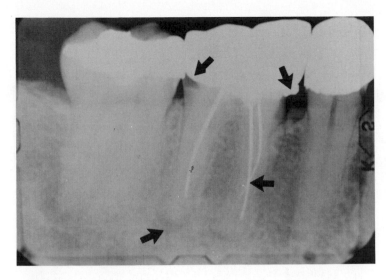

**Figure 14.10.** Preincident and postincident dental radiographs can be crucial evidence in the investigation and adjudication of fraud and malpractice cases. A radiograph shows marginal overhangs, marginal insufficiency or caries, inadequate endodontic therapy, and apical pathology. In identification cases, these features or even the unique contours of teeth and restorations, as in the second molar, are a "fingerprint" to that individual.

## CIVIL LITIGATION

A person might claim that improper dental care was rendered or that damage was sustained at the hands of another person (Fig. 14.10) or by food contaminated with a foreign body (glass, shell, etc.). Investigators of claimed malpractice and fraud often require examinations, comparisons, and testimony by expert witnesses. This may involve examining a person and studying records and radiographs from prior dentists. All of the techniques and careful comparisons described previously are useful.

## BITE MARKS

Numerous homicides and attack cases have been solved by bite mark identification, analysis, and comparison (Figs. 14.11 through 14.14). Many bites are severe and leave telltale marks long after an assault. One of several techniques of comparison and analysis is shown here, comparing bite mark tracings to the suspect's or defendant's tooth imprint pattern tracings (Figs. 14.12 and 14.13). Dental casts (Fig. 14.14) and photographs from the suspect are made after obtaining a court-ordered search warrant. These techniques can be useful in solving some child abuse cases in addition to many assaults and homicides. The forensic dentist must first establish the mark as a human bite mark, then identify, if possible, the teeth involved in the mark. Possibilities may involve missing, extruded, hypoerupted, rotated, tilted, and anomalous teeth. The chapter in this text on anomalies should be reason enough to remain open-minded and diligent when considering bite marks! The dental forensic examiner must also consider the possibility of animal bites, victim self-bites, and marks from foreign objects that might be mistaken for a bite mark. Separate analysis of those markings may be useful to law enforcement agencies by connecting the victim's injuries to a tool or instrument owned by a suspect.

Law enforcement agencies are becoming increasingly aware of potential identifications from the dental profession. In a landmark bite mark case in California, *State vs. Marx,* Dr. G. Vale, a forensic dentist, recognized bite marks on the autopsy photograph of a nose. After alerting investigators, the body was exhumed and studied with the resultant identification and conviction of the murderer based on the victim's nose bite mark and the suspect's dentition! An appeal was made to the Supreme Court on the grounds that the dental techniques were unique, untested and not scientific. The appeal was denied, making this the first United States bite mark case to withstand the appellate process. Thus, the reliability of this method of identification was legally verified. People (of California) versus Marx, 54 Cal. App. 3rd 100, 126 Cal. Reptr.

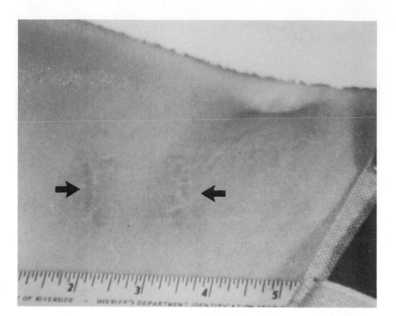

**Figure 14.11.** A bite mark was found on the abdomen of a crime victim. Color and black and white photographs were taken with a reference rule along side the mark. Other investigative techniques include saline swab washing for residual saliva blood-typing and a free-flowing, high-detail silicone impression of both the bite mark and the surrounding area.

350, Dec. 29, 1975. The outcome of the decision in this landmark case has been cited in fifteen states, before the military justice system and in Federal Court of Appeals (3rd Circuit Court).

The notorious mass murderer Ted Bundy (executed January 1989) was positively identified as the responsible person by his bite marks found on the buttocks of one of his young female victims.

John Wayne Gacy of Chicago, convicted of 33 counts of murder, became a real test of the vital role forensic dentistry plays in the identification of the involved victims. Only five of the human remains found still had soft tissue, making the identification process a nightmare. However, 20 of the 33 victims were identified through dental records.

One particular disaster highlights vividly the unique skills and tremendous value of a forensic dental team in the accurate identification of bodies. Few can ever forget the horror that

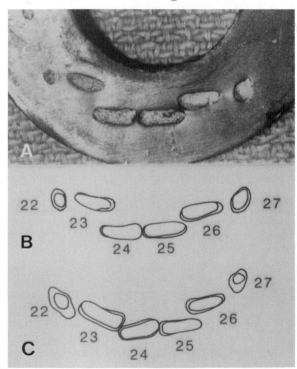

**Figure 14.12.** Wax test imprints from casts of a suspect's teeth can be made at various penetration levels (**A**). A composite overlay tracing of the suspect's 1 mm and 2 mm wax penetrations (**B**) can be compared to the tracing from another cast of "very similar" teeth and then both compared to a tracing of the bitemark as in Figure 14.13.

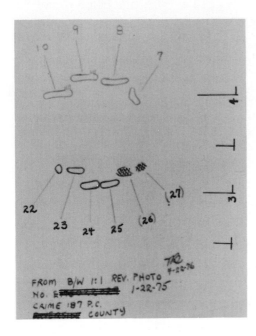

**Figure 14.13.** A bite mark tracing of a black and white photograph, taken in direct frontal position to the victim's bite mark and printed in 1:1 scale referenced to a ruler included in the photograph, can be compared to 1:1 scale tracings from test bites and wax penetrations as in Figure 14.12. The mandibular teeth marks are highly consistent with the defendant's tooth marks (Fig. 14.12**B**) but do not match with the other "suspect" (Fig. 14.12**C**). (Tracings in these illustrations are not reproduced here in 1:1 scale.)

occurred at 8:30 p.m., 17th July 1996 off East Moriches, New York: the explosion of a 747 airplane, TWA flight 800 bound for Paris, France, with two-hundred-thirty passengers aboard.

Within the first twelve hours, a team of thirty dentists, headed by Dr. B. K. Friedman, D.D.S., American Board of Forensic Dentistry, began the painstaking work of identifying the recovered bodies which were devoid of clothing. Two and a half weeks later, two hundred and eight of the two hundred and ten recovered bodies and body parts had been positively identified. Identification of ninety-five was by dental records alone, another sixty by dental records along with medical records (radiographs, MRI's, etc.), medical anomalies, fingerprints, etc.

For the first time ever, all relatives were screened for DNA samples to compare with the more than four hundred recovered body parts, enabling the return of each to the families for an appropriate resting place. Nuclear DNA samples were extracted from both bone and dental pulps, which was all that remained after the first week. Mitrocondrial DNA was also extracted from ground tooth structure, but it is only effective in matching females.

Altogether, sixty-one dentists and twenty-two auxillary dental personnel participated in this important forensic project. Thirty-five to forty of these dentists had worked with Dr. B. K. Friedman as part of his forensic dentistry team for five and a half years. Such dedication and professionalism by these dentists was a great service to the community and the families of the victims.

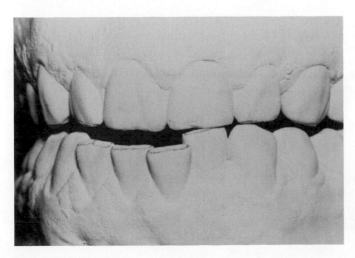

**Figure 14.14.** Potential occlusal positions with articulated casts of the suspect/defendant might suggest bite pattern potentials and possible orientation of the defendant when a bite was made. Casts can be compared to 1:1 scale photographs and compared to replicas of the bitemark in stone and silicone.

## CONCLUSION

Even if the average dentist does not intend to be involved in forensic dentistry, the probability is that eventually he or she may be contacted regarding questions about quality of care, observed injuries (such as suspected child or spousal abuse), or from law enforcement agencies requesting help. A valuable contribution can be made by understanding the role of dentistry in forensic science, by recognizing dental evidence or a bite mark, and by helping to properly preserve crucial evidence for later analysis.

You will find dental anatomy the foundation or basis for any forensic dentistry investigation. The references offered with this chapter were selected to give the novice a practical and representative introduction to the field and techniques of forensic dentistry.

The most recent and current well illustrated information to be found on this subject is in the May 1996 issue of the Journal of the California Dental Association (Vol. 2, No. 5, pp28–66). The general title is "True Forensics" and it includes seven concise articles: overview, bite marks, crime investigation, child abuse, photography, computers, and mass disasters. The authors are G. L. Vale, D. Sweet, J. A. DiZinno, D. E. Spencer, G. S. Golden, R. D. Rawson, and W. M. Morlang respectively.

## Acknowledgments

This chapter was contributed by Theodore Berg, Jr., D.D.S., who is Clinical Professor Emeritus, Section of Removable Prosthodontics, at the School of Dentistry, University of California, Los Angeles; Diplomate, American Board of Prosthodontics; member of the American Society of Forensic Odontology and the Forensic Odontology Team of the Los Angeles Coroner's Department, Los Angeles, California.

For the most part, photographs and tracings were made by the author while serving with the Los Angeles County Coroner's Forensic Odontology Team under Dr. G. Vale. The author thanks the staff of the UCLA School of Dentistry's Photography and Illustration Departments for help in preparing the materials for publication.

## General References

American Board of Forensic Odontology. Guidelines for bite mark analysis. JADA 1986;(Mar).
American Society of Forensic Odontology's information source via the Internet World Wide Web: http://www.together.net/~daverill/asfo.html.
Bowers CM, Bell GL, eds. Manual of forensic odontology. American Society of Forensic Odontology, 3rd Ed. 1995. This manual can be obtained from: Forensic Science Foundation, PO Box 1669, Colorado Springs, CO 80901–0669.
Cottone JA, Standish SM. Outline of forensic dentistry. Chicago: Year Book Medical Publishers, 1982.
Harvey W. Dental identification and forensic odontology. London: Henry Kimpton Publishing, 1976.
Journal of California Dental Association: Dec. 1974 (Sognnaes: M. Bormann mystery); May 1975 (Vale: SLA shootout); March 1984 (Vale and others: several areas covered; a good short overview).
Krogman W. The human skeleton in forensic medicine. Springfield, IL: Charles C. Thomas, 1973.
Lampe H, Roetzcher K. Age determination from adult human teeth. Med Law 1994;13(7–8):623–628.
Luntz L, Luntz P. Handbook for dental identification. Philadelphia: J.B. Lippincott, 1973.
Nuckles DB, Herschaft EE, Whatmough LN. Forensic odontology in solving crimes: dental techniques and bite mark evidence. Gen. Dent. 1994;42(3):210–214.
Rothwell BR. Bitemarks in forensic dentistry: a review of legal, scientific issues. 1995;126(2):223–232.
Sopher M. Forensic dentistry. Springfield, IL: Charles C. Thomas, 1976.
Standish SM, Stimson PG. Symposium on forensic dentistry: legal obligations and methods of identification for the practitioner. Dent Clin North Am 1977;21.

# Index

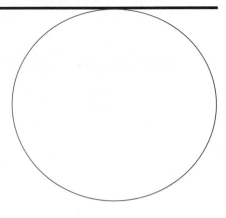

Page numbers in *italics* refer to illustrations; numbers followed by t indicate tables.

# Appendix

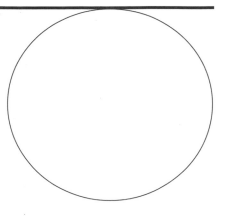

This Appendix includes numerous drawings of permanent and primary teeth which are labeled (with letters) to highlight features of each tooth. Traits represented by each letter are described on the back of each page after the same letter used on the drawings.

The pages in this Appendix are designed to be torn out to facilitate study for chapters 4 through 9 thus minimizing page turns.

# General Characteristics of All Incisors
## ( Using the maxillary right lateral incisor #7 as an example )

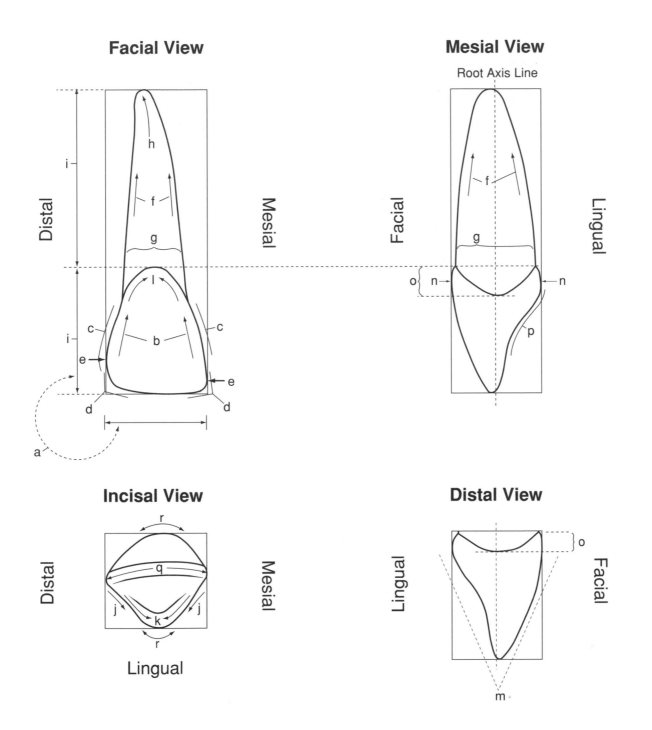

**Facial View**

**Mesial View**

**Incisal View**

**Distal View**

**Refer to letters a - r on back which describe each feature.**

# General Characteristics of All Incisors (Class Traits)

a. Crown shapes are rectangular; longer incisogingivally than mesiodistally (facial views).

b. Crowns taper from the contact areas to cervical lines (facial views).

c. Crown outlines on the distal are more convex than on the mesial (facial views) EXCEPT mandibular central incisors, which are known for their symmetry.

d. The mesioincisal angles are more square (or acute) than the distoincisal angles which are more obtuse (facial views).

e. Mesial contact areas are in the incisal third; distal contact areas are more cervical (facial view) EXCEPT on mandibular central incisors where mesial and distal contacts are at same height due to their symmetry (facial views).

f. Roots taper from the cervical line toward the apex (facial and proximal views) and from the facial toward the lingual (best seen on an actual tooth or model).

g. Roots are wider faciolingually than mesiodistally (comparing proximal to facial view) EXCEPT maxillary central incisors where dimensions are about equal.

h. When bent, roots often bend to the distal in the apical third (facial views).

i. Roots are slightly to considerably longer than crowns (facial and proximal views).

j. Crowns taper from proximal contact areas toward the lingual (incisal views).

k. The mesial and distal marginal ridges converge toward the lingual cingulum (lingual and incisal views).

l. Cervical lines on the facial (and lingual) surfaces are convex (curve) toward the apex (facial and lingual views).

m. Proximal outlines are wedge shaped (proximal views).

n. Facial and lingual crests of curvature are in the cervical third (proximal views).

o. Proximal cervical lines are convex (curve) toward the incisal AND more so on the mesial than on the distal surfaces (compare mesial versus distal views).

p. Lingual outlines are "S" shaped with a concave lingual fossa and convex cingulum, with the lingual outline of the marginal ridges more vertical than horizontal (proximal views).

q. Incisal edges terminate mesially and distally at the widest portion of the tooth crown (incisal views).

r. Facial outlines are less convex (broader) than lingual outlines (incisal views).

# Incisors

## Maxillary

Lateral (#7)   Central (#8)

## Mandibular

Lateral (#26)   Central (#25)

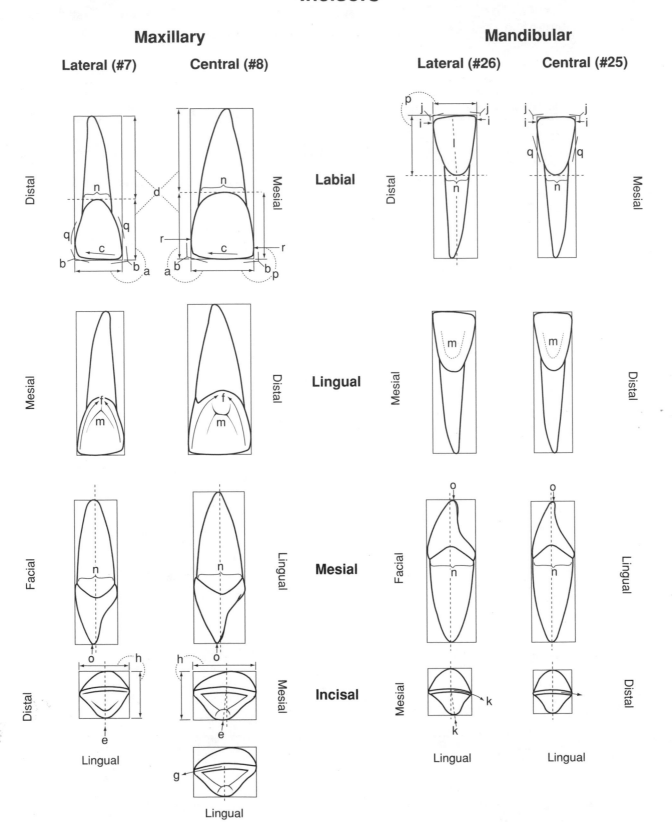

Labial

Lingual

Mesial

Incisal

Refer to letters a - r on back which describe each feature.

## Type Traits That Distinguish the Maxillary Central Incisor from the Maxillary Lateral Incisor

a. Although both have larger cervicoincisal dimension than mesiodistal, maxillary central incisors are closer to square. Lateral incisors are more oblong cervicoincisally (facial views).

b. On both maxillary incisors, the mesioincisal angles are close to 90°; the distoincisal angles are more rounded (facial views), but both angles are more rounded on the lateral versus central incisor (facial views).

c. Incisal edges slope cervically toward the distal (facial views); more so on lateral incisors (facial views).

d. The roots of maxillary central incisors have crowns and roots closer to the same length. Lateral incisors have proportionately longer roots relative to crowns (facial views).

e. When the incisal edges are aligned horizontally, cingula of maxillary central incisors are off-center to the distal versus cingula of lateral incisors which are centered (incisal views).

f. Mesial marginal ridges are longer than the distal marginal ridges (in central incisors due to the distally displaced cingulum, and in lateral incisors, due to the cervical slope of the incisal edge to the distal) (lingual views).

g. From the incisal view, when the crest of curvature of the cingulum is positioned directly downward, the incisal edge of maxillary central incisors have a slight distolingual twist with the distoincisal corner more lingual than the mesioincisal corner. Lateral incisor ridges run mesiodistally with no twist (incisal and mesial views).

h. Mesiodistal dimensions on central incisors are considerably wider than faciolingual dimensions (rectangular shaped). On lateral incisors these dimensions are more nearly equal (closer to square) (incisal views).

## Type Traits That Distinguish the Mandibular Central Incisor from the Mandibular Lateral Incisor

Mandibular central incisors are very symmetrical versus lateral incisors which are not. Examples of asymmetry in lateral incisors include the following:

i. Lateral incisors have the distal proximal contacts more apical than the mesial contacts. Central incisor contacts are at the same level (facial views).

j. Lateral incisors have the distoincisal angles more rounded than the mesioincisal angles. On central incisors the mesio- and distoincisal angles are quite similar (facial views).

k. Incisal edges of lateral incisors have a slight distolingual twist (relative to a line bisecting the cingulum). Central incisors have their incisal edges at right angles (with no twist) to this bisecting line (incisal views).

l. The crown of the mandibular lateral incisor tips slightly to the distal relative to the root (facial views).

## Arch Traits That Distinguish Maxillary from Mandibular Incisors

m. Lingual fossae are more pronounced on maxillary incisors (often with a lingual pit, especially on the maxillary lateral incisor). Mandibular incisors have smoother lingual anatomy without grooves and pits (lingual views).

n. Maxillary incisors have roots that are more round in cross-section. Mandibular incisors have roots that are more ribbon like (i.e., are thin mesiodistally and much wider faciolingually). Compare proximal views to facial views.

o. Incisal edges of maxillary incisors are labial to the root axis line. Mandibular incisal edges are lingual to the root axis line (proximal views).

p. Mandibular crowns are smaller and narrower mesiodistally relative to the length versus maxillary incisors which are wider (facial views).

q. Mandibular crowns have outlines mesially and distally that are flatter than on maxillary incisors (facial views).

r (compared to i). Proximal contact points (crests of curvature) are closer to the incisal edge on mandibular incisors (i) than on maxillary incisors (r) (although all incisor proximal contacts are in the incisal third of the crowns) (facial views).

# General Characteristics of All Canines
( Using the maxillary right canine #6 as an example )

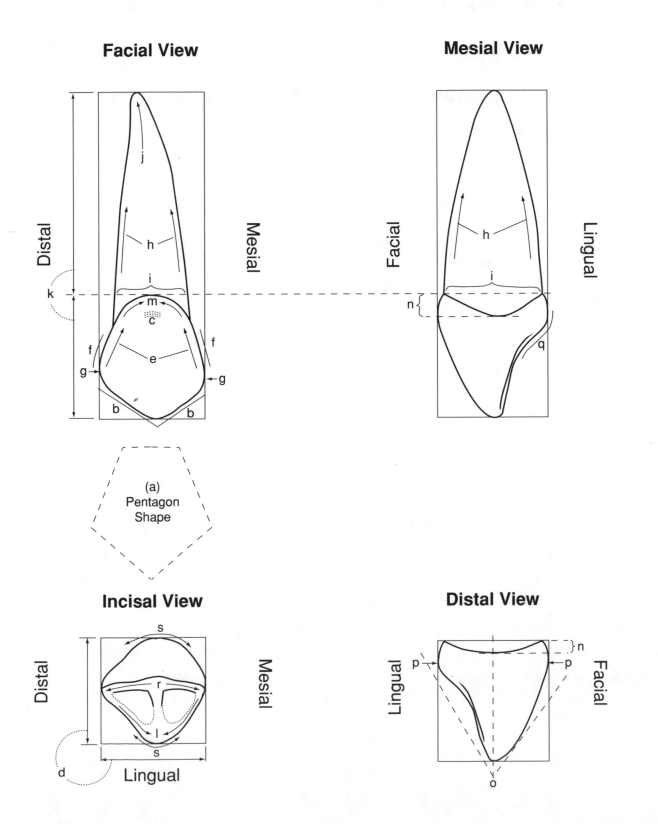

**Facial View**

**Mesial View**

**Incisal View**

**Distal View**

(a)
Pentagon
Shape

**Refer to letters a - s  on back which describe these features.**

## General Characteristics of All Canines (Class Traits)

a. Crowns are pentagon shaped (facial views).

b. Cusps have mesial ridges shorter than distal ridges (facial views).

c. Vertical labial ridges are prominent (more so on maxillary canines) (facial views).

d. Crowns are wider faciolingually than mesiodistally (similar to mandibular incisors) (incisal views).

## General Canine Characteristics Similar to Incisors

e. Crowns taper from contact areas to cervical line (facial views).

f. Crown outlines are more convex on the distal and flatter on the mesial (facial views).

g. Mesial contact areas are located in the incisal third of the crown; distal contact areas are more cervically positioned (facial views).

h. Roots taper from the cervical line toward the apex (facial and proximal views), and from facial toward lingual (which is best viewed on an actual tooth or model).

i. Roots are wider faciolingually than mesiodistally (compare proximal to facial views).

j. When bent, roots more often bend toward the distal in the apical third (facial views).

k. Roots are considerably longer than crowns (facial views).

l. Crowns taper from the proximal contacts toward the lingual (incisal views), so the mesial and distal marginal ridges converge toward the cingulum (incisal views).

m. Cervical lines on the facial (and lingual) surfaces are convex (curve) toward the apex (facial and lingual views).

n. Proximal cervical lines are convex (curve) toward the incisal, more so on the mesial than on the distal surface (proximal views).

o. Canines (like incisors) are wedge-shaped when viewed from the proximal.

p. Facial and lingual crests of curvature are in the cervical third (proximal views).

q. Lingual outlines are "S" shaped with a concave lingual fossa and convex cingulum; the marginal ridges are oriented more vertically than horizontally (proximal views).

r. Incisal edges run toward the mesial to the distal contact areas (incisal views).

s. Facial outlines are less convex (broader) than lingual outlines (incisal views).

# Canines

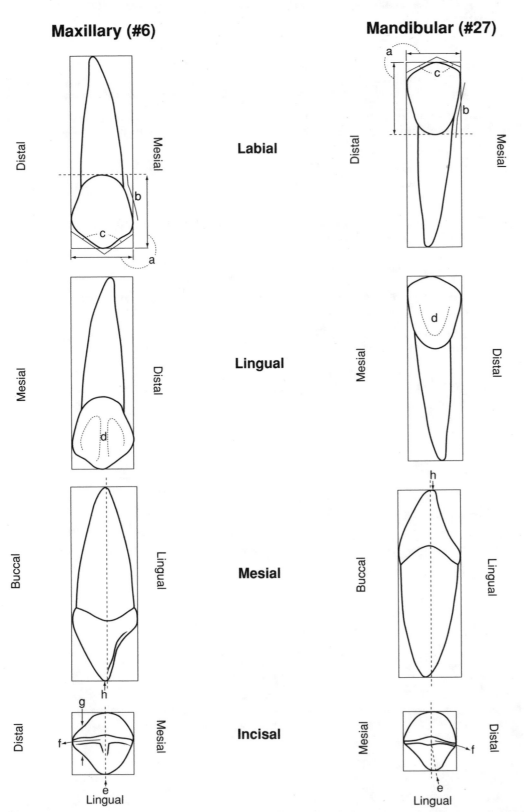

**Maxillary (#6)**

**Mandibular (#27)**

Labial

Lingual

Mesial

Incisal

**Refer to letters a - h on back which describe these features.**

## Type (and Arch) Traits That Distinguish the Maxillary Canine from the Mandibular Canine

a. Both maxillary and mandibular canine crowns are oblong with the mesiodistal dimension less than the incisocervical dimension, but the mesiodistal dimension of mandibular canines is more narrow than on maxillary canines (facial views).

b. Maxillary canines have mesial crown contours convex to flat cervically versus mandibular canines which have mesial crown contours more in line with the contour of the root (facial views).

c. The angles of the cusp slopes for maxillary canines are more acute and average about 105° versus the broader angle in the mandibular canine which averages 120° (facial views).

d. Lingual ridges with mesial and distal fossae are less prominent on mandibular canines than maxillary canines (lingual views).

e. Cingula on maxillary canines are large and centered mesiodistally. On mandibular canines they are often slightly to the distal (incisal views).

f. Incisal ridges on maxillary canines are straighter mesiodistally. On mandibular canines the distal cusp ridge bends distolingually (incisal views).

g. The distal half of the crown of maxillary canines is compressed (squeezed) faciolingually more than on mandibular canines (incisal views).

h. The cusp tip of the maxillary canine is on or labial to the root axis line whereas the mandibular cusp tip is lingual to this line (proximal and incisal views).

# General Characteristics of All Premolars
( Using the maxillary right second premolar #4 as an example )

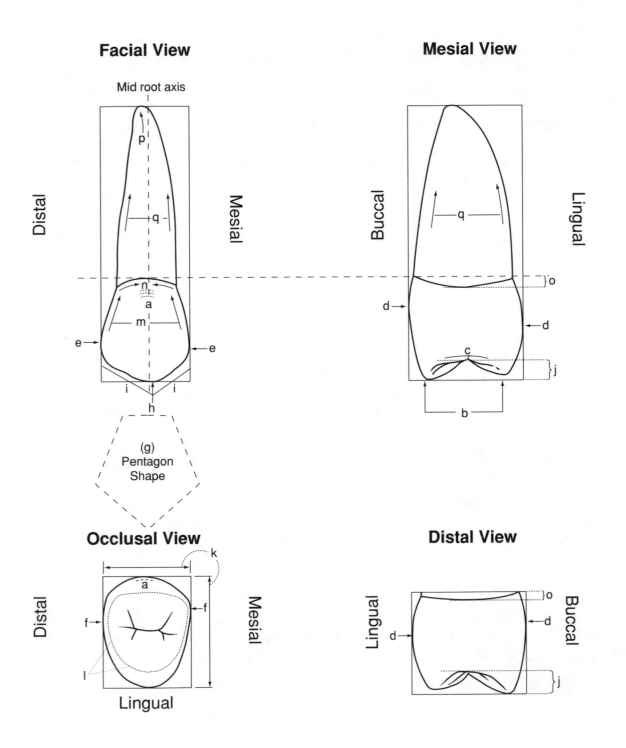

**Facial View**

Mid root axis

p

q

Distal

Mesial

n
a
m
e → ← e
i i
h

(g)
Pentagon
Shape

**Mesial View**

Buccal

Lingual

q

} o
d →
← d
c
} j
b

**Occlusal View**

k

Distal

Mesial

a
f → ← f
f →
l

Lingual

**Distal View**

Lingual

Buccal

} o
← d
d →
} j

Refer to letters a - q on back which describe these features.

# General Characteristics of All Premolars (Class Traits)

a. Buccal ridges are present (similar to canine labial ridges) (facial and occlusal views).

b. Usually premolars have two cusps: one buccal and one lingual cusp (EXCEPTION is the mandibular second premolar which often has two lingual cusps) (proximal views).

c. Marginal ridges are aligned relatively horizontally (EXCEPT on mandibular first premolars where the mesial marginal ridge is closer to a 45° angle from horizontal) (proximal views).

d. Buccal and lingual crests of curvature are more occlusal than on anterior teeth (still in cervical third on the facial, but in the middle third on the lingual) (proximal views).

e. Mesial proximal contacts are near the junction of the occlusal and middle thirds and the distal contacts are often slightly more cervical in the middle third (EXCEPT on the mandibular first premolar where the mesial contact is more cervical than its distal contact) (facial views).

f. Proximal contacts from the occlusal view are buccal to the center faciolingually (occlusal views).

g. From the facial, premolars are roughly pentagon shaped (similar to canines) (facial view).

h. The buccal cusp tip is mesial to the mid-root axis (EXCEPT on the maxillary first premolar where the cusp tip is distal to the mid-root axis) (facial views).

i. The Mesial cusp ridge of the buccal cusp is shorter than the distal cusp ridge (EXCEPT on the maxillary first premolar where the mesial cusp ridge is longer) (facial views).

j. Mesial marginal ridges are generally more occlusal than distal marginal ridges which are more cervical, EXCEPT on mandibular first premolars where distal marginal ridges are in a more occlusal position (compare both proximal views).

k. Crowns are oblong from the occlusal view: wider faciolingually than mesiodistally relative to anterior teeth. (Maxillary premolars are decidely oblong, whereas mandibular premolars are closer to square in shape.) (occlusal views.)

l. Cusp slopes and marginal ridges form the boundary of the occlusal surface (occlusal views).

m. Crowns taper from proximal contact areas toward the cervical (facial views).

n. Cervical lines are convex, curving apically on the facial and lingual sides (facial and lingual views).

o. Cervical lines curve occlusally on the proximal sides, with the mesial cervical line more convex than the distal (proximal views).

p. The apical third of roots bend distally more than mesially (facial views).

q. Roots taper toward the apex (both proximal and facial views).

# Premolars

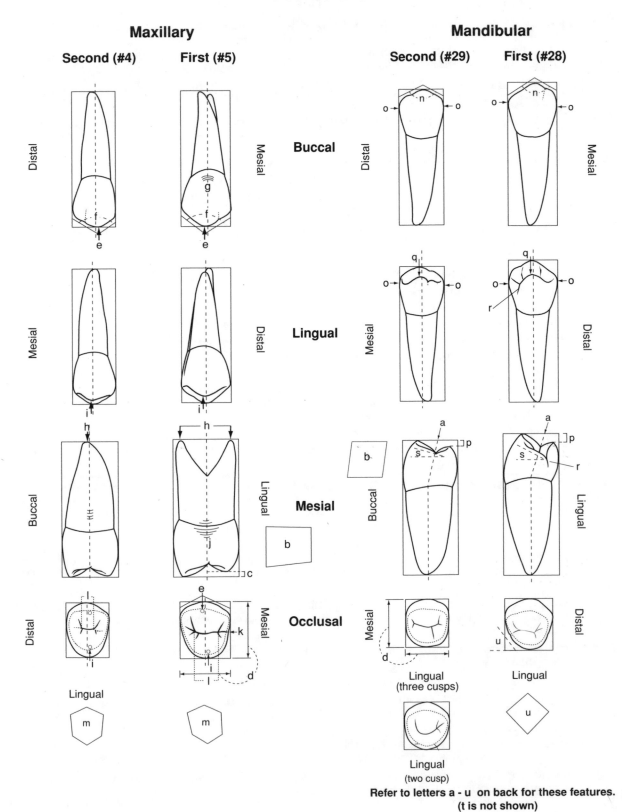

## Maxillary

### Second (#4)    First (#5)

## Mandibular

### Second (#29)    First (#28)

**Buccal**

**Lingual**

**Mesial**

**Occlusal**

Lingual
(three cusps)

Lingual

Lingual
(two cusp)

Lingual    Lingual

Refer to letters a - u  on back for these features.
(t is not shown)

# Arch Traits of Premolars That Distinguish Maxillary from Mandibular Premolars

a. Mandibular premolar crowns tilt to the lingual so mandibular lingual cusp tips may be lingual to the root (proximal views).

b. The outline of the mandibular premolars are rhomboid in shape, and the maxillary premolars are trapezoidal (proximal views).

c (compared to p). Although lingual cusps are shorter than buccal cusps for all premolars, the mandibular lingual cusps are relatively *much* shorter than buccal cusps (p) compared to maxillary lingual cusps which are closer to the same length (c) (maxillary second premolar cusps are almost equal in length) (proximal views).

d. Mandibular premolars are more square from the occlusal view; maxillary premolars are more rectangular (relatively wider buccolingually) (occlusal views).

## Type Traits Distinguishing Maxillary First from Second Premolars

e. Buccal cusps of maxillary first premolars are tipped more to the distal with mesial cusp slopes longer than distal cusp slopes. (THESE ARE THE ONLY PREMOLARS WITH THESE CHARACTERISTICS.) (Facial and occlusal views.)

f. Buccal cusps of maxillary first premolars are more pointed (average: 105°) versus on second premolars where they are more obtuse (120°) (facial views).

g. Buccal ridges are more prominent on maxillary first premolars (occlusal and facial views).

h. Maxillary first premolars *usually* have a divided root versus second premolars which usually have one root (proximal views).

i. Maxillary premolars have their lingual cusps tipped (bent) toward the mesial (lingual and occlusal views).

j. Both maxillary premolars have mesial and distal *root* depressions but only the maxillary first premolars exhibit a mesial *crown* concavity (mesial views).

k. Mesial marginal ridge grooves are almost always present on maxillary first premolars and are less common on second premolars (occlusal views).

l. The central developmental grooves on maxillary first premolars are longer (from mesial to distal pit) than those of second premolars where they are only one-third or less of the mesiodistal dimension (occlusal views).

m. Occlusal outlines of maxillary first premolars are more *a*symmetrical with the lingual cusp tip bent mesially, and mesial marginal ridge straight to concave, versus second premolars which are more symmetrical overall. (occlusal views)

## Type Traits Distinguishing Mandibular First from Second Premolars

n. Mandibular first premolar buccal cusps are more pointed (110°) versus on second premolar where they are more obtuse (130°) (facial views).

o. Mesial proximal contacts (and marginal ridges) of mandibular second premolars are more occlusal than distal contacts (following the general rule), whereas the reverse is true on mandibular first premolars (EXCEPTION) where mesial contacts and marginal ridges are more cervical (facial views).

p. Lingual cusps of mandibular first premolars are very small and nonfunctional. On second premolars the lingual cusps function and are relatively longer (proximal views).

q. Lingual cusps of mandibular second premolars are positioned to the mesial (or, if there are two lingual cusps, the mesiolingual is the more prominent) (lingual views).

r. Mandibular first premolars have a mesiolingual groove separating the mesial marginal ridge from the lingual cusp. Second premolars do not (lingual and mesial views).

s. Mesial marginal ridges of first premolars slope cervically toward the lingual at about 45° from horizontal. On second premolars they are more horizontal (mesial views).

t. The mesial root surfaces of mandibular second premolars are the only premolar root surface (maxillary and mandibular, mesial and distal) not likely to have a mid-root depression (best seen on models or actual teeth, not labeled in drawings).

u. Mandibular first premolars are the only premolars that have the mesiolingual corner, with its mesiolingual groove and low marginal ridge, pinched or squeezed in, forming about a 45° angle with the lingual surface. This makes the occlusal outline somewhat diamond shaped (occlusal views).

# General Characteristics of All Molars
( Using the second mandibular molar #31 as an example )

## Facial View

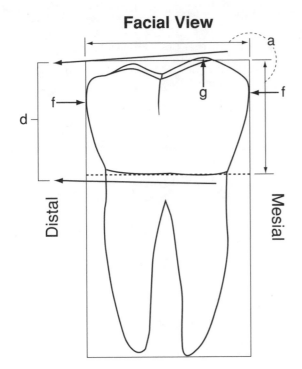

## Mesial View
Midline

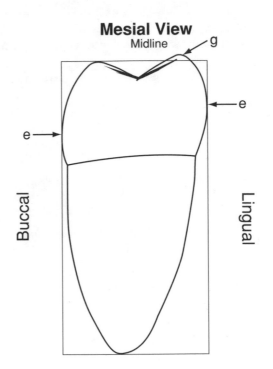

## Occlusal View

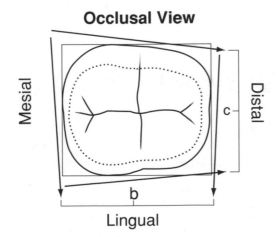

## Distal View

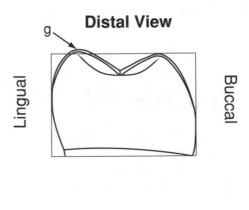

**Refer to letters a - g  on back.**

## General Characteristics for All Molars

a.  Crowns are wider mesiodistally than cervico-occlusally (facial views).

b.  Crowns taper (get narrower) from the buccal to the lingual, i.e., the mesiodistal width on the buccal half is wider than on the lingual half (EXCEPT some maxillary first molars with large distolingual cusps where crowns taper to the buccal, i.e., the mesiodistal dimension on the lingual is greater than on the buccal) (occlusal view).

c.  Crowns taper (get narrower) from the mesial to the distal (i.e., the buccolingual width is less on the distal half than on the mesial half (occlusal view).

d.  Crowns taper (get shorter) from mesial to distal (i.e., the crown height on the distal half is less than on the mesial half) (facial view).

e.  As with premolars, the buccal crests of curvature of crowns are in the cervical one-third and the lingual crests of curvature are in the middle third (proximal views).

f.  Proximal contacts on the mesial are at or near the junction of the occlusal and middle thirds; distal proximal contacts are more cervical, in the middle third near the middle of the tooth (facial views).

g.  Lingual cusps (particulary mesiolingual) are longer than buccal cusps when mandibular molars are oriented on a vertical axis (facial, mesial and distal views).

# Molars

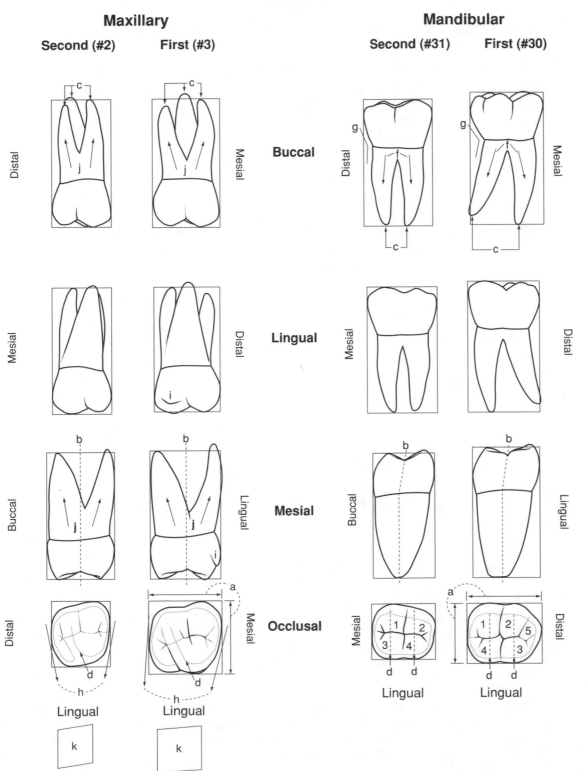

## Maxillary

### Second (#2)    First (#3)

## Mandibular

### Second (#31)    First (#30)

**Buccal**

**Lingual**

**Mesial**

**Occlusal**

**Refer to letters a - k on back describing these features.**

## Arch Traits That Distinguish Maxillary from Mandibular Molars

a. Mandibular crowns are wider mesiodistally than faciolingually resulting in a more rectangular or pentagon outline. Maxillary molar crowns have the faciolingual dimension slightly greater than the mesiodistal dimension and are more square or rhomboid in outline (k) (occlusal views).

b. Mandibular molar crowns tilt lingually at the cervix (proximal views).

c. Mandibular molars usually have two roots (a larger mesial and a smaller distal root) versus maxillary molars which have three roots (the shortest distobuccal, then mesiobuccal, and the longest lingual root) (facial or lingual views).

d. Maxillary molars have oblique ridges that run diagonally across the tooth from the mesiolingual to the distobuccal cusp versus mandibular molars which primarily have two transverse ridges that run directly buccolingually (occlusal views).

## Type Traits That Distinguish Mandibular First from Mandibular Second Molars

e. Mandibular second molars have four cusps (MB = 1, DB = 2, ML = 3, and DL = 4) with a "cross" pattern of occlusal grooves versus first molars which have five cusps, the same four cusps as the second molar plus a smaller distal cusp (D = 5) with a zigzag occlusal groove pattern. (facial or occlusal views; see corresponding numbered cusps, not labeled as "e")

f. First molar roots are more divergent and widely separated versus second molars roots which are more parallel and closer together (facial and lingual views).

g. There is more taper (narrowing) from the distal proximal contact to the cervical line on first molars than on second molars due to the presence of the distal cusp on first molars (facial views).

## Type Traits That Distinguish Maxillary First from Maxillary Second Molars

h. There is more taper (narrowing) from the buccal to lingual on second molars due to the smaller distolingual cusp versus less taper on maxillary first molars with their wider, prominent distolingual cusps (occlusal views).

i. First molars are more likely to have a fifth cusp, the cusp of Carabelli (located on the mesiolingual cusp). Second molars rarely have the cusp of Carabelli (occlusal, lingual, and mesial views).

j. Roots of first molars are more spread apart than on second molars (facial and proximal views).

k. The parallelogram outline shape of maxillary molars (with more acute mesiobuccal and distolingual angles and more obtuse distobuccal and mesiolingual angles) is more twisted on second molars than on first molars (i.e., acute angles are more acute and obtuse angles are more obtuse) (occlusal views).

# Primary Anterior Teeth

## Maxillary

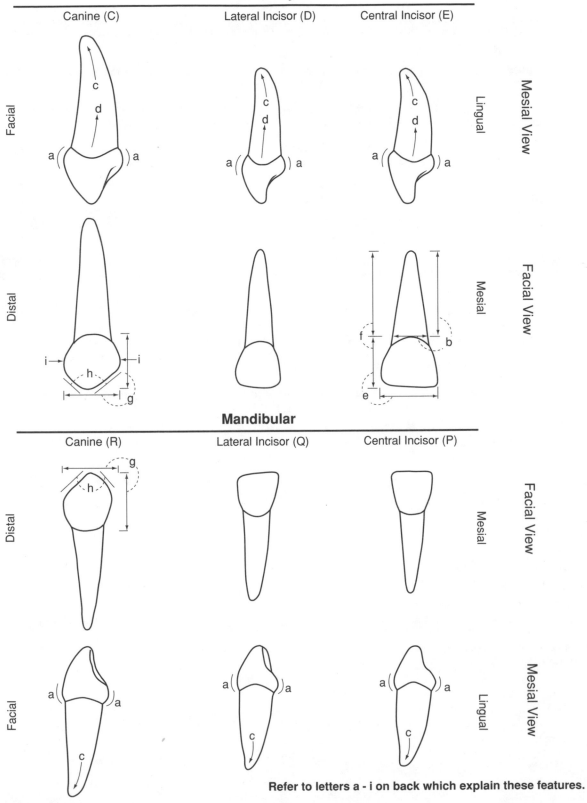

Canine (C)  Lateral Incisor (D)  Central Incisor (E)

## Mandibular

Canine (R)  Lateral Incisor (Q)  Central Incisor (P)

**Refer to letters a - i on back which explain these features.**

## Unique Properties of Anterior Primary Teeth

a. Primary anterior tooth crowns have a bulge labiolingually in their cervical third. This bulge is seen lingually as a relatively large cingulum which occupies up to one-third of the cervicoincisal crown length and is seen labially as a prominent convex cervical ridge (proximal views).

b. Roots are long in proportion to crown length and narrower mesiodistally than permanent anterior teeth (facial view).

c. Roots of maxillary and mandibular primary anterior teeth bend as much as 10° labially in their *apical* third, less so in mandibular canines (proximal views).

d. Roots of maxillary incisors bend lingually in the *cervical* third to half, whereas the mandibular incisors are straight in their cervical third (proximal views).

e. Primary central incisors are the only incisors, primary or permanent, that are wider mesiodistally than incisocervically (facial views).

f. Primary central incisor crowns are shorter relative to the root length compared to permanent teeth (facial views).

g. Primary maxillary canines are about as wide mesiodistally as they are long incisogingivally. Mandibular canines are longer incisocervically and narrower mesiodistally (facial views).

h. Primary maxillary canine cusps have their mesial cusp slope longer than the distal cusp slope (which is the **exception** to the rule for permanent teeth with one facial cusp which have a shorter mesial slope). Primary mandibular canines have their distal cusp slopes longer than on the mesial (as do all permanent canines and premolars except the maxillary first premolar) (facial views) .

i. Primary maxillary canines have mesial proximal contacts more cervical than the distal (which is **unique** to this tooth *and* the permanent mandibular first premolar) (facial views). All other primary and permanent teeth have the distal contact area more cervically located than on the mesial.

# Primary Molars

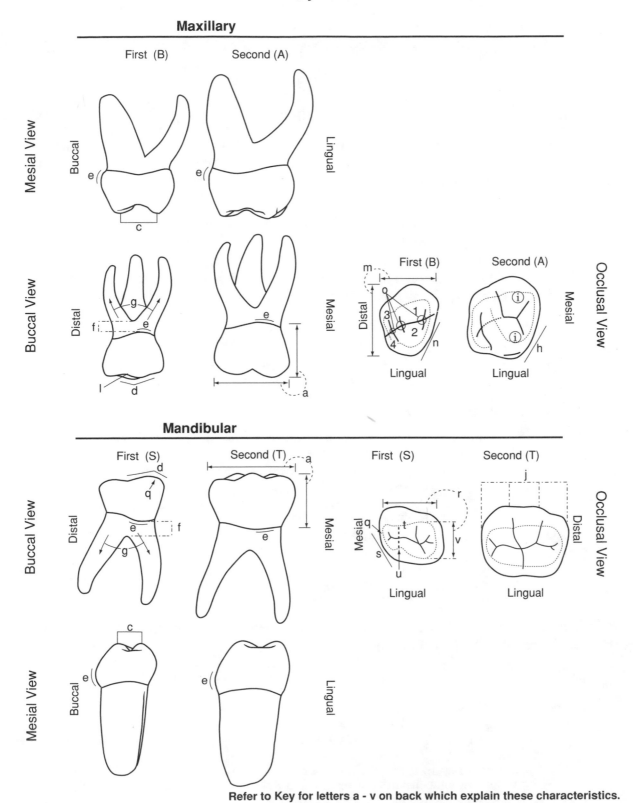

## Maxillary

First (B)     Second (A)

Mesial View

Buccal View

First (B)     Second (A)

Occlusal View

## Mandibular

First (S)     Second (T)     First (S)     Second (T)

Buccal View

Occlusal View

Mesial View

**Refer to Key for letters a - v on back which explain these characteristics.**

## General Characteristics of All Primary Molars

a. Primary molars crowns are wider mesiodistally and shorter cervico-occlusally (buccal views).

b. Primary first molars are decidedly smaller than primary second molars (versus permanent molars where the first molars are larger) (all views, not labeled as "b").

c. Primary molar crowns have a narrow chewing surface, or occlusal table, buccolingually (proximal views).

d. Buccal cusps are not sharp; cusp slopes meet at a wide (obtuse) angle (buccal views).

e. Mesial cervical ridges are prominent (proximal views) with curved cervical lines positioned more apically on the mesial (buccal views).

f. Root furcations are nearer to the crown with little or no root trunk (buccal views).

g. Roots are thin, slender, and widely spread (buccal views).

## Additional Characteristics Unique to Primary Maxillary Second Molars (Which Most Closely Resemble the Permanent Maxillary First Molars)

h. Mesiolingual corner of the occlusal surface is compressed toward the distal (occlusal views).

i. Primary mesiobuccal cusp is about equal in size to the mesiolingual cusp (versus permanent where the mesiolingual cusp is larger than the mesiobuccal cusp) (occlusal views).

## Additional Characteristics Unique to Primary Mandibular Second Molars (Which Most Closely Resemble the Permanent Mandibular First Molar)

j. The three buccal cusps are of nearly equal size, versus permanent first molars where the distal cusp is usually considerably smaller. (buccal views)

## Additional Characteristics Unique to Primary Maxillary First Molars (Which Somewhat Resemble A Permanent Maxillary Premolars)

k. There are often four cusps: two larger cusps (like a maxillary premolar), the mesiobuccal cusp (1) is widest and longest, the mesiolingual cusp (2) is smaller but sharpest; and two smaller cusps, the distobuccal (3) and the inconspicuous, sometimes absent, distolingual (4) (occlusal views; see corresponding numbered cusps).

l. A notch (distal to center) divides the large mesiobuccal cusp from the indistinct distobuccal cusp (buccal views).

m. The crown is wider faciolingually than mesiodistally like a maxillary premolar, but unlike other primary molars (occlusal views).

n. The mesial marginal ridge is directed distolingually (occlusal views).

o. There are three fossae: a large mesial triangular fossa, a medium central fossa, and minute distal fossa (occlusal views).

p. The grooves form an "H" pattern (somewhat similar to a maxillary premolar) (no letter; seen on occlusal views).

## Additional Unique Characteristics of Primary Mandibular First Molars (Resembling No Other Tooth)

q. The mesial marginal ridge is overdeveloped, almost resembling a cusp (buccal and occlusal views).

r. The occlusal table is wider mesiodistally than buccolingually like permanent mandibular molars (occlusal views).

s. The mesial surface converges to the lingual with an acute and prominent mesiobuccal angle of the occlusal table (occlusal views).

t. The mesiobuccal cusp is the largest and longest cusp covering nearly two-thirds of the buccal surface (occlusal views), but is not wide buccolingually (occlusal views).

u. A transverse ridge runs between the mesiobuccal and mesiolingual cusp (occlusal views).

v. The occlusal table is larger distal to the transverse ridge with a larger distal fossa and a smaller mesial triangular fossa (no central fossa) (occlusal views).